SKIN, HEREDITY, AND MALIGNANT NEOPLASMS

By

HENRY T. LYNCH, M.D.

Professor and Chairman

Department of Preventive Medicine
and Public Health
Creighton University School
of Medicine
Omaha, Nebraska

MEDICAL EXAMINATION PUBLISHING COMPANY, INC.
65-36 Fresh Meadow Lane
Flushing, New York 11365

Library of Congress
Catalog Card Number
79-163617

ISBN 0-87488-744-5

March 1972

PREFACE

The idea for writing this book began when I encountered a family with xeroderma pigmentosum wherein a plastic surgeon, knowledgeable in genetics was able to establish a diagnosis of this disease in two of the proband's siblings (and in two subsequent born identical twin sibs); in turn through instituting a program of meticulous sunlight avoidance, he was able to achieve a remarkable degree of skin cancer control in the affected members of this kindred. The idea was rekindled in greater force when a short time later I treated a patient who at that time had a far–advanced posterior fossa neurofibrosarcoma secondary to neurofibromatosis. He had been followed by his family physician for over a year during which time his neurological signs progressed under the very eyes of this doctor who had failed to correlate the significance of *café au lait* spots in his patient, with significant cutaneous evidence of neurofibromatosis in the pa-

tient's relatives. Prolonged medical and genetic experience with both of these families was sobering and whetted the thirst to explore the subject in as much depth as possible.

This book is the result of the efforts of several colleagues in the field with similar interests, all of whom are concerned with opening up new avenues for cancer control through knowledge of genetic principles in context with critical evaluation of dermatologic signs which when integrated, might bespeak the presence of cancer or a risk for subsequent development of this disease.

Many excellent books are available on dermatology, genetics, and on cancer. However, we have been unable to find any single resource which has integrated these disciplines in such a way that the practicing physician could apply this knowledge to his busy clinical practice. It is our fervent hope that this book might in a small measure achieve this goal.

DEDICATION

TO THE FACULTY OF CREIGHTON UNIVERSITY SCHOOL OF MEDICINE: A HUB OF HUMANITARIANISM, INSPIRATION, SCIENTIFIC REFLECTION, AND TEACHING.

ACKNOWLEDGEMENTS

One of the pleasures of writing and editing a multi–authored book is the realization that extremely busy authorities are willing to devote their time and effort to the preparation of material toward the goal that the editor has set forth for his book. Unfortunately, this grand feeling of appreciation can only be felt fully by the editor and his expression of gratitude can never sufficiently do justice to his true inner feelings. Therefore, with this limitation, I wish to humbly state my gratitude and appreciation to the several contributors to this book. Without their help this manuscript very definitely could not have been written.

There are colleagues behind the scenes in many writings who contribute in a variety of ways without fanfare in the quest for scientific truth and for the betterment of humanity. My colleague, Anne Krush, M.S., Assistant Professor of Preventive Medicine is a dedicated associate and has played a major role in the many editings of this manuscript and she has provided numerous insights into the content and direction that the book has taken.

My secretary, Katherine Dyhrberg, has labored over this entire manuscript from its inception and has coddled and nurtured it almost as her own. Her painstaking efforts at technical accuracy and precision were constantly evident to me; the knowledge that these matters were under efficient control relieved me of considerable anxiety and provided me confidence.

A deep sense of gratitude is felt toward Creighton University School of Medicine which has provided me with comfortable physical facilities and a wealth of spiritual and moral backing in this endeavor.

TABLE OF CONTENTS

Chapter 1

INTRODUCTION

by Henry T. Lynch, M.D.

The skin is readily accessible to critical observation and appraisal for both patient and physician. When a patient's integument is studied in context with his environmental background and genetic endowment and/or their interaction, much useful information about skin aberrations might be forthcoming. All too frequently, however, hereditary factors have been overlooked in etiologic evaluations of the skin and surprisingly little attention has been given to skin signs and genetic factors associated with cancer. Therefore, this book is being written to focus attention primarily upon skin lesions which are related directly or indirectly to hereditary factors in context with their probable or known association with cancer of the skin and cancer of underlying organs or viscera.[1,2]

The skin contains a variety of components which are genetically determined. Most apparent, of course, is skin color and hair color, which are closely controlled by genetic and/or "racial" factors. Other characteristics of hair, such as texture, quantity, etc. are often racially or genetically determined. Hereditary pattern baldness and premature graying of hair occur in certain families and are also under genetic control. Such skin features as Mongolian spots, i.e., a cutaneous–subcutaneous pigmentation, often found in the sacral area of newborn children, are also due to racial or hereditary factors in that these occur regularly in members of oriental races, but are rarely found among caucasians. Many discrete genetic anomalies of skin such as piebaldness (autosomal dominant), vitiligo (autosomal dominant), ichthyosis congenita (autosomal recessive), ichthyosis simplex (autosomal dominant or sex–linked recessive in some families), keratosis pilaris (autosomal dominant), pityriasis rubra pilaris (autosomal dominant and incomplete dominance in some families), cutis laxa (autosomal recessive, though autosomal dominant has been reported rarely), alopecia areata (autosomal dominant), and acrodermatitis enteropathica (autosomal recessive), are just a few of a large group of skin lesions which, while not associated with cancer, are nevertheless controlled by simple genetic factors.[3] However, it will not be in the realm of this book to discuss the many hereditary skin disorders which are unrelated to cancer, rather we shall restrict ourselves to lesions of known or presumed genetic etiology which are associated with *cancer* of the skin or underlying organs and tissues.[1]

Skin signs must be evaluated in context with multiple factors including age, sex, race and occupational exposures. For example, one must use caution and discretion when ascribing cutaneous signs in aged individuals to the presence of genetic factors and/or to an underlying malignant neoplasm. As a point of fact, many normal aging effects of skin disorders in the elderly are completely unrelated to visceral cancer. However, such rare disorders as acanthosis nigricans or the sudden sprouting of lanugo hair over the face of an adult may herald an underlying cancer. Unfortunately, when a sign such as acanthosis nigricans makes its first appearance in an adult the underlying malignancy is often advanced beyond the possibility of a surgical or radiological cure. Thus the clinician must evaluate critically the entire issue. In the case of acanthosis nigricans he should evaluate the possibility that this is the hereditary form which has an *early* onset and is *not* associated with cancer (see below). He should evaluate the integument from a variety of perspectives in order to appraise signs of genetic or unknown etiology which may provide advance notice of the possibility of cancer development, signs which indicate that cancer has already developed and may even be advanced such as in the case of acanthosis nigricans, and finally, skin signs which normally occur with aging and which do not necessarily have any cancer association.

The clinician must also differentiate skin lesions which have a definite cancer association from those which may have a similar appearance but which are not associated with cancer. In certain circumstances, the family history may prove invaluable for this differentiation. For example, in acanthosis nigricans a hereditary variety of this lesion occurs at a very young age and behaves as an autosomal dominant.[4] Thus, this benign form characterized by early age of onset and autosomal dominant inheritance is distinguished from the same lesion which appears in adulthood and is almost invariably associated with visceral carcinoma. More specifically, about 90 percent of the carcinomas associated with acanthosis nigricans arise in the abdomen and about 61 percent involve the stomach. The clinical course of such patients is often highly malignant and rapidly fatal.[4] A variant of acanthosis nigricans is the occurrence of seborrheic wartlike lesions with minimal or absent change at the flexures. These lesions may be interspersed with café–au–lait spots and are frequently associated with an underlying cancer.[5] This rare clinical cutaneous sign is apparently well known in the European literature having been described in 1890 by the French surgeon Ulysse Trelat and is called the sign of Trelat.

Another skin sign which may be confused with acanthosis nigricans which is associated with malignancy, is a benign condition known as pseudoacanthosis nigricans. The lesion is relatively common and consists of pedunculated skin tags occurring in the axillae and perineum of obese patients.

We believe that physicians have always been intrigued with internal manifestations of skin diseases in spite of their frequent diagnostic complexity. However, with the advent of modern diagnostic laboratory technology, physicians of the present era are probably not as adept at the physical diagnosis and characterization of dermatologic signs as their brethren of past generations. This is unfortunate because a wealth of diagnostic and prognostic information might be acquired through critical appraisal of the skin, and this might be further embellished through correlation of genetic information. Wiener[6] called attention to the importance of the skin as a clue to internal manifestations of diseases and referred to these as *dermadromes,* a term which denotes the skin portion of a particular syndrome which is known to be a manifestation of an internal disorder. Interestingly, when Dr. Weiner wrote his book in 1947, he stated the following in context with the potential yield from critical observation of the skin: "And yet, it seems that the tremendous wealth of clinical observations on cutaneous phenomena accompanying internal disease has, in our time, not found the attention it deserves." Unfortunately in spite of the efforts of many, with an elapse of almost 25 years since Weiner's admonishment of this problem, the present author could make virtually the same statement; moreover, with the informational explosion of genetic knowledge, it must also be stated that appropriate utilization of genetic information with specific cutaneous implications is abysmally ignored by many. Thus, we hope in a small way, to be able to call attention to these matters and will focus our attention upon an extension of the problem to include cancer; we thus shall try to integrate the problem in context with skin, cancer, and heredity!

Objectives

The primary objective of this book is to present a trilogic approach to cancer comprehension and control through the application of the following: 1) physical clues manifested in the skin; 2) genetic information based on the significance of these clues and the family history; 3) diagnostic methods in the search for evidence of cancer. This approach is illustrated in Figure 1 which diagrammatically depicts an "equation" which when utilized systematically by the physician could lead to improved cancer control. Thus this

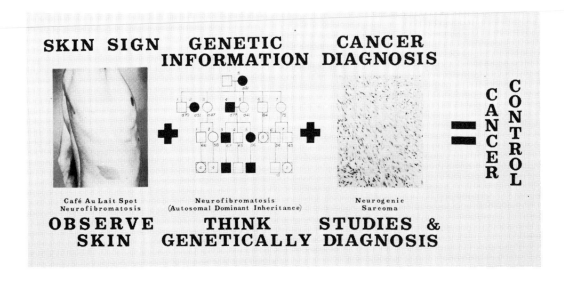

Figure 1. Diagrammatic formula for utilization of genetic information, physical signs, and diagnostic measures for cancer control.

equation provides an underlying philosophic and pragmatic approach which will be espoused throughout this book. Hopefully in pursuing this objective it will provide insight for the clinician as well as basic fundamental information for the use of the clinical investigator.

In order to provide the reader with a general perspective of the problem, scope, and intent of the book, we present the following tables (Tables 1 to 4) which list cancerous and pre-cancerous syndromes with cutaneous and genetic implications. These are inherited either under classical Mendelian control or are presumed to have a genetic etiology in certain families; *all* of these conditions are associated with cancer. Thus, Table 1 lists autosomal dominant, Table 2 — autosomal recessive, and Table 3 — sex-linked recessive inherited conditions. Finally, Table 4 lists conditions wherein the role of hereditary factors is less clear; nevertheless, while classical Mendelian inheritance patterns have not been delineated, there is empirical evidence for a genetic etiology in some families.

Chapter 2 is devoted exclusively to fundamentals of human inheritance. Because the science of human genetics has only recently been presented in a systematic fashion in some medical school curricula, many clinicians may not have had an exposure to this discipline. On the other hand, those physicians who may have had a lesser or greater formal background in genetics may not have had many opportunities to apply genetics in their busy clinical practices. This brief review may therefore be of interest.

Chapter 3 is included in order to cast light in a bold way upon the muddy waters in the area of integrating skin signs with the existence of cancer. Applicable genetic factors are given so that one might readily appreciate the ease of making diagnoses in families through anticipation of signs and symptoms following the diagnosis of the particular condition in the proband.

Chapter 4 presents a discussion of basic biochemical research as it has evolved recently in one of the genetic models used in this book, namely xeroderma pigmentosum (xdp). Specifically, the material in this chapter highlights basic metabolic pathways with emphasis upon one of these involving an enzyme known as endonuclease which is involved in DNA repair replication. However, it will be shown clearly in this chapter that this enzyme is lacking in patients with xeroderma pigmentosum. Furthermore, when patients with xdp are exposed to ultraviolet radiation their skin fails to undergo repair replication. An important point is that this information in time could provide important clues to carcinogenesis.

Subsequent chapters deal with a variety of clinical disorders of known genetic or in some cases presumed genetic etiology having cutaneous manifestations which could provide a beacon to the existence of an underlying cancer. The final chapter on genetic counseling represents an attempt to present a philosophy and methodologic approach toward the management of a number of problems of a genetic nature. We feel that the family physician is capable of assisting the patient and his family with most of these problems.[7]

Because of the potential importance of genetic counseling for cancer control, we have included an appendix with a listing of genetic units throughout the world which provide genetic counseling and/or are engaged in research in cancer genetics.[8]

References

1. Lynch, H.T.: Skin, Heredity, and Cancer, *Cancer 24*: 277–288, 1969.

2. Lynch, H.T. and Szentivanyi, J.: Genetics as a Guide to Early Diagnosis and Cancer Control – Cutaneous Syndromes, *Cutis 6*: 179–185, 1970.

3. Butterworth, T., and Strean, L.P.: *Clinical Genodermatology,* Williams and Wilkins, Baltimore, 1962, pp. 221.

4. Curth, H.O. and Aschner, B.M.: Genetics Study on Acanthosis Nigricans, *Arch. Derm. 79*: 55–66, 1959.

5. Snedden, I.B.: Cutaneous Manifestations of Visceral Malignancy, *Postgrad. Med. 46*: 678–685, 1970.

6. Wiener, K.: *Skin Manifestations of Internal Disorders (Dermadromes),* C.V. Mosby Company, St. Louis, 1947, pp. 690.

7. Lynch, H.T.: *Dynamic Genetic Counseling for Clinicians,* Charles C. Thomas, Springfield, 1969.

8. Lynch, H.T.: Editor, *International Directory of Genetic Services,* National Foundation, New York, 2nd Edition, 1969.

TABLE 1
AUTOSOMAL DOMINANT INHERITANCE

DISORDER	SKIN MANIFESTATIONS	MANIFESTATIONS OF OTHER SYSTEMS	PREDOMINANT CANCERS
Neurofibromatosis	café au lait spots, cutaneous neurofibromas, all sites, axillary freckle–like lesions, oral papillomatous tumors	multiple congential anomalies	sarcoma, acoustic neuroma, pheochromocytoma
Gardner's Syndrome	epidermoid inclusion cysts, sebaceous cysts, dermoid tumors	osteomas, polyposis coli	adenocarcinoma of the colon
Multiple Nevoid Basal Cell Carcinoma Syndrome	multiple nevoid appearing basal cell carcinomas, benign cysts, hypokeratinized area of palms, "palmar pits," and soles	jaw cysts, rib & vertebral anomalies, neurologic and ophthamologic anomalies, intracranial calcifications	multiple basal cell carcinomas
Cutaneous Malignant Melanoma	usually darkly and unevenly pigmented cutaneous growths, might be mistaken for junctional nevi	none	cutaneous malignant melanoma
Tylosis & Esophageal Carcinoma (Keratosis Palmaris et Plantaris)	tylosis of palms and soles	none	esophageal cancer
Tuberous Sclerosis (Bourneville's Disease)	adenoma sebaceum of Pringle, *café au lait* spots, periungual fibromata, shagreen patch, fibromatous plaques	epilepsy, mental retardation, hamartomas in brain, kidneys, and heart	intracranial neoplasms (astrocytomas, glioblastomas)
von Hippel–Lindau's Syndrome	vascular nevi of the face, angiomatosis of the retina, cystic lesions	cerebellar angiomatosis	hemangioblastoma of cerebellum, hypernephroma, & pheochromocytoma

DISORDER	SKIN MANIFESTATIONS	MANIFESTATIONS OF OTHER SYSTEMS	PREDOMINANT CANCERS
Peutz–Jegher's Syndrome	distinctive pigmentation (melanin spots) of nose, face, and distal portions of fingers, of mucous membranes and lip	polyposis coli of intestinal tract except esophagus	adenocarcinoma of duodenum and colon
Epidermolysis Bullosa Dystrophia (Congenital Traumatic Pemphigus)	vesicles, bullae, epidermal cysts, extensor surfaces & sites exposed to trauma with disabling scarring	bullae and ulcers of mucous membranes	carcinoma of mucous membranes, multiple basal & squamous cell carcinoma of skin*
Kaposi's Sarcoma (Multiple Idiopathic Hemorrhagic Sarcoma of Kaposi)	reddish, purplish, or bluish brown nodules, rubbery or firm consistency, often unilateral, predominantly on extremities along veins or lymphatics	lesions may occur in gastrointestinal tract or genitalia	sarcoma; high incidence of coexistent leukemia or lymphoma
Porphyria Cutanea Tarda	photosensitivity, bullae on areas exposed to trauma, hyperpigmentation, sclerodermatous thickening with calcification	systemic disease (may be similar to acute intermittent porphyria and precipitated by barbiturates)	basal cell carcinoma of skin, hepatoma*
Generalized Keratoacanthoma	red macules with rapid progression to papules and nodules; circular, firm, pearly, rolled, notched rim surrounding an umbilicated crater; may show exceedingly rapid involution	none	rare occurrences of squamous cell carcinoma*
Pachynychia Congenita	thickening of the nails, subungal hyperkeratosis, keratoderma of the palms and soles	occasionally may encounter hyperhidrosis, abnormalities of hair, teeth, and bone development, bulla formation, and mental deficiency.	carcinoma of mucous membranes
Syndrome of Bilateral Pheochromocytoma; Medullary Thyroid Carcinoma and Multiple Neuromas	true neuromas which may occur on the eyelids, lips, tongue or the nasal and laryngeal mucosae	parathyroid adenomas, hypertension secondary to pheochromocytoma	pheochromocytoma (often bilateral) medullary thyroid carcinoma

*Rare, but neverthless definite, cancer association

TABLE 2
AUTOSOMAL RECESSIVE INHERITANCE

DISORDER	SKIN MANIFESTATIONS	MANIFESTATIONS OF OTHER SYSTEMS	PREDOMINANT CANCERS
Xeroderma Pigmentosum	dry, scaling, hyperpigmentation and freckling, hyperkeratosis, and telangiectasia, basal and squamous cell carcinoma	multi-system involvement	basal and squamous cell carcinoma of skin and malignant melanoma
Werner's Syndrome (Progeria of the Adult)	premature aging of the skin, scleroderma-like findings, loss of subcutaneous fat, greying of the hair, baldness	juvenile cataract, diabetes mellitus, hypogonadism, short stature, arteriosclerosis	sarcomas, meningiomas
Ataxia-Telangiectasia (Louis-Bar Syndrome)	oculocutaneous telangiectasia temporal and nasal area of conjuntive, also of butterfly areas, ears, antecubital, popliteal, dorsum of hands and feet; telangiectasia are venous	cerebellar ataxia, mental and growth retardation, recurrent sinopulmonary infection; lymphopenia; deficiency in developing delayed hypersensitivity (gamma 1-A globulin defect)	acute leukemia & lymphoma
Bloom's Syndrome (Congenital Telangiectatic Erythema & stunted growth)	congenital telangiectatic erythema of face "butterfly distribution," photosensitivity; occasionally, *café au lait* spots, ichthyosis, acanthosis nigricans, hypertrichosis & lichen pilaris	short stature, fine featured face, dolicocephalic head	acute leukemia
Chediak-Higashi Syndrome	semi-albinism, hyperpigmentary response to sunlight, excessive sweating	hematologic (anomalous intracellular granulations); retinal albinism, photophobia, recurrent infections, lymphadenopathy, and neurologic manifestations	lymphoma
Albinism	partial or total absence of pigmentation of skin, hair, eyes ("pink eye"). premature aging of skin as noted by actinic chelitis, telangiectasia, keratosis, and cutaneous horns	several phenotypic varieties, including impairment of vision, hearing, and mental retardation	basal and squamous cell carcinoma of skin
Fanconi's Aplastic Anemia	spotty or patchy brown pigmentation	pancytopenia, bone marrow hypoplasia, congenital abnormalities including hypoplasia of thumbs, absent radius	leukemia
Glioma-Polyposis Syndrome* (Turcot's Syndrome)	*café au lait* spots	none	brain tumors, most commonly glioblastoma multiforme (one patient had medulloblastoma) and adenocarcinoma of colon secondary to polyposis coli

*Condition restricted to siblings (males and females) in two unrelated families strongly suggesting autosomal recessive inheritance.

TABLE 3
SEX-LINKED RECESSIVE INHERITANCE

DISORDER	SKIN MANIFESTATIONS	MANIFESTATIONS OF OTHER SYSTEMS	PREDOMINANT CANCERS
Aldrich syndrome (Wiskott–Aldrich syndrome)	chronic eczema, erythroderma, petechiae, purpura, furuncles	thrombocytopenia, recurrent infections, pyoderma, purulent otitis media; death often due to overwhelming infections	leukemia, lymphoma
Bruton's agamma globulinemia	Pyodermas, furunculosis, cellulitis, conjunctivitis	multiple recurrent infections; defect in formation of immunoglobulin–producing system	acute leukemia

TABLE 4

POSSIBLE GENETIC ETIOLOGY—MODE OF INHERITANCE UNKNOWN

DISORDER	SKIN MANIFESTATIONS	MANIFESTATIONS OF OTHER SYSTEMS	PREDOMINANT CANCERS
Scleroderma	"stiffness of skin" with loss of lines of normal facial expression, history of Raynaud's phenomenon	esophageal involvement with decreased peristalsis, dilation, dysphagia, alteration of pulmonary function	Bronchiolar carcinoma, malignant carcinoid
Dermatomyositis	inflammatory changes of skin and muscle, erythema, puffy edematous swelling of eyelids "heliotrope bloating" minute telangiectasia	serum enzyme and electromyographic changes; may be preceded by Raynaud's phenomenon	adenocarcinoma of viscera
Sjögren's syndrome (keratoconjunctivitis sicca)	dryness of skin and mucous membranes, hyperpigmentation, café au lait spots, purpura and telangiectasia of lips and fingertips	rheumatoid arthritis	lymphoma
Systemic lupus erythematosus	malar erythema of "butterfly area", macules; variety of cutaneous vascular changes	intermittent fever, arthritis, arthralgia, arteritis, phlebitis, CNS and renal disease (lupus nephritis) biologic false-positive serology, positive LE preps	thymic tumors, leukemia and lymphoma
Giant pigmented nevi* (bathing trunk nevi)	nevi covering extensive cutaneous surface; variable manifestations ranging from flat to angiomatous, verrucous, and hairy nevi	none	Melanomas in children
Nevus Sebaceous of Jadassohn	hamartoma often present at birth primarily on scalp, face or neck. Several centimeters or more, circumscribed, round on irregular, slightly raised, waxy, hairless which at puberty, becomes verrucous & nodular & later may be complicated by benign or malignant nevoid tumors	variable, may find convulsive disorder, focal EEG abnormalities, mental deficiency & brain dysplasia; ocular abnormalities have included colobomas of the irides & choroid, conjunctival lipodermoids, and nystagmus	Basal cell epithelioma (15% to 20%), sebaceous epithelioma, salivary gland adenocarcinoma, syringocystadenoma papilliferum (apocrine duct stage differentiation), and keratoacanthoma

*Hereditary etiology has not yet been established, but the congenital basis and known hereditary factors of certain melanomas raise suspicion about genetic etiology.

Chapter 2

FUNDAMENTALS OF GENETICS

by Arnold R. Kaplan, Ph.D.

INTRODUCTION

The etiology of a pathological condition may be evaluated in terms of the combination of constitutional predisposition and exposure to precipitating factors. Individual differences in predispositions to acquire a particular disorder in any specific environment are the consequences of individuals being different from each other. The variations in such liabilities are manifestations of individual differences in the effects of interacting genetic and nongenetic variables. A given property of an organism depends on series of complex biochemical reactions and biochemically–determined developmental processes. Interference with these at any of many different levels may affect the final end–product. The complexity of metabolic activities within each cell is such that vast numbers of genes might be expected to exert some influence on almost any activity. A particular gene or group of genes determines an indefinite but limited assortment of effects, the different effects being associated with differences in environment and/or with differences in other aspects of the total genetic make–up. A first step toward understanding the etiologic role of biological heredity is achievement of the realization that one's genetic material,

which an individual has derived from his parents, is a set of potentialities and not a set of already–formed or predetermined characteristics.

Much of the controversy over the relevance of genetic differences in disease etiology relates to concern for the patients' prognoses and therapies. Involvement of genetically–determined constitutional differences in predisposition to a disorder does not necessarily imply a poor prognosis or negate therapy. The occurrence of a primary relevance of genetic differences for different predispositions to a disease does not mean that the disease is any less curable or any less amenable to any particular therapy than it would be if the principal etiological variables for the same disease were all environmental. A disease is a condition which may be an effect of, and may be affected by, genetic and/or environmental alterations. Theoretically, no disorder or disease is necessarily incurable, but the environmental changes which must be introduced in order to effect a cure may be unknown. The study of the genetics of a disease may facilitate its prevention or amelioration by purely environmental methods. The more it becomes possible to precisely characterize the genetic constitution of an individual, the more likely are we to learn how to modify or tailor

17

the environment according to the individual's needs.[1] In effect, it may be possible to determine the environmental differences between the predisposed individuals who develop the disease and those who do not. Then, if these environmental circumstances can be recognized, they can hopefully be adjusted for the genetically–predisposed individuals before development of the clinical abnormality.

PHENOTYPES, GENOTYPES,

PHENOCOPIES, and GENOCOPIES

The term, *phenotype,* refers to an individual's observable properties, physiological and pathological, structural and functional, which are effects of the interactions between his genotype and his environment. The sum total of an individual's genetic material, the total genetic constitution, is his *genotype.* The characteristics of an individual's development and growth, from conception to birth to maturity to death, are effects of the interactions of his genotype with his environment.

A trait or disorder which is usually associated with a particular gene or group of genes may, in response to particular environmental variables, be manifested without that gene or group of genes. Nonhereditary phenotypic modifications, which are caused by special environmental conditions, and which mimic similar phenotypes characteristically associated with particular genes, have been termed *phenocopies.*[2] Specific effects of genic action can be imitated by certain environmental influences, interacting with genotypes which norms of reaction (*i.e.,* phenotypic flexibilities) include the potentials for such manifestations, even though the genotypes do not include the particular gene(s) which is/are characteristically associated with these effects.

Series of grades of phenocopies may occur, to resemble effects characteristically associated with various combinations of multiple genes. A trait or disorder which is characteristically associated with a particular gene or group of genes may also occur in the absence of such gene(s), effected by other (*i.e.,* different) genes. The effects of such 'mimetic genes' have been termed *genocopies.*[3]

Certain phenocopies are only inducible when a particular environmental influence is applied during a specific, or within a limited, period of development. That is, for some effects, there is a limited sensitive or critical period during which the effects may be determined. This suggests that, during such critical stages in development, there exist alternative paths which lead to different effects, and the path which is to be followed may be determined by genetic and/or environmental factors.[4] The existence of a particularly sensitive period in development, during which a specific disorder is most easily initiated, means that induction of a phenocopy may depend upon the stage of development during which the environmental influence occurs, as well as upon the interacting genotype (*i.e.,* the potential responsiveness or norm of reaction of that genotype) and the nature and intensity and duration of the environmental influence. Only a part of the population segment consisting of individuals who are genetically predisposed to a particular pathology actually do develop that pathology. Identification of those individuals in the population, who are genetically predisposed, would provide a powerful tool for discovering the relevant critical environmental factors.

Many criteria have been studied for indications of the significance of genetic factors in etiologies of various pathologies, including: elevated morbidity risks in relatives of index cases compared with the general population; increasing morbidity risks associated with increasing degrees of genetic kinship to index cases; greater concordance in monozygotic than in dizygotic pairs of twins; and variation in frequencies of the disorders in different populations. These observations, alone, are not rigorous and conclusive evidence of genetic etiology.[5] Environmental factors common to relatives can simulate genetic determinants. It is not possible to conclusively prove that a trait is genetic except by showing that it could be due to one of several modes of inheritance. The genetic method consists in attempting to extract from a possibly heterogeneous trait one or more genetic entities due, in increasing order of refinement, to a single inheritance pattern, locus, or allele. Sometimes genetic traits depend on the presence of several genes (*i.e., complementary epistasis*). If the effect of each gene is recognizable, each component may be studied separately. Otherwise, the analysis may be beyond the limits of available methods in human genetics. The only unequivocally reliable approach to a nonexperimental system is to defer final determination of mode of inheritance until the reasonable genes are individually recognizable. Traits determined by many genes, not individually recognizable, are unfavorable for genetic analysis. The possible occurrence of multiple etiologies and consequent multiple morbidity risks may be masked by associating a trait with a single morbidity risk figure which was actually based on heterogeneous populations.[6] An alternative approach would be to divide individuals into those belonging to high–risk *versus* those in low–risk (sporadic) families, if such a division of available data were supported by segregation analysis.[7] The

dichotomy could be based, for example, upon familial *versus* nonfamilial index cases, or upon concordant *versus* discordant pairs of monozygotic twins. Even if the disorders in most or many of the affected individuals were associated with simple modes of genetic transmission, some cases could be sporadic due to occurrence of phenocopies, genocopies, diagnostic errors, *etc.* The assumption of the occurrence of sporadic cases may lead to recognition of heterogeneity in data previously regarded as homogeneous, and may even show that the risk in high–risk families is great enough to suggest a simple genetic hypothesis.[5] Genetic ratios within sibships may be utilized to test for Mendelian modes of genetic transmission, based upon observations of individuals in only a single generation. Pedigree analysis, which utilizes available data regarding individuals in various generations of the family tree, is far more informative and is the principal method of genetic study in man. Essentially, pedigree analysis involves utilization of the basic principles of Gregor Mendel,[8] for extrapolation of genotypes from information regarding phenotypes and the genetic relationships.

Pedigree Analysis

The term, *family,* is usually applied to a pair of parents and their children. The term may also be used to refer to a more extensive association of relatives, although a larger group of individuals who are related to each other genetically and through marriage is usually called a *kindred.*[9] Females are usually symbolized by circles, and males by squares (Fig. 1), but sometimes other symbols are used (*e.g.,* the symbol for Mars to indicate a male, the one for Venus to indicate a female). The symbols of a pair of parents

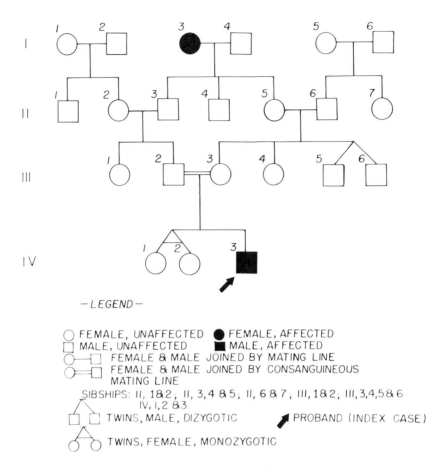

Figure 1. Pedigree showing use of symbols for communication of relationships within a kindred.

are joined by a horizontal mating line, and their offsprings' symbols are located in a horizontal row below that line. Double horizontal mating lines indicate a consanguinous combination. The off–springs' symbols are connected by vertical lines to a horizontal line above them, which is connected further above by a single vertical line to the horizontal mating line. The children of a parental pair form a *sibship*; and the children in a sibship, regardless of sex, are *siblings* or *sibs* of each other. Possession of the trait being examined in the pedigree is designated by shading the symbol (*e.g.*, circle or square) of the individual involved, and an unshaded symbol denotes absence of the character or disease. Twins are designated by lines extending, from the two symbols involved, to a common point on the horizontal sibship line. The affected individual with whom a particular pedigree study was initiated may be identified as the *index case* or *proband*, or *propositus*. Generations are customarily identified with Roman numerals, ranging from the earliest at the top of a pedigree schematic to the most recent at the bottom. Within each generation, the individuals are numbered from left to right with

Arabic numerals. Thus, each individual in a particular pedigree may be identified by the combination of a Roman number and an Arabic number.

Pedigree patterns characteristically provide information on the Mendelian principles of segregation and independent assortment, and they may also provide information on allelism and linkage.[10] A specific pedigree pattern depends upon whether effects of the gene involved are manifested in single dosage or only in double dosage, and upon whether the gene is located on one of the autosomes or on a sex chromosome. An individual who possesses an identical pair of genes on a particular locus of a pair of homologous chromosomes is *homozygous* for the locus; and an individual whose pair of genes on a particular locus are different from each other is *heterozygous* for the locus. In a heterozygous individual, if one of the pair of genes is recognizably manifested while the other one is suppressed, the former gene is termed *dominant* and the latter one is *recessive.* Genetic dominance is a manifestation of a gene's ability to be expressed in the phenotype of a genetically heterozygous individual. The failure of a gene to be expressed in the phenotype, when it occurs in a genetically heterozygous genotype, is genetic recessivity. A recessive gene may be carried and transmitted through innumerable generations without being manifested. A dominant gene, however, is characteristically manifested in the phenotypes of the individuals who possess either one (i.e., in the heterozygous individual) or a pair (i.e., in the homozygous individual) of them.

The manifestation of a trait transmitted by a single autosomal dominant gene with complete penetrance is indicated in a pedigree in which the trait does not "skip" generations. An individual with the trait has a parent with the trait, and approximately one–half the offspring of couples in which one of the parents is affected are similarly affected. A trait which is transmitted by a pair of autosomal recessive alleles, by contrast, may occur without any previous family history of the trait in either the maternal or the paternal side. Children born subsequent to an index case, establishing both parents as heterozygous carriers of the recessive gene for the trait, will include approximately one–fourth affected; and approximately two–thirds of the unaffected siblings will be heterozygous "carriers" of the recessive gene. In the case of a very rare trait (in the population) transmitted by a pair of autosomal recessive alleles, consanguinity may be expected to occur more frequently in affected families than in the general population.

Genes which are located on the X chromosome, like those on an autosome, may be dominant or recessive. A female, with two X chromosomes, may be either homozygous or heterozygous for a particular locus on the X chromosome. A male, with only one X chromosome, is *hemizygous* for any X–linked gene. Such a gene may be dominant or recessive in the female. In the hemizygous male, with no other gene at the locus, an X–linked gene is always expressed. X–linked genetic transmission is characterized by the absence of male–to–male transmission, because a son necessarily inherits a Y chromosome from his (XY) father and an X chromosome from his (XX) mother. The X chromosome of a male is characteristically transmitted to none of his sons but to all of his daughters.

One's sex may affect the expression of a gene, and a trait transmitted by a gene which is manifested differently in the two sexes is *sex–influenced*. That is, a sex–influenced trait is one in which phenotypic manifestations are different in the two sexes. If the gene is completely suppressed in one of the two sexes, then it is *sex–limited*. A sex–influenced or sex–limited gene (i.e., regarding its manifestation in the phenotype) may occur on an autosome or on an X chromosome.

Genetic *linkage* involves the occurrence of different genetic loci on the same chromosome. If two loci occur on separate nonhomologous (*i.e.,* not pairing at meiosis) chromosomes, then independent assortment occurs. If two loci occur on the same chromosome, and particularly if they occur relatively close to each other, then the genes occurring on the two loci would usually tend to be transmitted in the same combination (*i.e.,* without independent assortment) from generation to generation. Close genetic linkage of different loci may be difficult to distingusih from *allelism, i.e.,* occurrence of alternate gene forms at a single locus on a particular chromosome. The term, *X–linked,* refers to the location of a gene on the X chromosome. A gene whose locus occurs on the Y chromosome is termed *Y–linked* or *holandric.* Such a gene would characteristically affect only males, and would be transmitted only from father to sons.

PENETRANCE, EXPRESSIVITY, AND HERITABILITY

A disorder or trait for which individual differences are studied is a dependent variable resulting from interactions of independent variables and the organism with its intervening variables (*e.g.,* morphogenetic and neuroendocrine characteristics). The intervening variables do not remain constant, but are themselves modified by the independent variables which affect the organism. The *penetrance* of a gene or group of genes and the nature of its/their *expressivity*, observed as phenotypic manifestations, differ in different *milieux,* environmental and/or genetic. Thus, there are differences in penetrance of the gene(s) associated with predisposition to a disease, which are associated with different environmental *milieux* and different genetic *milieux* (*i.e.,* the complete genotypes). When the gene(s) is/are penetrant, these differences affect variability in expressivity. Complete penetrance is shown by a genotype which is always associated with a particular phenotype. Even when a genotype associated with predisposition to a pathology is penetrant, there may be clinical differences between different affected individuals. Thus, even when penetrant, a genotype may show variable expressivity. Environmental, as well as ancillary genetic, variables interpose numerous influences between primary gene products and the final mechanisms by which genetic manifestations are actuated. Environmental variables may affect reductions in correlations between genotypes and observable phenotypic effects, causing variable expressivity and/or incomplete penetrance.

Heritability determinations are estimates of the proportion of the total phenotypic variance (*i.e.,* individual differences), shown by a trait, that can be attributed to genetic variation in some particular population at a single generation under one set of conditions. The heritability of a particular pathology may be defined as the extent to which the variation in individual risk of acquiring the pathology is due to genetic differences. A trait will show a greater–than–

zero heritability if two or more segregating alleles, which manifest different effects upon the trait, occur on at least one genetic locus. A relevant genetic locus, which is associated with phenotypic variation in one population because it is represented there by two or more different segregating alleles, might show no variation in another population because the same locus involves only a single allele (*i.e.*, identical genes on homologous loci) in that other population. One environment may activate a particular gene, while another may not. Thus, a trait may show a particular greater–than–zero heritability in one allele–segregating population, but other heritabilities in other populations which involve population-genetic differences and/or environmental differences. The different heritabilities shown for a particular trait in different populations do not indicate that any particular gene manifests different degrees of heredity in the different populations involved. The ontogeny of an individual's phenotype (*i.e.*, observable outcome of development) has a norm or range of reaction which is not predictable in advance. Even in the most favorable investigations, only an approximate estimate can be obtained for the norm of reaction, when, as in plants and some animals, an individual genotype can be replicated many times and its development studied over a range of environmental conditions. The more varied the conditions, the more diverse might be the phenotypes developed from any one genotype. Different genotypes do not have the same norm of reaction. Therefore, the limits set by a particular gene or group of genes cannot be entirely specified. These limits are plastic within each individual but differ between individuals.

Extreme environmentalists have been wrong to hope that one law or set of laws might describe universal features of modifiability, and extreme hereditarians have been wrong to ignore the *norm of reaction.*[11] In its strictest sense, a heritability measure provides an estimate of the proportion of the variance which a specific population shows in trait (*i.e.*, phenotype) expression and which is correlated with segregation of independently–acting alleles of a relevant genetic locus or of relevant genetic loci. Heritability is a property of a specific population and not of a trait (*i.e.*, in all populations or in all *milieux*). In any particular population, heritability coefficients are based on observed correlations among individuals with different degrees of genetic kinship. Many published twin, family, twin–family and extended–pedigree studies of disease incidence have essentially been studies of heritability, because they have not indicated a clearly–defined mode of heredity (*i.e.*, a specific mode of genetic transmission). Heritabilities may vary between different groups because of different environmental contexts, as well as because of numerous secondary genetic (*i.e.*, in addition to the genetic factors predominantly associated with the liability to the pathology) differences. Thus, the findings from different studies of heritability, for any category of disorder which does not involve a clear and simple mode of genetic transmission with complete penetrance, may be expected to vary from each other. The demonstration of significant heritability for a pathology, in one particular group, indicates the major relevance of genetic differences for different predispositions to the pathology. The demonstration of lower heritability for the same pathology, in another group, may indicate that the effects of these genetic factors (*i.e.,* within the genetically–defined norm or range of reaction) may be profoundly modulated by other genetic factors and/or by nongenetic influences.[12] Different combinations of different genetic and nongenetic factors may manifest similar phenotypes. The same genetic or nongenetic factor affecting different individuals, who differ with regard to other genetic factors and/or environmental influences, may show different manifestations. Thus, different genes may be associated with the same phenotype, and different phenotypes may be associated with the same gene(s), depending upon the total interacting genetic and environmental contexts. If the incidence of a particular pathology varies from one population to another, and the difference is not due solely to diagnostic inconsistencies, the variance can be ascribed to differences of mean liability, or to differences of variance of liability, or to combinations of both.[13] If there is a difference between two populations in the pathology's heritability, then two or more (rather than only one) predisposing genotypes are involved, and/or the lower heritability is associated with environmental circumstances which increase the nongenetic differences of the liability. The relative contributions of heredity and environment for a trait may differ with different overall heredities (*i.e.,* total genotypes) and with different environments. The reaction–norm concept is of fundamental importance to an understanding of gene action. Modification of a gene's environment, either by nongenetic environmental influences or through the effects of other genes, may affect the expression of any specific gene within the limits characteristic of that gene's phenotypic potential.

Probability Analysis

Inference or reasoning is a mode of thinking by which one starts from something known and proceeds to form a belief that there exists a fact hitherto unknown. The basic assumption is that one's methods of reasoning are reliable and lead to conclusions which correspond with facts. Many of the reasoned conclusions can then be checked and verified by perceptions of objective investigations. Every perception is received by a mind already made up of memories, interests, expectations, and bias. Therefore, the resultant new state of consciousness is derived in part from the observations and in part (sometimes the larger part) from what is in the mind already. Even at the times of observations, there are natural tendencies to confuse one's preconceptions with what is actually perceived.[14] The most useful hypotheses are those which are testable, and testability is associated with simplicity and directness. As hypotheses increase in their complexity, and as they involve secondary hypotheses, their testabilities diminish. The contributions of additional hypotheses which cannot be subjected to conclusive tests, which cannot be proved or disproved, provide little more than exercises for their contributors. The many relevant variables cannot always be entirely controlled, and some of them may not even be recognized. One may measure the overall variation, which is due to all the uncontrolled variables, as well as the differences relatable to the factors one is evaluating. Then, by comparing the two, one may judge whether the latter are statistically significant to provide confidence that they are not just the misleading expression of some uncontrolled or even unrecognized source of variation.[15] Scientific conclusions necessarily emerge as statements of probability. There is always the risk that particular results do not facilitate a sound or unbiased basis for a general statement, as reflected in the statement of probability which the analysis yields. The conclusions drawn from any study or combination of studies are not immutable or certain but, as the body of observational experience grows, the level of uncertainty is decreased.

A deviation from the expected ratio, in the observed ratio of unaffected and affected individuals, may be due to chance or to some relevant variable. The meaning of the *statistical significance* of a deviation can be calculated in terms of statistical probability that it may occur due only to chance. Statistical probability, the mathematical evaluation of chance, may be defined as the ratio of the number of occurrences of a specified combination of events to the total number of all possible combinations of the events. The term, statistical significance, relates to whether or not some specific reason or reasons, and not only chance, underlies the observed deviation. The probability level which is regarded as significant is somewhat arbitrary and depends upon the judgment of the investigator involved. If the probability that a deviation may occur between two populations, or between the observed and expected findings, is lower than one percent, then the findings would generally be regarded as statistically significant. A probability level above one percent but below five percent is sometimes considered significant, but more conservative investigators tend to consider such a figure as only of doubtful or questionable significance. The choice of which statistical test might most appropriately be utilized for any particular evaluation depends upon many factors, including the sizes of the samples involved, the parametric or nonparametric character of the data distributions, *etc.* [16, 17] One of the simplest and most commonly used tests in genetics is the *chi-square test*: the value of chi-square equals the sum of the squares of the absolute differences between the observed and expected categories divided by the respective expected values being compared [9, 18]; and the probability value may be determined from a corresponding chi-square value listed in standard tables. [19] The happenings of nature involve probability laws rather than predetermined causality. [20] A scientific investigator only determines his best posits from the available information. The addition of more specifically relevant information facilitates more accurate judgments. A genetic factor may be manifested only by appropriate genotype–environment combinations. The determination of whether a gene is harmful or useful or indifferent is related to the bearer's environment. The genetic epidemiologist functions as a kind of ecologist seeking significant correlations between a disorder and one or another variable from the great array of environmental influences. His success in these efforts will be related to the uniqueness of the variable involved and the directness of its effect, to the frequency of the basic defect, and to the ease of detection of the disorder under consideration. [21]

The Hardy–Weinberg Principle

Hardy [22] and Weinberg [23] independently developed the principle that genotypic frequencies within a population in any generation depend solely upon the frequencies in the previous generation, if none of the genotypes was affected by selective factors and if the population was random–mating. The fundamental idea of gene distribution in populations, based on the assumption of random mating and no differential selection and no significant contribution from new mutations, is a deduction from the Mendelian principles of segregation and recombination. In a large population, if A_1 and A_2 are alleles for one particular locus, and the frequency of the gene A_1 in the population is p_1, and the frequency of the gene A_2 is p_2, then the genotypic frequencies after one or more random matings will be: for genotype $(A_1 A_1)$, $(p_1)^2$; for genotype $(A_1 A_2)$, $(2p_1 p_2)$; and for genotype $(A_2 A_2)$, $(p_2)^2$. The proportions may be determined by expansion of the binomial, $(p_1 + p_2)^2$. The genotypic frequencies may be determined for any number of alleles on a single locus, by expansion of the appropriate binomial. Thus, for three alleles $- -$ with the genes A_1, A_2 and A_3 occuring in the population, respectfully, at frequencies p_1, p_2, and p_3 $- -$ $(p_1 + p_2 + p_3)^2$ equals $p_1^2 + p_2^2 + p_3^2 + 2p_1 p_2 + 2p_1 p_3$. $+ 2p_2 p_3$. The frequencies, then, would be: for $(A_1 A_1)$, $(p_1)^2$; for $(A_2 A_2)$, $(p_2)^2$; for $(A_3 A_3)$, p_3^2; for $(A_1 A_2)$, $(2p_1 p_2)$; for $(A_1 A_3)$, $(2p_1 p_3)$; and for $(A_2 A_3)$, $(2p_2 p_3)$.

SELECTION, GENETIC DRIFT, AND MUTATION

If individuals of differing genotypes should differ in their viabilities or fertilities, then there would be differences in the proportionate contributions of individuals of different genotypes to the total offspring. That is, *selection* would occur in different degrees for the different phenotypes. The alleles in individuals whose genotypes are characterized by higher reproductive fitness will be represented in higher proportions than the alleles associated with the individuals of lower reproductive fitness. Selection can cause alterations in gene frequencies from one generation to the next.

The process of *genetic drift*[24] may lead to the establishment of a trait which is neutral and nonadaptive or even unfavorable. It involves the random fluctuation of gene frequencies due to chance, and is particularly important for small isolated populations. The probability of genetic drift affecting the gene frequencies of a population depends largely upon the size of the population: with a greater number of parents, the likelihood of loss and fixation are lower, because of the decreased probability that the same chance loss will occur consistently for the different parents. When an isolated population is small, the speed of drift may be high from one generation to the next; but, when a population is large, the process of drift would tend to be a slow one.

Mutations are changes in the genetic material, which are irreversible except for subsequent mutations. *Chromosomal mutations* involve genetic changes which are visible with present cytogenetic techniques and which involve duplication, deletion, or translocation of a complete chromosome or discernible chromosomal fragment. *Gene mutations* or *point mutations* involve changes which are not cytologically visible and which are identifiable only by their phenotypic manifestations. The estimated frequency of a gene mutation may be calculated. One method for such a calculation, primarily applicable to dominant mutations, is based simply on a census of the frequency of children with the particular dominant trait under study who are born to parents without the trait.[9] The underlying assumptions for such a direct calculation involve complete penetrance of the gene, and the occurrence of no other genetic locus or mode of genetic transmission associated with the trait. An indirect method for calculating a particular mutation rate has been based upon the hypothesis that recurrent mutations from normal to abnormal balance the loss in fitness associated with the mutation.[25, 26, 27] The number of new mutants depends on the total number of normal alleles and the frequency with which they can mutate.[9] For a dominant mutant, the mutation rate equals $\frac{1}{2}(1 - f)x$ when f equals the fraction of mutant genes which are 'lost' because of reduced reproductive fitness, and x is the frequency of the abnormality in the parent generation. The mutation rate for a recessive mutant may be approximated, using the same concept of equilibrium between new mutations and 'loss,' from the following formula: mutation rate equals $(1 - f)x$. An adaptation of the latter formula may be used for estimating the mutation rate for an X-linked recessive mutant. Since hemizygous males have one-third of the X-linked abnormal alleles in the population, one-third of the X-linked abnormal alleles are exposed to reduced reproductive fitness and some 'loss.' Thus, in an equilibrium between mutation and elimination, the mutation rate equals $(1/3)(1 - f)x_m$ when x_m is the frequency of the abnormality among the males of the parent generation.[9]

Polygenic Inheritance

The terms, *polygenic inheritance* and *multifactorial inheritance*, refer to traits associated with more than a single locus and a single pair of genes. There is, as yet, no conclusive proof for polygenic determination of alternative-trait development in man. Polygenic inheritance could account for many abnormal traits that seem to have a genetic basis but have no regular sequence of generations or clear-cut ratios. A polygenic theory may be involved in an attempt to account for inheritance of graded characters within a basic Mendelian framework, or in association with the concept of a genetic-threshold effect. Characteristically, such theories have been applied to problems which were obviously insoluble in terms of major genes. The principal fault associated with polygenic theories is the fact that they are not specifically testable or refutable. A polygenic device can be adapted to explain anything, with components which cannot be independently checked by observation.[28]

Concluding Remarks

Extrapolations are risky, but they are necessary interim steps in the process of acquiring firm knowledge. More research is needed. More examinations and critical interpretations of the available data and material are also needed.

References

1. Harris, H.: *The Principles of Human Biochemical Genetics.* New York, American Elsevier, 1970.

2. Goldschmidt, R.: *Physiolocigal Genetics.* New York, McGraw-Hill, 1938.

3. Nachtsheim, H.: Mutation and Phänocopie bei Saugetier und Mensch. Ihre theoretische und praktische Bedeutung für Genetik und Eugenik. *Experientia, 13*: 57, 1957.

4. Thoday, J.M.: Components of fitness. *Sympos. Soc. Exp. Biol.,* 7: 96, 1953.

5. Morton, N.E.: Segregation and linkage. In Burdette, W.J. (Ed.): *Methodol-*

ogy in Human Genetics. San Francisco, Holden–Day, 1962.

6. Kaplan, A.R.: Genetic counseling in mental retardation and mental disorders, In Lynch, H.T. (Ed.): *Dynamic Genetic Counseling for Clinicians.* Springfield, Thomas, 1969.

7. Morton, N.E.: Genetic tests under incomplete ascertainment. *Amer. J. Hum. Genet., 11*: 1, 1959.

8. Olby, R.C.: *Origins of Mendelism.* New York, Schocken, 1969.

9. Stern, C.: *Principles of Human Genetics,* Second Edition. San Francisco, Freeman, 1960.

10. McKusick, V.A.: *Human Genetics.* Englewood Cliffs, Prentice–Hall, 1964.

11. Hirsch, J.: Behavior–genetic analysis and its biosocial consequences. *Seminars in Psychiatry, 2*: 89, 1970.

12. Kaplan, A.R.: Concluding remarks: genetics and schizophrenia. In Kaplan, A.R. (Ed.): *Genetic Factors in "Schizophrenia." Springfield, Thomas*, in press.

13. Falconer, D.S.: The inheritance of liability to diseases with variable age of onset, with particular reference to diabetes mellitus. *Ann. Hum. Genet., 31*: 1, 1967.

14. Kohler, I.: *The Formation and Transformation of the Perceptual World.* Psychological Issues, Vol. III, No. 4, Monograph 12 (Translated from the German by Fiss, H.). New York, Int. Univ. Press, 1963.

15. Mather, K.: *Human Diversity.* Edinburgh, Oliver and Boyd, 1964.

16. Mather, K.: *Statistical Analysis in Biology,* Fourth Edition. London, Methuen, 1965.

17. Burdette, W.J. (Editor): *Methodology in Human Genetics.* San Francisco, Holden–Day, 1962.

18. Edwards, A.L.: *Statistical Analysis,* Revised Edition. New York, Holt, Rinehart and Winston, 1965.

19. Fisher, R.A. and Yates, F.: *Statistical Tables for Biological Agricultural and Medical Research,* Sixth Edition. New York, Hafner, 1963.

20. Reichenbach, H.: Predictive knowledge. In Jarrett, J.L., and McMurrin, S.M. (Eds.): *Contemporary Philosophy.* New York, Holt, Rinehart and Winston, 1954.

21. Francis, T., Jr.: Genetics and Epidemiology. In Neel, J.V., Shaw, M.W., and Schull, W.J. (Eds.): *Genetics and Epidemiology of Chronic Diseases, Publication No. 1163.* Washington, D.C., U.S. Dept. of Health, Education and Welfare, 1965.

22. Hardy, G.H.: Mendelian proportions in a mixed population. *Science, 28*: 49, 1908.

23. Weinberg, W.: Über den Nachweis der Vererbung beim Menschen. *Jahreshefte Verein f. vaterl. Naturk. in Württemberg, 64*: 368, 1908.

24. Wright, S.: Classification of the factors of evolution. *Cold Spring Harbor Symposium on Quantitative Biology, 20*: 16, 1955.

25. Danforth, C.H.: The frequency of mutation and the incidence of hereditary traits in man. *Eugenics, Genetics and the Family, 1*: 120, 1923.

26. Haldane, J.B.S.: The rate of spontaneous mutation of a human gene. *J. Genet., 31*: 317, 1935.

27. Gunther, M. and Penrose, L.S.: The genetics of epiloia. *J. Genet., 31*: 413, 1935.

28. 'Epinasse, P.G.: The polygene concept. *Nature, 149*: 732, 1942.

Chapter 3

CUTANEOUS CLUES TO INTERNAL MALIGNANT DISEASE

by Harold O. Perry, M.D., Joseph M. Kiely, M.D. and Charles G. Moertel, M.D.

Today the general population is concerned with cancer. Recent emphasis on health practices, such as smoking, in relationship to the subsequent development of cancer or the possibility of ingestants in some way altering the physical status so as to produce abnormalities in physiology, makes the average patient health conscious. As such, he becomes concerned about alterations in his physiognomy, particularly the development of skin lesions, some of which he may interpret as a form of cancer or as evidence of an internal malignancy.

The physician must thus be knowledgeable about cutaneous changes which may indeed indicate that a systemic malignant disease may be present. Careful inspection of the skin may reveal skin lesions which, taken in their proper perspective, may prompt the physician to undertake examination for the discovery of a systemic malignant disease.

At times, visual inspection of the skin alone may be sufficient, whereas, on other occasions, the microscopic examination of these lesions may be required to be certain that the cutaneous alterations are indicative of a systemic disease. Although there may be voids in our knowledge as to the mechanisms operating to elucidate the association between cutaneous change and visceral cancer, the physician, once alerted by recognized cutaneous changes, must be aggressive in his efforts to study the patient completely.

We would like to present briefly some cutaneous changes that have been recognized as important in alerting physicians to systemic malignant disease. It should be emphasized that these cutaneous changes, in themselves, are not malignant, but they present in a variety of morphologic forms. The specific distribution of what appears to be mundane lesions may produce clinical constellations as vulnerable to the patient as was the heel of Achilles to him.

We have classified the cutaneous changes into three general categories: (1) cutaneous changes that are indicative of a specific type of cancer; (2) cutaneous changes that might indicate the presence of malignant lesions of various organ systems; and (3) cutaneous changes that suggest the presence of lymphoreticular cancers. By clinical description, augmented at times by an illustration, we would like to emphasize the major cutaneous findings that we consider important in suggesting visceral malignant disease. Some of these diseases are based on a hereditary pattern, and when such exists, this will be mentioned. It is hoped that the physician will find in this chapter a ready reference to the most commonly accepted cutaneous signs of visceral malignant disease.

By choice we have eliminated from consideration those systemic malignant diseases in which the disease itself is manifested in the skin. Thus, not to be considered are cutaneous metastases, which at times may be the first sign of an underlying malignant lesion but which more often represent obvious extension to the cutaneous surface of an already recognized malignant lesion. Likewise, clinical and histologic cutaneous lymphoma will not be considered.

CUTANEOUS CLUES INDICATIVE OF A SPECIFIC MALIGNANT TUMOR

Paget's Disease

The presence of either a slightly elevated eczematous or smooth plaque about the areola of the nipple suggests the diagnosis of Paget's disease of the nipple which must be confirmed by histologic study of tissue (Color Plate 1–A). When typical clear Paget's cells are present, one must consider that an intraductal mammary carcinoma is present within the breast, even though this may not be perceptible on physical examination or by mammography. Mastectomy should be performed and careful histologic study of the entire breast should be carried out.

Extramammary Paget's Disease

Asymptomatic, sharply demarcated scaling and sometimes eczematoid plaques located around the lower part of the abdomen, the genitalia, or the inner regions of the thighs should suggest the possibility of extramammary Paget's disease (Fig. 1). Histologically, a biopsy of the skin lesions shows the presence of the same clear cells as seen in Paget's disease of the nipple and the implication is the same, namely, the presence of an underlying malignant tumor. Extramammary Paget's disease should suggest primary adenocarcinoma of the bladder, rectum, or one of the skin appendages. Rarely, a primary malignant process cannot be found.

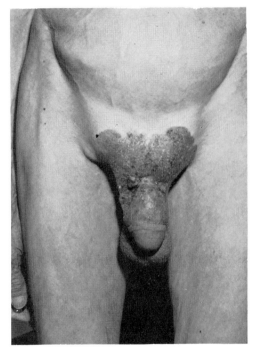

Figure 1. Superficial, erythematous, eczematoid, and scaling plaques in anogenital area are similar to those of Paget's disease of nipple and likewise may indicate underlying malignant disease. Note lymph node metastasis in right groin. (From Perry, H.O., Moertel, C.G., and Kiely, J.M.: Cutaneous Clues to Visceral Cancer. *Mod Med* 37:97–103 [Oct. 6] 1969. By permission.)

The Malignant Carcinoid Syndrome

The constellation of episodic cutaneous flushing, diarrhea, asthma, and valvular lesions of the right side of the heart provides a spectacular example of the peripheral manifestations of visceral neoplasia. Although this syndrome usually is produced by a carcinoid tumor primary to the small intestine and metastatic to the liver, it also may originate in bronchial carcinoids without liver involvement and in large bulky carcinoids limited to the ovary. Histologically identical neoplasms of the rectum will not produce the carcinoid syndrome, whereas wholly dissimilar oat cell carcinomas of the lung, adenocarcinomas of the pancreas, and medullary carcinomas of the thyroid may give rise to an identical clinical and laboratory picture.

Whereas initially serotonin was thought to be the sole mediator of the syndrome, more recent evidence has suggested that the kinin peptides also may play a major, or at least a contributory role. Carcinoid tumors of the stomach and bronchi may give rise to an intense florid flush associated with facial edema with evidence suggesting increased production of histamine and 5–hydroxytryptophane. The laboratory hallmark of the carcinoid syndrome in most cases, however, continues to be high urinary excretion of 5–hydroxyindolacetic acid, the metabolite of serotonin.

Gardner's Syndrome

The association of benign subcutaneous and osseous tumors with multiple polyposis of the large bowel has been recognized with increasing frequency since Gardner's initial report in 1962. The subcutaneous lesions include fibromas, lipomas, epidermoid cysts, and desmoid tumors (Fig. 2). Desmoid tumors generally occur in the anterior abdominal wall either coincident with pregnancy or in an operative scar. Osseous lesions are osteomas and osteochondromas with a particular predilection for the angle of the mandible.

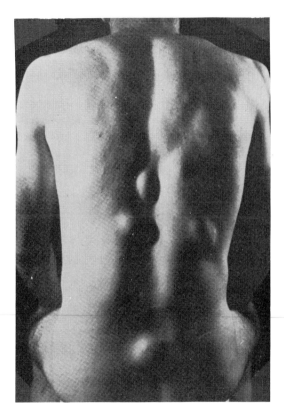

Figure 2. Numerous sebaceous cysts are among benign skin lesions that suggest possibility of Gardner's syndrome.

The polypoid lesions of the colon are typical adenomatous polyps, and symptoms are in every way typical of familial multiple polyposis. The polyps are generally first recognized in adolescence or young adulthood. It is likely that in all patients, adenocarcinoma of the large bowel will develop unless this organ is surgically removed.

The associated subcutaneous and osseous lesions may be observed sporadically among families with multiple polyposis and probably represent a less penetrant manifestation of the same genetic trait, namely, an autosomal dominant. They can, however, provide a valuable clue for early diagnosis and treatment and prevention of a potential fatal cancer of the bowel.

Multiple Mucosal Neuromas

An awareness of the predilection of patients with multiple mucosal neuromas to the development of pheochromocytoma and medullary carcinoma of the thyroid may save the life of the afflicted individual.

Mucosal neuromas are pink pedunculated nodules, usually first recognized on the lips and tongue (Color Plate 1–B); later they involve the conjunctiva and oropharyngeal mucous membrane. The cornea is frequently the site of medulated nerve fibers, and a number of these patients have a marfanoid build.

In this syndrome, medullary carcinomas of the thyroid (taking origin in the parafollicular cells derived from the ultimobranchial body) develop in patients who are younger than those in whom such lesions occur independently. Pheochromocytomas (taking origin in the adrenal medulla derived from the neural crest) have a striking tendency to multiplicity and bilateralism. Both of these tumors are capable of endocrine secretion—prostaglandins and pressor amines, respectively — that may produce additional clinical clues, such as diarrhea or hypertension, to their presence.

Tylosis Palmaris et Plantaris

Tylosis palmaris et plantaris is one of a large family of dyskeratoses characterized by severe thickening of the epithelium of the palms and soles. It is usually a familial condition apparently transmitted by a single autosomal gene with a high penetrance and a heterozygous effect. Howell–Evans and associates reported the association of squamous cell carcinomas of the esophagus in 18 of 48 tylotic members of two families and in only 1 of 87 nontylotic members. The literature also contains scattered reports of both esophageal and bronchogenic carcinomas in sporadic and apparently nonfamilial tylotic patients. No recognizable premalignant lesions have been found in the esophageal mucosa in patients with these associated conditions.

Melanosis

The sudden development over 2 to 3 months of a generalized slate gray or brown pigmentation of the skin and mucous membrane should suggest to the physician a rare complication of disseminated malignant melanoma (Fig. 3). The pigmentation may vary from a diffuse bluish gray to a brownish black so that the involved skin of a Caucasian can be mistaken for the coloration of a Negro. Mucous membranes also may be involved. The discoloration is caused by the pathologic deposition of melanin particles in histiocytes and extracellularly throughout the dermis.

Subcutaneous Fat Necrosis

Disseminated intra–abdominal and extra–abdominal fat necrosis has long been recognized as a classic physical sign in

COLOR PLATE 1

A   The sharply demarcated scaling or eczematoid plaque about the areola is almost pathognomonic of Paget's disease of the breast.

B   Asymptomatic firm nodules along lateral borders and tip of tongue as part of multiple mucosal neuromas can be seen on many mucosal surfaces. (From Perry, H.O., Kiely, J. M., and Moertel, C.G.: Cutaneous Clues to Visceral Cancer. *Minn Med* 51:1719–1726 [Dec.] 1968. By permission of the Minnesota State Medical Association.)

C   The cutaneous changes of dermatomyositis are edema, especially of the face, neck, arms, and upper trunk, and the pink–lavender heliotrope color of the skin most accentuated on the eyelids.

D   The hyperkeratotic warty lesions of the palms and soles should lead the physician to expect previous ingestion of arsenic.

E   The clue to the diagnosis of generalized bullous pemphigoid is not the individual vesicular or bullous lesions themselves but their grouping on the trunk and intertriginous areas. (From Perry, H.O., Kiely, J.M., and Moertel, C.G.: Cutaneous Clues to Visceral Cancer. *Minn Med* 51:1719–1726 [Dec.] 1968. By permission of the Minnesota State Medical Association.)

F   Red brown to violaceous papules and nodules are commonly seen over the dorsa of the fingers and hands in patients with multicentric reticulohistiocytoma. Note the deformities of the distal interphalangeal joints.

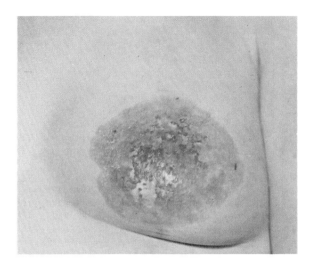

A
Paget's disease

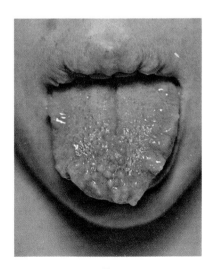

B
Mucosal neuromas

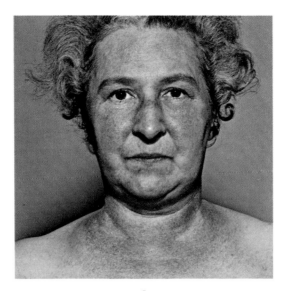

C
Dermatomyositis

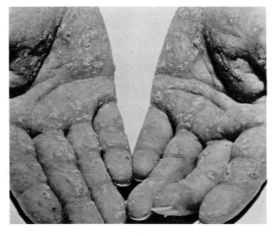

D
Arsenical keratoses

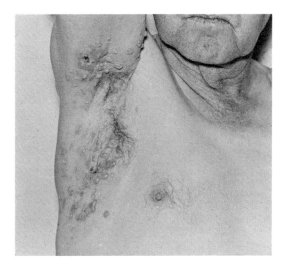

E
Bullous pemphigoid

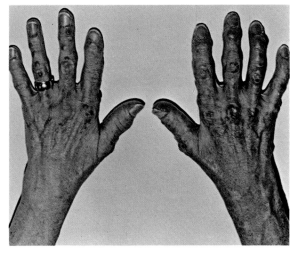

F
Reticulohistiocytoma

COLOR PLATE 2

G   The patient with chronic lymphatic leukemia may experience an unusually severe and necrotizing reaction to mosquito bites.

H   Systemized amyloidosis with its associated myeloma may be recognized initially by the ecchymotic reaction of the fragile tissues of the eyelids.

I   The photosensitive butterfly reaction of Bloom's syndrome is produced by the presence of numerous telangiectasias. The condition of such patients should be followed for the development of leukemia.

J   Generalized plane xanthomas impart a chamois yellow hue to the skin and are so superficial that they may be overlooked without careful inspection of the skin.

K   Grouped papules involving hair follicles in alopecia mucinosa may precede or be found in association with lymphoma. (From Perry, H.O., Kiely, J.M., and Moertel, C.G.: Cutaneous Clues to Visceral Cancer. *Minn Med* **51**:1719–1726 [Dec.] 1968. By permission of the Minnesota State Medical Association.)

L   Red–brown papulonodules, either singly or confluent, which urticate, may indicate that the patient has systemic involvement with mast cell disease and mast cell leukemia.

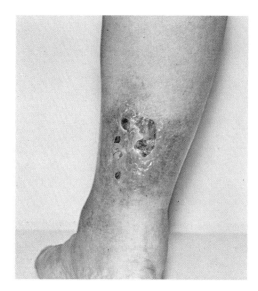

G
Mosquito Bites

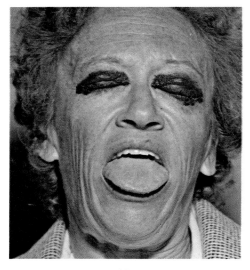

H
Amyloid

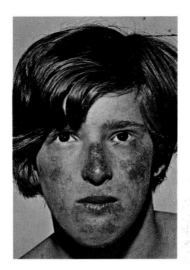

I
Bloom's Syndrome

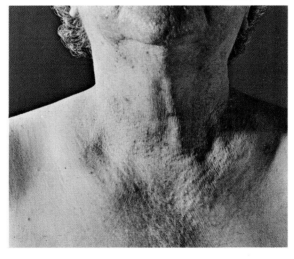

J
Plane Xanthoma

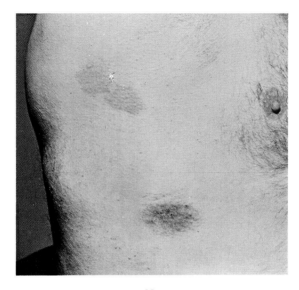

K
Alopecia Mucinosa

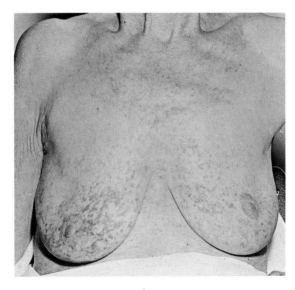

L
Urticaria Pigmentosa

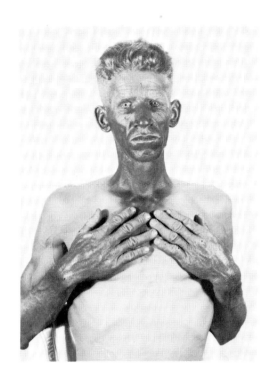

Figure 3. Sudden development of generalized hyperpigmentation accentuated on exposed areas. (From Odel, H.M., Montgomery, H., and Horton, B.T.: Diffuse Melanosis Secondary to Malignant Melanoma: Report of Case. *Mayo Clin Proc* 12:742–747 [Nov. 24] 1937. By permission.)

acute hemorrhagic pancreatitis. The subcutaneous lesions present as tender, indurated masses with inflammation of the overlying skin. Recognizable lesions seem to have a particular predilection for the lower extremities.

Far less commonly, similar lesions may be observed in patients with carcinoma of the pancreas, possibly resulting from mild episodes of obstructive pancreatitis. In our experience this phenomenon has been exceedingly rare.

CUTANEOUS CLUES SUGGESTIVE OF INTERNAL MALIGNANT TUMORS

Dermatomyositis

The early skin changes in dermatomyositis consist of suffusion and generalized erythema of the face, neck, and upper part of the trunk with edema of the face, especially the eyelids (Color Plate 1–C). Telangiectasias may develop subsequently, imparting a purple hue to the skin, and when the eyelids are involved, it may produce the characteristic "heliotrope change." The initial erythema over joints is replaced by erythematous, atrophic, and scaling plaques, some of which may ulcerate, especially when traumatized. The myopathy involves particularly the proximal muscles of the pelvic and shoulder girdles and the back.

A thorough general evaluation with appropriate laboratory tests may lead to the discovery of a primary malignant lesion in a patient presenting evidence of dermatomyositis. Less frequently, a patient presents with a malignant lesion, and only when metastatic disease develops does dermatomyositis make its appearance.

In large centers where many patients with this disease are referred for further evaluation and where the search for underlying malignancy is meticulous, the incidence of an associated malignancy may be as high as 50%, but its true incidence is probably closer to 15 to 25%.

Removal of the associated malignant lesion is often sufficient to produce a remission in the dermatomyositis; development of metastatic disease causes an exacerbation of the dermatomyositis.

Arsenical Keratoses

The ingestion of arsenic, whether prescribed or taken for some other reason, predisposes to the development of cancer of the skin and subsequently of the upper respiratory and urinary tracts.

Palmar and plantar punctate hyper-keratoses (Color Plate 1–D) and general-ized variegated pigmentation of the skin are the earliest changes occurring after a latent period, sometimes years after in-gestion of trivalent inorganic arsenic. The palmar and plantar keratoses, which ini-tially are barely palpable, gradually in-crease in size and can themselves evolve into squamous cell carcinoma. In addi-tion, scattered over the body are super-ficial erythematous macular and scaling areas, some of which become eroded and ulcerated and represent superficial basal cell epitheliomas.

In patients with cutaneous changes of chronic arsenism, independent primary tumors of the urogenital, oral, esophageal, and respiratory epithelia may occur. Kupffer's cell sarcoma (hemangiosar-coma) of the liver also is regarded as a rare complication of arsenism.

Generalized Bullous Pemphigoid

In patients of middle age or older, gen-eralized bullous eruptions that involve primarily the intertriginous regions should be suspected clinically as evidence of generalized bullous pemphigoid. The bullae (Color Plate 1–E) frequently are grouped on an erythematous somewhat urticarial plaque but may occur on nor-mal skin. Pruritus and sensations of local discomfort may be disabling.

Patients with generalized bullous pem-phigoid must be distinguished from pa-tients with pemphigus vulgaris, erythema multiforme, and dermatitis herpetiformis. Specific histologic study shows the bullae of generalized bullous pemphigoid to be located subepidermally. Thus, routine histologic studies afford ready differenti-ation of various forms of pemphigus. Of the various diseases characterized by sub-epidermal bullae, and these include ery-thema multiforme, dermatitis herpetifor-mis, and benign mucous membrane pem-phigoid, generalized bullous pemphigoid alone demonstrates the antibodies local-ized in the basement membrane of the epidermis as disclosed by fluorescent microscopy.

Patients with generalized bullous pem-phigoid must be evaluated for the possi-bility of underlying malignant disease. Skog has emphasized the relative fre-quency of lymphoreticular disease occur-ring in patients with generalized bullous pemphigoid.

Acanthosis Nigricans

This striking disease is characterized by hyper-pigmentation and papillary hyper-trophy observed most prominently in the axilla, the neck, the groins, and the peri-neum (Fig. 4). In adults, acanthosis

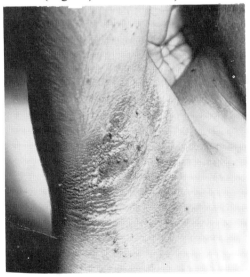

Figure 4. Verrucal hyperplasia and hy-perpigmentation of skin of in-tertriginous areas are well–rec-ognized hallmarks for acan-thosis nigricans.

nigricans is associated frequently with visceral carcinoma of various types—33% in a consecutive series of patients at the Mayo Clinic. Gastric adenocarcinoma probably is the neoplasm most frequently cited in the literature.

In addition, acanthosis nigricans may occur in patients receiving drug therapy or in association with simple obesity or a variety of endocrine diseases such as pituitary tumors, polycystic ovaries, diabetes mellitus, and adrenal insufficiency. Juvenile acanthosis nigricans has not been established as bearing any correlation to either malignant or endocrine disease.

Basal Cell Nevus Syndrome

The basal cell nevus syndrome is characterized by the appearance early in life of numerous pearly papules, some of which ulcerate and heal with atrophic scars over the face, neck, upper part of the trunk, and upper extremities (Fig. 5). Histologically, these lesions appear to be basal cell hamartomas; thus they are designated as "basal cell nevus syndrome." Other cutaneous findings are those of milia, epithelial and subcutaneous cysts, lipoma, and punctate dyskeratoses of the palms and soles. Patients present with a facies characterized by accentuated frontal bossing, a depressed nasal bridge, and a prominent jaw. Ocular findings including hypertelorism, dystrophia canthorum, cataracts, and congenital blindness have been recognized as a part of the problem. In association with these lesions are cysts of the jaw, particularly of the mandible, with resorption and loss of teeth and various congenital skeletal deformities. Soft tissue changes include calcification of the falx cerebri, ovarian fibromas with calcification, and lymphatic mesenteric cysts. Partial agenesis of the corpus callosum also has been noticed.

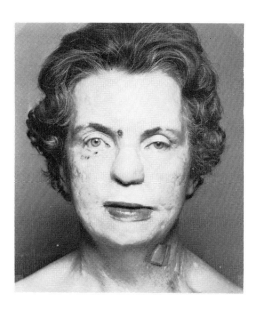

Figure 5. Basal cell hamartomas in basal cell nevus syndrome at times resolve with scar formation or at other times require surgical extirpation for complete removal.

Medulloblastomas are now being reported with such increasing frequency in these patients that their development can no longer be considered mere coincidence. Fibrosarcoma of the maxilla has also occurred.

Epiloia

The characteristic skin lesions in epiloia are yellowish verrucoid papular lesions over the central portion of the face, involving particularly the nose, nasolabial folds, and chin together with periungual and subungual fibromas (Fig. 6). Other cutaneous findings are connective tissue nevi of the lumbosacral area or of the neck and patches of alopecia and canities. These findings should prompt the physician to evaluate the patient neurologically for intracerebral lesions producing epilepsy and a peculiar potato-

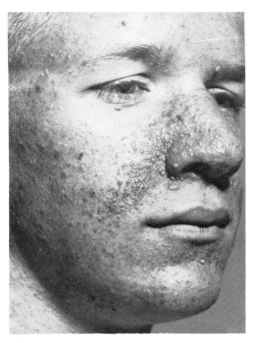

Figure 6. Verrucal papular adenoma sebaceum of central part of face indicates epiloia.

like nodularity of the cerebrum. This disease is transmitted as an autosomal dominant trait.

Hamartomas in the brain, liver, thyroid, pancreas, and testes have been reported. Approximately 20% of the patients have renal tumors that are usually bilateral, multiple, and varied in size. These are best classified as lipomyxosarcomas. Rhabdomyosarcomas of the heart are found in approximately 5% of the patients. Intracranial tumors composed of mixtures of spongioblasts and gemistocytic astrocytes have been associated with this condition.

Hippel–Lindau Syndrome

Hippel–Lindau syndrome is inherited as an autosomal dominant trait with incomplete penetrance often with the de- velopment of findings occurring earlier in each succeeding generation. The commonest finding suggesting this syndrome is that of angiomas of the retina, which are typically in the periphery of the visual field. As a part of the angiomatosis of the retina and cerebellum, vascular nevi of the face may be seen, though rarely. Those patients with exaggerated retinal angiomas are the patients in whom hemangioblastomas of the cerebellum usually develop. Hypernephromas may be found in other patients.

Werner's Syndrome (Progeria of the Adult)

Werner's syndrome, a hereditary familial disorder, is transmitted as a recessive trait. Consanguinity of parents and the occurrence of the syndrome in siblings are often reported.

Development is normal through late adolescence, but the patient fails to achieve full growth or weight and changes of premature aging develop during the third decade of life. Ulcerations over the soles and lower part of the legs, cataracts, endocrine disturbances, and a loss of tissue substance give the patients a characteristic facies. Atrophy of the subcutaneous tissue and musculature develops, producing a sclerodermoid-like appearance, particulary of the extremities and face. The patient presents a birdlike facies with a prominent beaked nose, a small mouth, and a receding chin. Ulcers may develop over the malleoli of the ankles, calves, heels, and toes; evidence of the premature senility consists of premature graying of the hair, premature baldness, early development of arteriosclerosis, and juvenile cataracts.

Since these patients age prematurely, various malignant tumors that include carcinoma of the liver, fibrosarcoma, uterine sarcoma, malignant melanoma, and osteogenic sarcoma, develop at an earlier age than usual.

Leser–Trelat Sign

The sudden appearance and rapid increase in number and size of freckles and keratoses with severe pruritus (Fig. 7) on a skin previously blemish–free may be a manifestation of visceral cancer. This cutaneous manifestation of cancer has been called "the sign of Leser–Trelat."

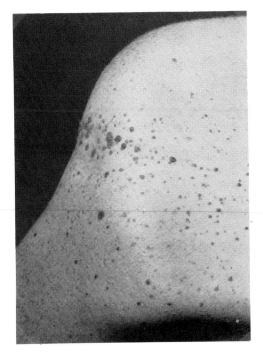

Figure 7. Verrucal keratoses of Leser-Trelat sign are characterized by rapid development and large numbers.

Acquired Universal Hypertrichosis Lanuginosa (Malignant Down)

The sudden development of long, silky, reddish–blonde lanugo hair in an adult is so frequently associated with development of an internal cancer that the growth of hair has been referred to as "the development of malignant down." The hair tends to be shorter on the face and longer as one progresses toward the trunk, thus imparting an animal–like appearance to the patient. The palms, soles, upper eyelids, distal phalanges, and penis may be spared. The excessive growth of hair is to be differentiated primarily from that which occurs in the congenital forms of hypertrichosis with an onset early in life, the hypertrichosis associated with drug ingestion (that is, Dilantin), and with metabolic and hormonal disturbances such as porphyria cutanea tarda and tumors with masculinizing syndromes.

The development of malignant down has been associated with cancer of the breast, bladder, lung, and gallbladder at a time when the primary tumor has metastasized diffusely. The cause of this rapid growth of hair remains unknown.

Pachydermoperiostosis

This syndrome is characterized by digital clubbing, periosteal bone changes, furrowing of the skin, and over–activity of the sebaceous glands. The forehead and scalp especially may show deep horizontal lines, and the condition may be associated with oily skin and acne. Bronchogenic carcinoma and pleural mesothelioma are the most frequent tumors found in patients with this condition.

This secondary type of pulmonary hypertrophic osteoarthropathy should be distinguished from the benign, idiopathic familial form of the disorder. The benign form starts earlier in life, the cutaneous signs tend to be more pronounced, and musculoskeletal pain is less prominent.

Bowen's Disease

A cluster of flesh–colored to pink papules or a single erythematous cutaneous plaque which, on histologic study, proves to be a squamous cell epithelioma in situ has become known as "Bowen's disease" (Fig. 8). These lesions occur during middle and later life on any areas of the body.

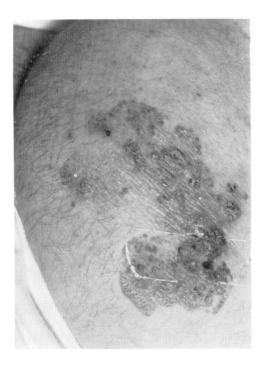

Figure 8. Note the superficial quality of the erythematous scaling papules and plaques of Bowen's disease.

It was not until 1959 that Graham and Helwig emphasized the association of Bowen's disease with a primary internal cancer. These authors emphasized that half of their patients had other cutaneous premalignant or malignant lesions and that 80% had either a primary cutaneous tumor with metastasis or a primary internal cancer. These tumors involved squamous cell carcinoma of the hypopharynx, larynx, and lung, bronchogenic carcinoma, squamous cell carcinoma of the esophagus, adenocarcinoma of the stomach, urinary bladder, and prostate, and malignant disease of the lymphoreticular system. Recent studies show that in Bowen's disease, lesions on covered areas of the body frequently are associated with an internal cancer, whereas lesions on exposed areas of skin are not. Our own unpublished studies seem to indicate that internal malignant disease does not occur any more frequently in patients with Bowen's disease than in a control group of the same age.

Erythema Perstans

"Erythema perstans" is the preferred term employed to denote erythema previously described under such names as "erythema gyratum perstans," "erythema figuratum perstans," "erythema chronica migrans," "erythema annulare centrifugum," and "erythema gyratum repens." Gammel first emphasized the importance of such a cutaneous pattern in association with carcinoma of the breast. Appreciation that fixed, persistent urticarial lesions in a gyrate pattern (Fig. 9) might be associated with a malignant lesion prompted us to review our experience at the Mayo Clinic with erythema perstans. A comparison of a group of patients with erythema perstans with a controlled group with psoriasis seen during the same period did not show a statistical difference in the incidence of malignant disease in the two groups. Thus, an asso-

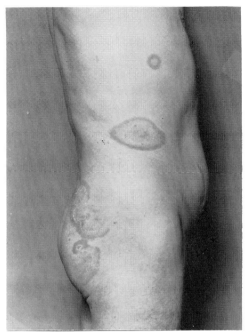

Figure 9. Persistant gyrate urticarial plaques characterized erythema perstans.

ciation between erythema perstans and underlying malignant disease seems unlikely to us.

Multicentric Reticulohistiocytosis

This rare systemic disease of middle-aged adults is manifested by the gradual development of red or copper colored nodules on the face, scalp, ears, hands, arms, and sometimes the oral mucosa (Color Plate 1–F). Xanthelasma has been noted in about a third of the reported cases. In addition, the patients have severely disfiguring destructive joint changes simulating those of rheumatoid arthritis. The terminal interphalangeal finger joints are involved and the fingers are shortened but stretchable, thus giving rise to the term "telescope fingers" or "opera glass hands." Biopsy of skin, mucous membrane, or synovium reveals lipid-filled histiocytes and multinucleated giant cells.

A variety of epithelial visceral cancers were reported in 6 (18%) of the 33 documented cases in the world literature.

CUTANEOUS CLUES SUGGESTIVE OF MALIGNANT LYMPHORETICULAR DISEASE

Pruritus

Severe generalized itching without visible skin lesions may be the earliest sign of visceral cancer (Fig. 10) and is especially characteristic of Hodgkin's disease. The intense pruritus usually is unrelieved by local therapy.

Bath pruritus is a common manifestation of myeloproliferative syndromes, especially polycythemia vera. Objective signs of mycosis fungoides may be preceded for years by localized or generalized

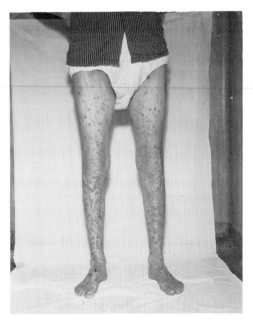

Figure 10. Severe excoriation and multilation of the skin of a patient with Hodgkin's disease in an effort to relieve intense pruritus.

itching. Patients with malignant disease of the viscera associated with acanthosis nigricans also may have intractable pruritus.

Herpes–Varicella Infections

The incidence of herpes simplex (Fig. 11) and herpes zoster (Fig. 12) infections in patients with chronic lymphocytic leukemia, lymphoma, and myeloma is con-

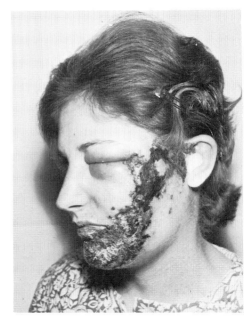

Figure 12. Herpes zoster may be extremely severe and gangrenous in patients with lymphoma because of their altered immunologic status.

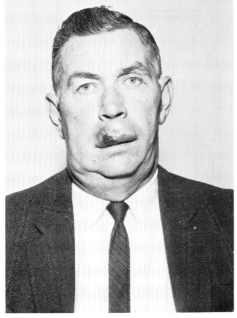

Figure 11. Herpes simplex infections in patients with lymphoma tend to be frequent and unusually severe.

siderably higher than in the general population. These infections are more likely caused by reactivation of latent virus than by reinfection. The cutaneous reaction in herpes zoster is frequently unusually severe in such persons and necrosis and scarring of the skin are common. Generalized eruptions are especially frequent in patients with advanced Hodgkin's disease with immunologic deficits and about 50% of such patients are dead within a year.

Exaggerated Delayed Hypersensitivity to Mosquito Bites

This unusual cutaneous sign may be noted in patients with chronic lymphocytic leukemia and more rarely with malignant lymphoma (Color Plate 2–G). The reactions to bites develop slowly, reaching a peak in 12 to 24 hours, and usually resolve within 2 to 14 days. The lesions are characterized by induration, edema, erythema, intense pruritus, and sometimes bullae. Delayed cutaneous reactions to other antigens are usually normal in these subjects, and no correlation has been found with serum immunoglobulin levels. This exaggerated response to mosquito bites may be related to the same abnormal immune mechanism that results in the severe reaction to smallpox vaccination in similar patients.

Purpura

Intracutaneous bleeding accompanying thrombocytopenia may be the presenting symptom of hematopoietic malignancies, especially acute leukemia. Lympho-plasmocytic malignant diseases such as multiple myeloma may present with purpura as a prominent sign, perhaps because the abnormal proteins produced in these disorders interfere with the coagulation mechanism. The paramyloidosis associated with myeloma may be responsible for extensive purpura, especially in the loose skin around the orbits (Color Plate 2-H). Purpura also may herald a circulating fibrinolysin or the defibrination syndrome seen in patients with bony metastasis, especially from prostatic carcinoma. Patients with extensive hepatic metastasis also may have purpura secondary to hypoprothrombinemia. Rarely, purpura with cutaneous infarction secondary to an embolus arising from nonbacterial verrucal endocarditis may be seen in patients with carcinoma.

Congenital Telangiectatic Erythema With Stunted Growth (Bloom's Syndrome)

Low birth weight, stunted growth, and a sunlight–sensitive telangiectatic erythema in the butterfly area of the face characterize this disease (Color Plate 2-I). The facies is small with sharp features. It is inherited as an autosomal recessive trait and consanguinity is frequent among the patients' parents. The disease is most frequent in families of Jewish ancestry. A high frequency of chromosomal breakage and rearrangement has been found in cultured blood cells of the patients. A high frequency of malignant diseases especially leukemia, is associated with this disorder.

Ataxia Telangiectasia

In children with this disorder of autosomal recessive immunologic deficiency, progressive cerebellar ataxia develops during the second year of life. Preceding ataxia, telangiectasia is common and dilated blood vessels appear on the sclerae and on the skin of the eyelids, earlobes, neck, and popliteal and antecubital areas (Fig. 13). They regularly show striking deficiencies of cell–mediated immune responses, lymphocytopenia, and delayed rejection of homografts. Recurrent respiratory infections are associated with immunoglobulin deficiencies of both IgA and IgE. If survival is long enough, fatal lymphoma or reticuloendotheliosis frequently develops.

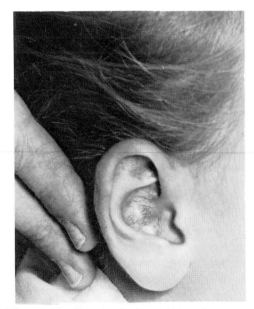

Figure 13. Particularly striking in ataxia telangiectasia are the prominent vessels of the ears. (From Siekert, R.G., Keith, H.M., and Dion, F.R.: Ataxia-Telangiectasia in Children. *Mayo Clin Proc* 34:581–587 [Dec. 9] 1959. By permission.)

Wiskott–Aldrich Syndrome

Infants with this sex–linked recessive disorder exhibit eczematoid dermatitis, thrombocytopenic purpura, and intense susceptibility to infections (Fig. 14). No patients with this syndrome have lived to adulthood and most die before they are 5 years of age. The eczematoid dermatitis usually begins on the scalp, face, flexural surfaces of the extremities, or about the buttocks and occasionally progresses to exfoliative erythroderma. Eczematous regions often become secondarily infected and appear crusted and impetiginous. A progressive deletion of circulating lymphocytes develops as well as a deficiency of lymphocytes in the thymic-dependent regions of lymphatic tissues. Immunoglobulins of all major classes are produced although concentrations of serum IgM are usually low. As in patients with ataxia telangiectasia, lymphoreticular malignant diseases are likely to develop and rapidly become widespread.

Chediak–Higashi Syndrome

This disorder appears to be inherited as an autosomal recessive trait. It is characterized by progressively impaired resistance to infections, hepatosplenomegaly, lymphadenopathy, terminal leukopenia, and thrombocytopenia and varying degrees of mental retardation. The leukocytes in this anomaly contain giant lysosomal granules that appear refractile and stain greenish gray with Wright's satin. The cutaneous hallmark is partial oculocutaneous albinism. These patients have an increased incidence of lymphoma.

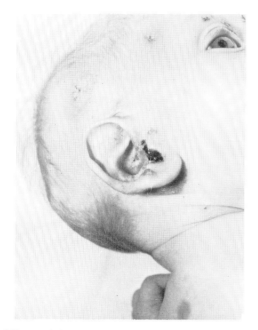

Figure 14. Eczematoid plaques, at times secondarily infected, are common in Wiskott–Aldrich syndrome. (From Johnson G.M., Burke, E.C., and Burgert, E.O., Jr.: Wiskott–Aldrich Syndrome: Report of an Additional Case. *Mayo Clin Proc* **39**: 258–262 [Apr.] 1964. By permission.)

Generalized Plane Xanthoma

Recent work on the xanthomas has dealt primarily with characterizing the associated types of hyperlipidemia. It is well to keep in mind, however, that some forms of cutaneous xanthomas without hyperlipidemia may be associated with internal malignant neoplasms, especially myeloma. Such is the case of generalized plane xanthoma in which the skin, particularly of the face, neck, upper part of the trunk, and proximal upper extremities, is involved with macular areas of yellowish discoloration that represents a superficial xanthomatous process (Color Plate 2–J). Tangential lighting of the skin is often required to visualize the lesions; otherwise, one may overlook the slight yellowish tint of the tissues.

Alopecia Mucinosa

A recently recognized dermatologic entity, that of follicular mucinosa, has assumed importance in patients more than 40 years of age as a cutaneous marker of lymphoreticular disease. The disease can be diagnosed with ease clinically because of the degenerative process of the hair follicles resulting in areas of alopecia that involve primarily the face, trunk, and upper extremities (Color Plate 2–K). Local symptoms are usually minimal, although pruritus may be present. Histologically, one can readily demonstrate mucinous degeneration of the hair follicles by biopsy and staining for mucopolysaccharides. Alopecia mucinosa may occur at any age in either sex. In young patients, the lesions usually consist of grouped follicular papules, which are of only local importance. In older patients this same pattern may be interspersed with elevated plaques studded with follicular papules and the incidence of lymphoma is increased.

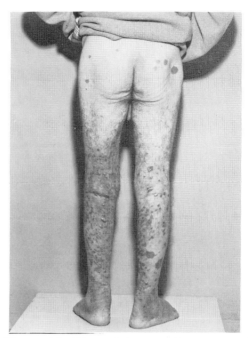

Figure 15. Blue–violet vascular tumors of feet and legs associated with lymphedema are characteristic of Kaposi's sarcoma and may be coexistent with systemic lymphoma.

Kaposi's Sarcoma

This rare cutaneous sarcoma is characterized by multiple tender reddish brown or bluish red nodules that usually appear first on the feet and legs and are associated with varying degrees of infiltration sometimes reaching the point of elephantiasis (Fig. 15). In many studies its coexistence with leukemia or lymphoma has been extraordinarily high. In Caucasians the incidence of this association has ranged from 8 to 17%; and in Africa, where both lymphoma and Kaposi's sarcoma are more common, a similar association has been documented. Various stages of histologic transition between typical lymphoma and typical Kaposi's sarcoma in different specimens from the same patient also have been observed and suggest that the coexistent neoplasms may not represent a coincidence of two distinct disease processes but rather another example of the pleomorphism of reticuloendothelial malignant disease.

Systemic Lupus Erythematosus

Patients with systemic lupus erythematosus may present a variety of cutaneous signs, including the classic sun–sensitive erythema in the so–called butterfly area of the face (Fig. 16). Immunologic abnormalities and immunoproliferative disorders commonly are associated with this disease. Neoplasia of the lymphore-

Systemic Mast Cell Disease

Abnormal proliferation of tissue mast cells in the skin and visceral organs characterizes this disorder. Its most prominent cutaneous manifestation is urticaria pigmentosa (Color Plate 2–L). The typical, multiple hyperpigmented skin lesions are easily mistaken for freckles; however, mild trauma such as scratching produces a characteristic erythematous halo and urtication of the macule often accompanied by pruritus. Frequent findings in addition to the skin lesions include dermatographism, bone lesions, hepatosplenomegaly, and peptic ulcer. Release of histamine stored in the mast cells may produce the so-called mastocytosis syndrome characterized by episodic erythematous flushing, tachycardia and hypotension, upper gastrointestinal distress, diarrhea, and pruritus.

Few reports indicate that mast–cell leukemia is fatal. In occasional patients with lymphosarcoma of the marrow and with Waldenstrom's macroglobulinemia, there may be secondary mastocytosis with humoral symptoms similar to those in primary mast cell disease.

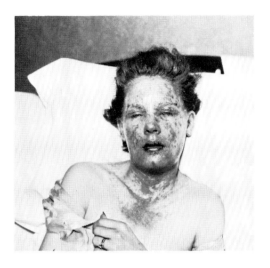

Figure 16. Superficial erythematous scaling and macular and plaquelike lesions of the face should suggest the diagnosis of systemic lupus erythematous.

ticular system as well as thymomas of the spindle cell type occasionally develops, perhaps as an expression of disturbed immunity.

SUBJECT BIBLIOGRAPHY

Paget's Disease
Fardal, R.W., Kierland, R.R., Clagett, O.T., and Woolner, L.B.: Prognosis in Cutaneous Paget's Disease. *Postgrad Med 36*:584–593 (Dec.) 1964.

Extramammary Paget's Disease
Helwig, E.B., and Graham, J.II.: Anogenital (Extramammary) Paget's Disease: A Clinicopathological Study. *Cancer 16*:387–403 (Mar.) 1963.

The Malignant Carcinoid Syndrome
Moertel, C.G., Beahrs, O.H., Woolner, L.B., and Tyce, G.M.: "Malignant Carcinoid Syndrome" Associated With Noncarcinoid Tumors. *New Eng J Med 273*:244–248 (July 29) 1965.

Thorson, A., Biörck, G., Björkman, G., and Waldenström, J.: Malignant Carcinoid of the Small Intestine With Metastases to Liver, Valvular Diseases of the Right Side of the Heart (Pulmonary Stenosis and Tricuspid Regurgitation Without Septal Defects), Peripheral Vasomotor Symptoms, Bronchoconstriction, and an Unusual Type of Cyanosis: A Clinical and Pathologic Syndrome. *Amer Heart J 47*:795–817 (June) 1954.

Gardner's Syndrome
Gardner, E.J.: Follow–up Study of a Family Group Exhibiting Dominant Inheritance for a Syndrome Including Intestinal Polyps, Osteomas, Fibromas and Epidermal Cysts. *Amer J Hum Genet 14*:376–390 (Dec.) 1962.

Multiple Mucosal Neuromas
Gorlin, R.J., Sedano, H.O., Vickers, R.A., and Cervenka, J.: Multiple Mucosal Neuromas, Pheochromocytoma and Medullary Carcinoma of the Thyroid: A Syndrome. *Cancer 22*:293–299 (Aug.) 1968.

Tylosis Palmaris et Plantaris
Parnell, D.D., and Johnson, S.A.M.: Tylosis Palmaris et Plantaris: Its Occurrence With Internal Malignancy. *Arch Derm* (Chicago) *100*: 7–9 (July) 1969.

Melanosis
Fitzpatrick, T.B., Montgomery, H., and Learner, A.B.: Pathogenesis of Generalized Dermal Pigmentation Secondary to Malignant Melanoma and Melanuria. *J Invest Derm 22*: 163–172 (Mar.) 1954.

Subcutaneous Fat Necrosis
Szymanski, F.J., and Bluefarb, S.M.: Nodular Fat Necrosis and Pancreatic Diseases. *Arch Derm* (Chicago) *83*:224–229 (Feb.) 1961.

Dermatomyositis
Williams, R.C., Jr.: Dermatomyositis and Malignancy: A Review of the Literature. *Ann Intern Med 50*: 1174–1181 (May) 1959.

Arsenical Keratoses
Sommers, S.C., and McManus, R.G.: Multiple Arsenical Cancers of Skin and Internal Organs. *Cancer 6*: 347–359 (Mar.) 1953.

Generalized Bullous Pemphigoid
Skog, E.: Cutaneous Manifestations Associated With Internal Malignant Tumours With Particular Reference to Vesicular and Bullous Lesions. *Acta Dermatovener* (Stockholm) *44*: 114–117, 1964.

Acanthosis Nigricans

Brown, J., and Winkelman, R.K.: Acanthosis Nigricans: A Study of 90 Cases. *Medicine (Balt)* 47:33–51 (Jan.) 1968.

Basal Cell Nevus Syndrome

Berlin, N.I., Van Scott, E.J., Clendenning, W.E., Archard, H.O., Block J.B., Witkop, C.J., and Haynes, H.A.: Basal Cell Nevus Syndrome: Combined Clinical Staff Conference at the National Institutes of Health. *Ann Intern Med* 64:403–421 (Feb.) 1966.

Epiloia

Kapp, J.P. Paulson, G.W., and Odom, G.L.: Brain Tumors With Tuberous Sclerosis. *J Neurosurg* 26:191–202 (Feb.) 1967.

Lagos, J.C., and Gomez, M.R.: Tuberous Sclerosis: Reappraisal of a Clinical Entity. *Mayo Clin Proc* 42:26–49 (Jan.) 1967.

Hippel–Lindau Syndrome

Christoferson, L.A., Gustafson, M.B., and Petersen, A.G.: Von Hippel-Lindau's Disease. *JAMA* 178:280–282 (Oct. 21) 1961.

Werner's Syndrome (Progeria of the Adult)

Thannhauser, S.J.: Werner's Syndrome (Progeria of the Adult) and Rothmund's Syndrome: Two Types of Closely Related Heredofamilial Atrophic Dermatoses With Juvenile Cataracts and Endocrine Features: A Critical Study With Five New Cases. *Ann Intern Med* 23:559–626 (Oct.) 1945.

Leser–Trélat Sign

Ronchese, F.: Keratoses, Cancer and "The Sign of Leser-Trélat." *Cancer* 18:1003–1006 (Aug.) 1965.

Aquired Universal Hypertrichosis Lanuginosa (Malignant Down)

Hensley, G.T., and Glynn, K.P.: Hypertrichosis Lanuginosa as a Sign of Internal Malignancy. *Cancer* 24:1051–1056 (Nov.) 1969.

Pachydermoperiostosis

Herman, M.A., Massaro, D., Katz, S., and Sachs, M.: Pachydermoperiossis: Clinical Spectrum. *Arch Intern Med* (Chicago) 116:918–923 (Dec.) 1965.

Bowen's Disease

Faber, J.W., and Perry, H.O.: Unpublished data.

Graham, J.H., and Helwig, E.B.: Bowen's Disease and Its Relationship to Systemic Cancer. *Arch Derm* (Chicago) 80:133–159 (Aug.) 1959.

Erythema Perstans

White, J.W., and Perry, H.O.: Erythema Perstans. *Brit J Derm* 81:641–651 (Sept.) 1969.

Multicentric Reticulohistiocytosis

Barrow, M.V., and Holubar, K.: Multicentric Reticulohistiocytosis. *Derm Digest*, August, 1970, pp. 55-60.

Pruritus

Fromer, J.L., and Geokas, M.C.: Cutaneous Manifestations in Lymphomas. *New York J Med* 63:3222–3228 (Nov. 15) 1963.

Zoster–Varicella Infections

Sokal, J.E., and Firat, D.: Varicella-Zoster Infection in Hodgkin's Disease: Clinical and Epidemiological Aspects. *Amer J Med* 39:452–463 (Sept.) 1965.

Exaggerated Delayed Hypersensitivity to Mosquito Bites
  Weed, R.I.: Exaggerated Delayed Hypersensitivity to Mosquito Bites in Chronic Lymphocytic Leukemia. *Blood 26*:257–268 (Sept.) 1965.

Congenital Telangiectatic Erythema With Stunted Growth (Bloom's Syndrome)
  Sawitsky, A., Bloom, D., and German, J.: Chromosomal Breakage and Acute Leukemia in Congenital Telangiectatic Erythema and Stunted Growth. *Ann Intern Med 65*: 487–495 (Sept.) 1966.

Ataxia Telangiectasia
  Peterson, R.D., Copper, M.D., and Good, R.A.: Lymphoid Tissue Abnormalities Associated With Ataxia-Telangiectasia. *Amer J. Med 41*: 342–359 (Sept.) 1966.

Wiskott–Aldrich Syndrome
  Cooper, M.D., Chase, H.P., Lowman, J.T., Krivit, W., and Good, R.A.: Wiskott–Aldrich Syndrome: An Immunologic Deficiency Disease Involving the Afferent Limb of Immunity. *Amer J Med 44*:499–513 (Apr.) 1968.
  Mills, S.D., and Winkelmann, R.K.: Eczema, Thrombocytopenic Purpura, and Recurring Infections: A Familial Disorder With Report of Four Families. *Arch Derm* (Chicago) *79*:466–472 (Apr.) 1959.

Chediak-Higashi Syndrome
  Tan, C., Etcubanas, E., Lieberman, P., Isenberg, H., King, O., and Murphy, M.L.: Chediak–Higashi Syndrome in a Child With Hodgkin's Disease. *Amer J Dis Child 121*:135–139 (Feb.) 1971.

Generalized Plane Xanthoma
  Lynch, P.J., and Winkelmann, R.K.: Generalized Plane Xanthoma and Systemic Disease. *Arch Derm (Chicago) 93*:639–646 (June) 1966.

Alopecia Mucinosa
  Plotnick, H., and Abbrecht, M.: Alopecia Mucinosa and Lymphoma: Report of Two Cases and Review of Literature. *Arch Derm (Chicago) 92*:137–141 (Aug.) 1965.

Kaposi's Sarcoma
  Moertal, C.G.: Multiple Primary Malignant Neoplasms. New York, Springer–Verlag, 1966, pp. 44–47.

Systemic Lupus Erythematosus
  Andreev, V.C., and Zlatkov, N.B.: Systemic Lupus Erythematosus and Neoplasia of the Lymphoreticular System. *Brit J Derm 80*:503–508 (Aug.) 1968.

Systemic Mast Cell Disease
  Mutter, R.D., Tannenbaum, M., and Ultman, J.E.: Systemic Mast Cell Disease. *Ann Intern Med 59*: 887–906 (Dec.) 1963.

Chapter 4

TISSUE CULTURE EXPERIMENTS IN HEREDITARY SKIN CANCER: DNA REPAIR SYNTHESIS

by *Vincent M. Riccardi, M.D. and*
James E. Cleaver, Ph.D.

When genetic factors seem to be critical or paramount in the etiology of cancer, we speak of "familial" or "hereditary" cancer. In a more restricted sense, "hereditary skin cancer" refers to those inherited disorders in which cancer of the skin regularly occurs in a proportion of affected individuals. This frequently used reference implies a "unity", purely semantic in nature, which obscures the diversity among these disorders: not only are there numerous types of tumors, but their presentations and associated clinical features are extremely varied.

For some of these disorders cancer is a *sine qua non* for diagnosis (e.g. familial malignant melanoma). For others, cancer is a variable feature among affected patients. Appropriate diagnosis would then depend on the presence of other characteristic features, both clinical and per the laboratory (e.g. xeroderma pigmentosum, dyskeratosis congenita, neurofibromatosis). The integument may be abnormal in more than one way, and other organs or tissues may be involved. Some abnormalities may be present at birth, such as the dental and bone anomalies in the basal cell nevus syndrome; or, they may develop in the course of the disease. Among these entities more than one mode of inheritance is seen[1]: most frequently the disorder is transmitted as an autosomal dominant (e.g. basal cell nevus syndrome, cutaneous malignant melanoma, giant pigmented nevi, Kaposi's sarcoma and multiple generalized keratoacanthoma), and less frequently as an autosomal recessive (e.g. xeroderma pigmentosum and oculocutaneous albinism); a sex–linked recessive pattern has been considered, though not established, for dyskeratosis congenita[2]. At times an increased familial occurrence of malignancies does not conform to these Mendelian patterns of inheritance (e.g. in dermatomyositis), and the role of inheritance is not clear. The cancers themselves comprise a heterogeneous group, including squamous cell carcinoma, basal cell carcinoma, malignant melanoma, sarcoma and neurofibrosarcoma, although any given disorder is usually associated with one type of cancer. An exception is xeroderma pigmentosum where squamous cell carcinoma, basal cell carcinoma, malignant melanoma and other cancers occur. Finally, there are considerable differences as to the frequency of cancer, and as regards its pattern of onset; occasionally, environmental factors are of importance (e.g. the adverse effect of ultraviolet light in xeroderma pigmentosum).

Emphasis on the diversity and heterogeneity among the hereditary skin cancer disorders serves to point up two fundamental principles relating to carcinogenesis: 1) the cancer is not usually present at birth, but rather develops during the lifetime of an affected individual; and 2) the development of skin cancer in such varied patterns probably indicates that there is more than one pathogenetic mechanism. In this context, hereditary skin cancer may be construed as a final development, the consequence of an inherited aberration of one or more common cellular processes. But how does the development of cancer result from an inherited gene? How could the person-to-person transmission of a gene, via the germ cells, lead to cancer, followed by consistent cell-to-cell transmission of this new trait? The remainder of this chapter deals with how an inherited biochemical defect appears to underlie the development of at least some skin cancers: recent investigations with xeroderma pigmentosum cells have elucidated a strategic biochemical defect, which in turn suggests one pathogenetic mechanism responsible for cancer on an inherited basis.

Cancer at the cellular level.

Cancer cells proliferate abnormally; they continue to grow and divide where normal cells would not. This and other characteristic traits of neoplastic cells are constant from one cell generation to another: daughter cells are endowed with these properties from the parent cell. A leading theory of carcinogenesis accounts for this phenomenon by suggesting that the initial event in cancer development is a mutation in the DNA of a somatic cell (3) and that the transmission of these features is mediated by the cell's genetic material (chromosomes, genes, DNA). This theory accounts for the observations that particular portions of the DNA molecule correspond to specific functional units (for specifying the synthesis of more DNA, or for specifying the synthesis of a particular protein, etc.). On the one hand, maintenance of the structural integrity of the DNA through all phases of the cell cycle appears to be the basis for the constancy of genetic information, and, on the other hand, certain changes in a cell's DNA structure can lead to aberrant behavior in those cells derived from it.

Tissue culture techniques and their application.

These aspects of cell-to-cell inheritance are amenable to study *in vitro*. In this regard, tissue cultures derived from patients with a skin cancer diathesis provide unique opportunities.

Organ cultures of full thickness skin samples include all cell types which contribute to the skin, including those of the epidermis, dermis and skin appendages (hair follicles, sweat and sebaceous glands). Certain biochemical functions which reflect each cell type and their inter-relationships are most suitably examined with this *in vitro* system. In this way the skin is studied as an organized tissue, which may be important in understanding its response (s) to various agents, including drugs, hormones, ultra-violet light, etc. However, the tissue fragments are usually short-lived, and their limited cell proliferation may be a disadvantage.

Cell cultures afford another approach to studying biochemical and genetic mechanisms, especially those which entail cell

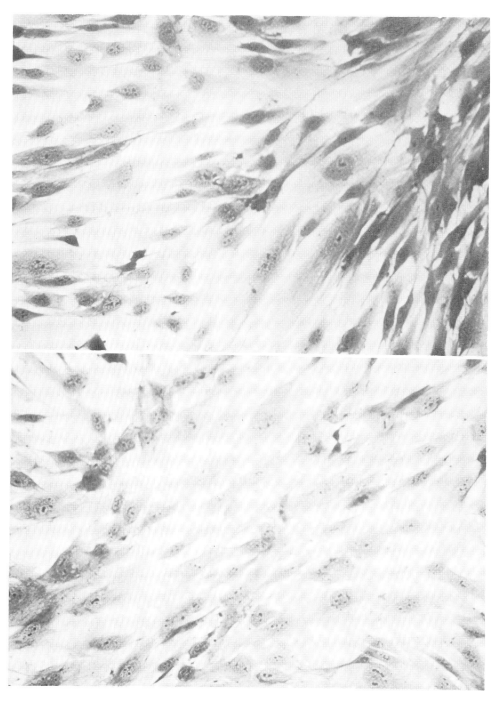

Figure 1. Fibroblasts cultured from skin biopsies of a normal individual (top) and a patient with xeroderma pigmentosum (bottom) (x400, approximately). As seen here, there is no significant difference in these cultures under ordinary conditions.

replication or large numbers of cells. A small piece of full or partial thickness skin obtained as a punch biopsy or surgical specimen is the source of the cells. The specimen is minced and the pieces secured to the surface of a culture vessel. The original outgrowth from these explants usually comprises epithelial cells which regress and are finally superceded by fibroblasts. Occasionally, fibroblasts represent the only outgrowth of cells. After two or three weeks, or about 15 cell divisions, a large number of fibroblasts have grown as a monolayer around the explant (Fig. 1). Although it is not clear from precisely which cell type (s) these are derived, this is not a practical limitation to studying processes common to all actively dividing cells. The advantages of such cell cultures include: 1) the fibroblasts represent a relatively uniform cell population; 2) the cells are essentially normal through about 50 division cycles, after which they deteriorate; 3) after a small number of generations, the fibroblasts can be arrested at that stage by freezing. They can be thus stored and later thawed to be used as needed.

Characteristics of cultured cells from patients with skin cancer diatheses.

Fibroblasts cultured from these patients do not seem to be unusual as regards cell-to-cell inheritance of various traits. Chromosome preparations from lymphocytes or skin fibroblasts from these patients have not revealed significant abnormalities (2, 4). This is in contrast to some other inherited disorders which show a proclivity to non–cutaneous malignancies (e.g. Bloom's syndrome (5, 6), Fanconi's anemia (7), ataxia–telangiectasia (8), etc.).

Efforts to characterize the inherited tendency to develop skin cancer under routine culture conditions have been unrewarding. The use of various mutagenic or carcinogenic agents to overtly manifest such a tendency has been more fruitful. Fibroblasts from certain patients may show such a heightened sensitivity to the deleterious effects of these agents, which include ionizing and ultraviolet radiation, a variety of chemicals and certain viruses (9, 10). Fibroblasts from patients with xeroderma pigmentosum show such a heightened sensitivity to far ultraviolet (UV) light; moreover, among these patients, in areas of sun–exposed skin, cells develop abnormal patterns of growth, including neoplasia (11–18). In a number of families showing frequent spontaneous carcinogenesis, representative fibroblast cultures have been exposed to the oncogenic virus SV–40; in these cultures malignant transformation occurs with a significantly higher efficiency than in cultures from control families (19). In both of these examples the fibroblasts show an excessive sensitivity to alterations in their genetic material: either from irradiation or from integrated viral DNA. The precise relationship between carcinogenesis *in vivo* and these laboratory observations is unclear, however.

Carcinogenesis and alterations in the genetic material (DNA).

The sensitivity of a given individual, or his cells to mutagenic or carcinogenic agents varies, depending on the agent and on inherent cellular abilities to offset the effects of the agent. Consistent with the somatic mutation theory (3) such effects may involve damage to DNA. Under ordinary circumstances, most damage would seem to be of minor significance because it can be "repaired"* or otherwise nullified. However, to the extent that the damage involves certain critical alterations in DNA structure and function, the cell's innate ability to actually "repair" this damage becomes paramount (10, 20). If the cell's ability to minimize damage to its DNA is overwhelmed– – either because the amount of damage is excessive, and/or because its repair mechanisms are imparied — then such a cell would be more liable to demonstrate mutations.

Cells of almost every organism from mycoplasma (21) and bacteria (22, 23) to plants (24) and mammals (12, 25) have biochemical processes which enable them to repair damage to DNA from radiation and various chemicals (26). There are several distinct repair processes (23, 24, 27, 28), all of which attempt to restore the original structure to DNA. The mechanistic basis for repair is the double-stranded structure of DNA. Genetic information is present in duplicate on opposite strands such that damage to one strand does not eradicate the genetic information in that region of the molecule: the structure of the intact strand allows for the specific complementary reconstitution of the damaged strand. Of the various repair processes that exist, the most wide-spread and best understood is the one known as "excision-repair" (20, 23, 24, 28). This process is defective in xeroderma pigmentosum (13–17, 28), which, as noted previously, is associated with a marked excess of actinic skin cancer (18, 29, 30).

Excision–repair and the defect in xeroderma pigmentosum.

As its name implies, excision-repair in-

volves the removal of a damaged region from a strand of DNA (12, 15, 16, 22) and resynthesis of the excised region (13, 14, 17, 23, 25) (Fig. 2). The latter step, wherein new bases are inserted into DNA is known as "repair synthesis", "repair replication", or "unscheduled synthesis." (The use of the terms may vary with the investigator, as a reflection of the various experimental techniques which are used.) A direct measure of "repair synthesis" or "repair replication" involves the analysis of repaired DNA on cesium chloride density gradients (12, 13, 23, 25). "Unscheduled synthesis" is measured by the incorporation of an isotope-labelled DNA precursor, such as tritiated–thymidine (^{3}HTdR), into DNA during excision-repair, as determined by radio autography (31). The word "unscheduled" is used here to emphasize two important characteristics of excision-repair: 1) it can occur at any and all stages of a cell's growth and differentiation and 2) is normally seen promptly after irradiation. This is in contrast to the limited period of "scheduled" DNA synthesis when the chromosomes are replicated (S-phase of the cell cycle). Thus, excision-repair can be easily assessed, as a result of the characteristic incorporation of labelled DNA precursors into DNA at times other than the S-period of the cell cycle. More specifically, if H^3-TdR is provided following UV irradiation, and radioautographs are prepared, the number of grains over lightly labelled (non-S-phase) cells can be counted (Fig. 3, 4). The average number of grains per cell is thereby a measure of the amount of ^{3}HTdR incorporated during excision–repair.

This mode of assessment can be applied

---

*Repair is a word that has many meanings in current usage. We use it here to refer to those changes in DNA, following damage by radiation or chemicals, which restore the original structure and function wholly or in part. More specific terms are introduced later to describe specific biochemical mechanisms.

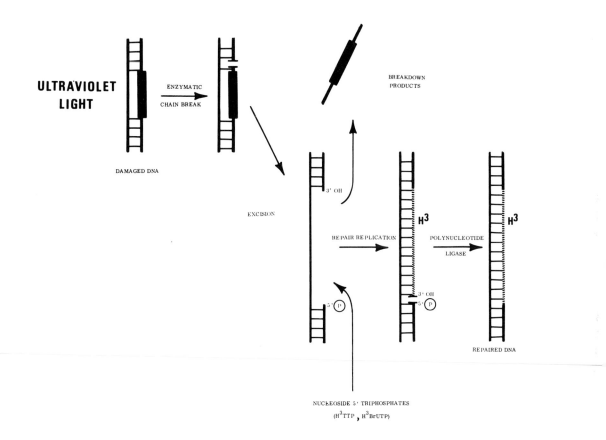

Figure 2. Hypothetical scheme for repair of UV damage in human cells. The steps involved include an enzymatic chain break, excision of the UV damage, replacement of the excised region by repair replication, and enzymatic joining of the final single strand gap. This scheme represents necessary steps for repair, although the precise sequences and details are as yet unknown. In particular, it is unlikely that any large regions of single strand DNA would ever be exposed *in vivo,* as shown above; excision and repair replication most probably proceed in concert such that no single strand regions are ever exposed. The initial step, involving enzymatic chain breakage, is probably defective in xeroderma pigmentosum.

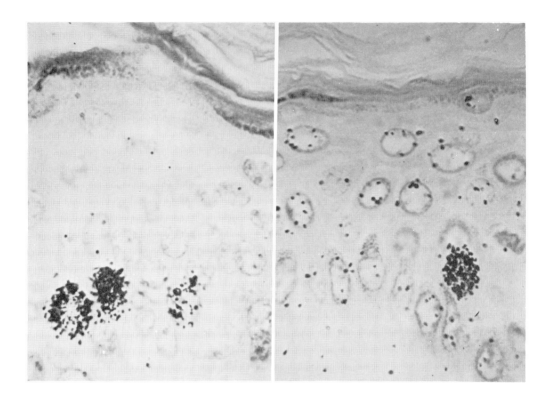

Figure 3. These autoradiographs represent the incorporation of intradermally injected ³HTdR into DNA of epidermal cells *in vivo* before and immediately after local UV irradiation (H and E; x1500, approximately).

left: *before irradiation*–in germinative basal cells of normal human epidermis *in vivo,* ³HTdR is incorporated into DNA only during the period of DNA replication (S–phase), as demonstrated by the combination of dense labeling in 3 basal cells and the absence of any other labeling.

right: *immediately after irradiation*–unscheduled DNA synthesis in non–dividing granular malphighian cells as well as in the basal cells is demonstrated by sparse accumulation of silver grains over most of these nuclei. In addition, 1 basal cell shows dense labeling, indicative of S–phase DNA replication. (These radioautographs were obtained through the courtesy of Drs. J.H. Epstein, K. Fukuyama and W.L. Epstein in their studies reported in References 32 and 33).

in vivo or *in vitro*. With the *in vivo* technique, the [3]HTdR is injected intradermally. Under ordinary circumstances, in skin epithelium DNA synthesis is confined to cells in the basal layers, and their incorporation of [3]HTdR is limited to the S-phase of the cell cycle (Fig. 3). Cells do not normally synthesize DNA once they have migrated from the basal layer (Fig. 3). However, irradiation of the skin with far UV light* damages the DNA of cells throughout the epidermal layer and these cells then undergo unscheduled synthesis to repair the damage (32, 33, 34). *In vitro,* lymphocyte or fibroblast cultures are used. In fibroblast cultures all the cells are actively growing, and DNA replication is confined to the S-phase of the cell cycle (33) (Fig. 4). Other processes such as RNA and protein synthesis occur throughout the cell cycle. As in the skin, irradiation with UV light normally causes all of the cultured cells to perform unscheduled synthesis (Fig. 4).

Comparative data for normal and xeroderma pigmentosum cells show that the latter are very low in their ability to repair (Fig. 4, Table I). This low level of repair synthesis is seen in various cells from patients with xeroderma pigmentosum: peripheral lymphocytes (36, 37), fibroblasts in culture (13, 14) and in epidermal cells and dermal fibrocytes *in vivo* (32–35). A low level of unscheduled synthesis is detectable in xeroderma pigmentosum cells, but there is considerable variation in the amounts actually measured. Both of the two clinical forms of xeroderma pigmentosum show similar skin involvement but in one (the de Sanctis-Cacchione syndrome (38) there are also severe neurological abnormalities. In cultured skin fibroblasts, representing both

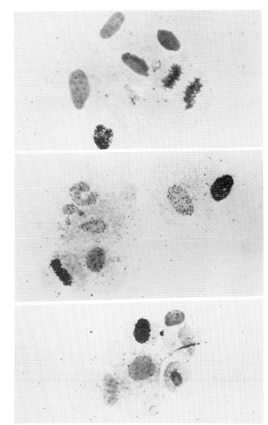

Figure 4. Radioautographs of human skin fibroblasts labeled for 2 hours with [3]HTdR (10 Ci/ml 12 Ci/mmole). (Top) xeroderma pigmentosum fibroblasts showing one cell labeled during DNA replication and one cell in mitosis. (Center) normal human fibroblasts labeled after 630 ergs/ mm^2 UV light. (Bottom) xeroderma pigmentosum fibroblasts labeled after 630/ergs mm^2 UV light. Note difference between cells lightly labeled by unscheduled synthesis in center (normal fibroblasts) and absence of such labeling in bottom (xeroderma pigmentosum fibroblasts).

*i.e. UV light of wavelength 254 nm, conveniently provided by low pressure mercury discharge tubes.

forms, the defect in excision–repair appears to be similar; the neurological complications typical of one form may be unrelated to the skin abnormalities and defective excision–repair (12, 16). Cells from the parents (heterozygotes) of xeroderma pigmentosum patients show little, if any, detectable aberration in this repair ability (14).

In the sequence of biochemical reactions of excision-repair, it is the initial step which appears to be defective in both forms of xeroderma pigmentosum (14–

Table I. Levels of Excision-Repair (Measured as the "unscheduled" uptake of ^3HTdR in the 4 hours following one dose of UV light (254 nm, @220 ergs/mm^2); values are given as percentages of the uptake in normal fibroblasts.

Normal skin fibroblasts	100%
Fibroblasts (from amniotic fluid)	103%
HeLa (cervical carcinoma)	94%
xeroderma pigmentosum female heterozygote)	77%
xeroderma pigmentosum (female heterozygote)*	100%
xeroderma pigmentosum (homozygotes)	6%
xeroderma pigmentosum (homozygotes)	25%
xeroderma pigmentosum (homozygotes)	5%
xeroderma pigmentosum (homozygotes)*	9%
xeroderma pigmentosum (homozygotes)*	25%
xeroderma pigmentosum (homozygotes)*	0
xeroderma pigmentosum (homozygotes)*	0
xeroderma pigmentosum (homozygotes)*	0

*de Sanctis–Cacchione syndrome

16). This step involves an enzyme (endonuclease) which cleaves a damaged but unbroken DNA chain and thus begins the excision of the damaged regions (Fig. 2). When cleavage does not take place, subsequent steps in the excision–repair process cannot be carried out. However, since the other enzymes for excision-repair are present in xeroderma pigmentosum, any damage which involves a break in the DNA chain circumvents this biochemical defect and is consequently repaired (14). Such broken–strand DNA damage has been shown to be repaired in normal and XDP cells; damage of this kind includes that from X–rays and radiomimetic agents such as methyl methane sulfonate and nitrogen mustard.

Xeroderma pigmentosum cells are very sensitive to killing by UV light, apparently in consequence to their low level of excision-repair. Their growth is markedly depressed by UV which *does* have little effect on normal cells (Fig. 5): the ability of individual cells to survive and form large colonies shows a sensitivity to UV light 4 to 5 times greater than for normal cells (i.e. a dose of 30 ergs/mm^2 to normal cells is equivalent in effect to a dose of 6 to 7.5 ergs/mm^2 to xeroderma pigmentosum patients). One of the direct effects of sunlight on the skin is probably an excessive killing of cells in the proliferative basal layers.

Summary and Conclusions.

These findings in xeroderma pigmentosum cells are consistent with previous expectations: parallel to their defective excision-repair mechanism, non-excessive UV irradiation is associated with a decrease in cell proliferation (*in vitro*), or the development of new growth patterns-- dysplasia and neoplasia--(*in vivo*). How-

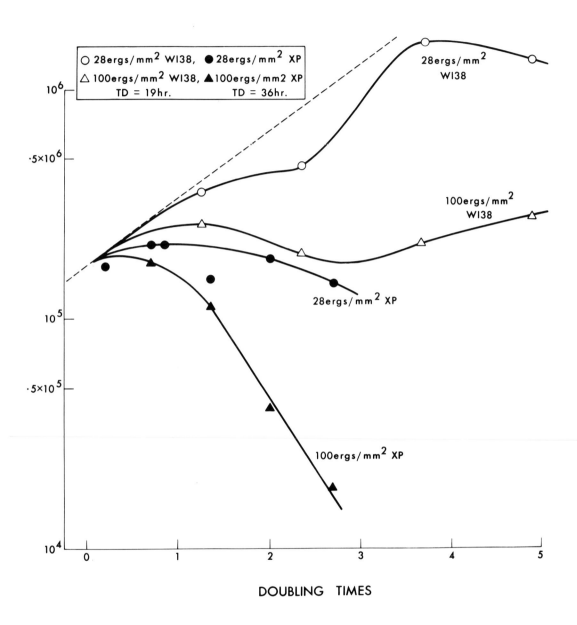

DOUBLING TIMES

Figure 5. The change in the ability of cells to proliferate following irradiation with various doses of UV light: cell number (ordinate) as a function of time (expressed in units of "doubling time" for each cell type); normal human fibroblasts (WI 38) and xeroderma pigmentosum fibroblasts (XP). Dashed (– –) line represents the curve for both cell types without irradiation.

ever, xeroderma pigmentosum patients and their cells do appear to represent a special case. In view of this, it would be misleading to use the defect in XDP as a general model to account for the development of many forms of cancer. For example, cells cultured from neoplasma--such as HeLa cells, derived from a cervical carcinoma--have normal levels of excision–repair (Table II). Nonetheless, this defect will likely continue to be informative in the understanding of certain aspects of carcinogenesis, and possibly other modes of pathology.

The level of unscheduled synthesis or repair replication can be determined for many other disorders, with or without skin involvement, in the same way as in normal and xeroderma pigmentosum cells. This is important since other diseases may be shown thereby to reflect mutations for other steps in DNA repair. A number of diseases have been evaluated in this manner (Table II). However, no distinctive changes in excision-repair (12)

have been shown among these entities, including those associated with excessive malignant neoplasia (e.g. dyskeratosis congenita, Bloom's syndrome, Rothmund–Thompson syndrome, etc., Table II).

References

1. Lynch, H.T.; "Skin, Heredity and Cancer," *Cancer 24*:277, 1969.

2. Bryan, H.G. and Nixon, R.K.; "Dyskeratosis Congenita and Familial Pancytopenia," *JAMA 192*:203, 1965.

3. Szilard, L.: "The Ageing Process," *Proc. Nat. Acad. Sci.* U.S. *45*: 30, 1959.

4. Berlin, N.I., Van Scott, J., Clendenning, William E., Archard, Howell O., Block, Jerome B., Witkop, Carl J., Haynes, Harley A.; "Basal Cell Nevus Syndrome," *Ann Intern Med 64*: 403, 1966.

Table II. AMOUNTS OF REPAIR REPLICATION IN HUMAN FIBROBLASTS FROM VARIOUS DISORDERS (measured after 200 to 400 ergs/mm^2)

	Skin Affected	Repair
normal skin	- - -	normal level
fetal lung (WI 38)	- - -	"
HeLa (malignant)	yes	"
Rothmund–Thompson syndrome	yes	"
Progeria	yes	"
Bloom's syndrome	yes	"
lupus erythematosus	yes	"
ataxia telangiectasia	yes	"
dyskeratosis congenita	yes	"
acanthosis nigricans	yes	"
Darier's Disease	yes	
xeroderma pigmentosum	yes	5 to 25% (3 cases)
xeroderma pigmentosum (De Sanctis–Cacchione syndrome)	yes	0 to 25% (4 cases)

5. Rauh, J.L. and Soukup, S.W.; "Bloom's Syndrome," *Amer. J. Dis. Child.* 116:409, 1968.

6. Sawitsky, A., Bloom, D. and German J.; "Chromosomal Breakage and Acute Leukemia in Congenital Telangiectatic Erythema and Stunted Growth," *Ann Intern Med* 65:487, 1966.

7. Bloom, G.E., Warner, S., Gerald, P.S. and Diamond, L.K.; "Chromosome Abnormalities in Constitutional Aplastic Anemia," *New Eng. J. Med.* 274:8, 1966.

8. Pfeiffer, R.A.; "Chromosomal Abnormalities in Ataxia–Telangiectasia (Louis Bar's Syndrome)," *Humangenetik* 8: 302, 1970.

9. Black, P.H.; "The Oncogenic DNA Viruses; A Review of In Vitro Transformation Studies," *Ann. Rev. Microbiol.* 22: 391, 1968.

10. Cleaver, J.E.; in Proceedings of the Second International Symposium on Radioprotective Drugs, 1969.

11. Goldstein, S; "Survival of Cultured Fibroblasts from Xeroderma Pigmentosum and Normals After Ultraviolet Irradiation," *J. Clin. Invest.* 49:36a, 1970. (Abstract).

12. Cleaver, J.E.; "DNA Damage and Repair in Light—Sensitive Human Skin Disease," *J. Invest. Derm.* (In Press, 1970.)

13. Cleaver, J.E.; "Defective Repair Replication of DNA in Xeroderma Pigmentosum," *Nature* 218:652, 1968.

14. Cleaver, J.E.; "Xeroderma Pigmentosum: A Human Disease In Which an Initial Stage of DNA Repair is Defective," *Proc. Nat. Acad. Sci.* U.S. 63:428, 1969.

15. Setlow, R.B., Regan, R.D., German, J. and Carrier, W.L.; "Evidence that Xeroderma Pigmentosum Cells Do Not Perform the First Step in the Repair of Ultraviolet," *Proc. Nat. Acad. Sci.* U.S. 64: 1035, 1969.

16. Cleaver, J.E. and Trosko, J.E.; Photochem. Photobiol. (In Press, 1970.)

17. Reed, W.B., Landing, B., Sugarman, G., Cleaver, J.E. and Melnyk, J.; "Xeroderma Pigmentosum," *JAMA* 207:2073, 1969.

18. Rook, A., Wilkinson, D.S. and Ebling, F.J.G.; Textbook of Dermatology, Vol I, Blackwell Scientific Publications, Oxford and Edinburgh, 1968, page 62.

19. Miller, R.W. and Todaro, G.J.; "Viral Transformation of Cells from Persons at High Risk of Cancer," *Lancet* 1: 81, 1969.

20. Wittein, E.M.; "Ultraviolet–Induced Mutation and DNA Repair," *Ann. Rev. Genet.* 3:525, 1969.

21. Smith, D.W. and Hanawalt, P.C.; "State of Aggregation of the Growing Point in the Bacterial Chromosome," Biophys. J. 7: 78, 1967. (Abstract).

22. Setlow, R.B. and Carrier, W.L.; "The Disappearance of Thymine Dimers from DNA: An Error–Correcting Mechanism," *Proc. Nat. Acad. Sci.* U.S. 51:226, 1964.

23. Pettijohn, D. and Hanawalt, P.C.; "Evidence for Repair–Replication of Ultraviolet Damaged DNA in Bacteria," *J. Molec Biol* 9:395, 1964.

24. Trosko, J.E. and Mansour, V.H.; "Response of Tobacco and Haplopappus Cells to Ultraviolet Irradiation After Posttreatment with Photoreactivating Light," Rad. Res. 36: 333, 1968.

25. Painter, R.B. and Cleaver, J.E.; "Repair Replication, Unscheduled DNA Synthesis, and the Repair of Mannalian DNA," *Radiol Res* 37:451, 1969.

26. Okada, S.; in Radiation Biochemistry, Vol I: Cells; Academic Press, New York and London, 1970.

27. Setlow, J.K.; in Current Topics in Radiation Research, Vol II; North Holland Publishing Co., Amsterdam, 1966. page 195.

28. Lett, J.T., Caldwell, I., Dean, C.J. and Alexander, P.; "Rejoining of X–ray Induced Breaks in the DNA of Leukemia Cells," *Nature 214*:790, 1967.

29. Lynch, H.T., Anderson, D.E., Krush, A.J. and Mukerjee, D.; "Cancer, Heredity and Genetic Counseling," *Cancer 20*: 1796, 1967.

30. Lynch, H.T., Anderson, D.E., Smith, J.L., Jr., Howell, J.B. and Krush, A.J.; "Xeroderma Pigmentosum, Malignant Melanoma, and Congenital Ichthyosis," *Arch. Derm. 96*:625, 1967.

31. Djordjevic, B. and Tolmach, L.J.; "Responses of Synchronous Populations of HeLa Cells to Ultraviolet Irradiation at Selected Stages of the Generation Cycle," *Radiol Res 32*:327, 1967.

32. Epstein, J.H., Fukuyama, K. and Epstein, W.L.; "An In Vivo Study of a Defect in DNA Synthesis in Xeroderma Pigmentosum," *J. Clin. Invest. 48*:23a, 1969. (Abstract).

33. Epstein, J.H., Fukuyama, K. and Epstein, W.L.; "UVL Induced Stimulation of DNA Synthesis in Hairless Mouse Epidermis," *Dermatologica (Basel) 51*:445,

34. Epstein, J.H., Fukuyama, K., Reed, W.B. and Epstein, W.L.; "Defect in DNA Synthesis in Skin of Patients with Xeroderma Pigmentosum Demonstrated in Vivo," *Science 168*:1477, 1970.

35. Cleaver, J.E.; Thymidine Metabolism and Cell Kinetics, North Holland Publishing Co., Amsterdam, 1967.

36. Burk, P.G., Lutzner, M.A. and Robbins, J.H.; "Decreased Incorporation of Thymidine into the DNA of Lymphocytes from Patients with Xeroderma Pigmentosum After Ultraviolet Irradiation In Vitro," *Clinical Res. 17*:614, 1969.

37. Burk, P.G., Levis, W.R., Lutzner, M.A. and Robbins, J.H.; "Decreased Rate of Thymidine Incorporation into DNA of Some Xeroderma Pigmentosum Patients' Lymphocytes After Ultraviolet Irradiation in Vitro."

38. Desanctis, C. and Cacchione, A.; "L'idiozia Zero Dermica," *Riv. Sper. Freniat. 56*:269, 1932.

Chapter 5

XERODERMA PIGMENTOSUM*

by Henry T. Lynch, M.D.

INTRODUCTION

Xeroderma Pigmentosum (XDP) is an exceedingly rare and chronically progressive multisystem disease. It is inherited as an autosomal recessive. The skin is the principal target organ and XDP manifestations are dependent in part upon the patient's age and environmental exposures, particularly solar radiation. Pathologic changes of the skin vary but include disturbances of pigmentation and maturation of epidermal cells, leading eventually to the formation of malignant skin tumors, usually basal and squamous cell carcinomas.[1] Malignant melanoma appears to have an increased association with this disease.[2] Neurologic manifestations may include speech disturbances, mental deficiency, and convulsive disorders.[3] Ocular manifestations may include photophobia, conjunctivitis, keratitis, blepharitis, ectropion, and basal and squamous cell carcinomas.[4] Endocrinologic aberrations have been reported, including aminoaciduria, prolonged erythrocyte glucose–6–phosphate dehydrogenase (G–6–PD) activity with suggestion of erythrocyte glutathione deficiency, and possible pituitary adrenal abnormalities.[5] Congenital anomalies, including short stature, microcephaly, and joint abnormalities[6], have also been reported.

In the usual clinical setting, XDP occurs in context with one or more of the above sequelae. However, XDP, like any other hereditary disease may, on rare occasions, occur in association with another hereditary disease; in such circumstances, as will be shown shortly, one cannot be absolutely certain that he is dealing with *two* distinct hereditary diseases or whether, on the other hand, he is observing a widening clinical spectrum of one of the particular genetic diseases, i.e. so–called variable expressivity of the gene. Such occurrences provide a unique opportunity to study the interactions of the particular diseases in a common constitutional and environmental milieu. One of the purposes of this chapter is to present detailed clinicogenetic and pathologic findings in a family with XDP and congenital ichthyosis, who in addition showed malignant melanoma. In addition, XDP will be discussed in context with skin cancer including its occasional, but nevertheless significant association with malignant melanoma.

*Portions of this paper are reprinted by permission of *Archives of Dermatology* from Lynch, H.T., *et, al*: *Arch. Derm. 96*: 625–635, 1967.

Family Study

The proband, a 17 year–old white boy, had previous histologically confirmed diagnosis of XDP and malignant melanoma. He was admitted to the University of Texas M.D. Anderson Hospital and Tumor Institute where detailed medical, genetic, and endocrinologic studies were performed.

Because of a history of other similarly affected siblings, a "field trip" was made to the patient's home, approximately 1,200 miles away, after his hospital discharge. Participants in the field trip included an internist, a dermatologist, and a geneticist. Complete physical examinations were performed on six siblings of the patient, his mother, and his father. Skin biopsies were done on each individual except the oldest brother.

The proband's (Fig. 1, II–4 and Fig. 2) birth and gestational history were normal. Lentigines and areas of pigmentation were visible over the entire integument by 4 to 5 months of age. The skin was extremely dry with scaling, accentuated during the winter months. At 7 years of age, a diagnosis of XDP was made, and at the same time the disease was recognized in an older sister. After this, the patient and his affected siblings were assiduously protected from exposure to solar radiation. At age 13, a dark mole, which proved to be malignant melanoma, was excised from the right cervical triangle. The following year, a basal cell carcinoma was removed from the right supraorbital region. When the patient was 17, a metastatic malignant melanoma was excised from the volar surface of the

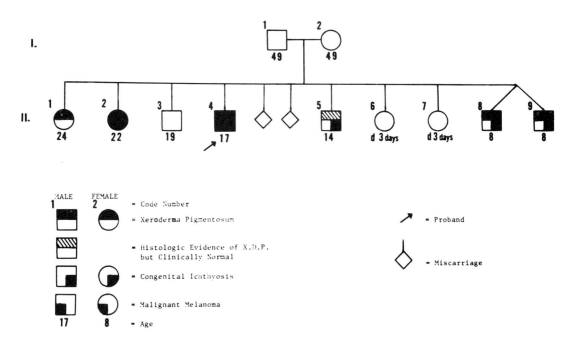

Figure 1. Pedigree of a family with xeroderma pigmentosum, congenital ichthyosis, and malignant melanoma.

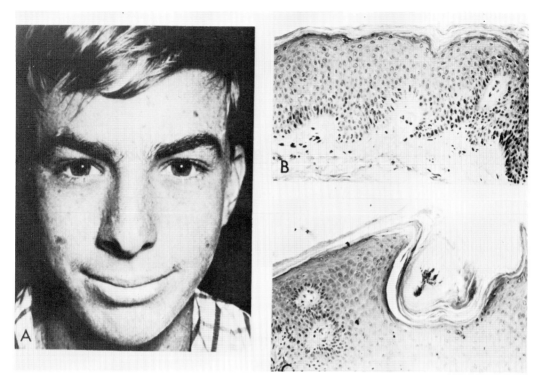

Figure 2. **A.** Front–face view of the 17–year–old proband. Note the multiple lentigines.
B. Epidermis shows absence of the granular cell layer, and a dense overlying keratin layer. Melanin pigmentation is patchy and early dyskeratotic changes are noted.
C. Follicular plugging of the granular cell layer is absent.

right arm. The remainder of the medical history was unremarkable. Physical examination revealed an alert well–developed boy. Vital signs were normal. Results of examination of the head and neck, heart, lungs, abdomen, and neurologic system were within normal limits. The only abnormalities on physical examination were confined to the integument. This showed obvious XDP of moderate severity. The skin of the exposed area was only slightly more freckled and pigmented than the unexposed areas of skin. The scalp was almost as hyperpigmented and freckled as the face. Freckling of the upper eyelids and dorsa of the feet was noteworthy. Only a few moles (nevus cell nevi) were observed. An unexpected finding was ichthyosis. This was characterized by generalized dryness, scaling of the scalp, face, diffusely hyperkeratotic soles and palms, and horizontally hyperkeratotic folds or ridges of skin over the knees, elbows, and Achilles tendon areas. The skin of the legs, especially the pretibial site, was dry, fissured, and resembled fish skin.

Histologically, biopsies from these

areas exhibited features of both ichthyosis and XDP. Those of ichthyosis included an absent granular cell layer, keratin layer which was slightly thickened, more dense and homogenous than normal, keratin plugging of hair follicles and eccrine sweat pores. A few scattered parakeratotic foci were encountered. In addition to the features of ichthyosis the epidermis also exhibited irregular patches of melanin pigmentation, some represented by areas of lentigo, others by increased numbers of melanocytes and melanin pigment in cells of the basal and lower malpighian layers without an increase in the number of melanocytes. Focal areas of the non-pigmented epidermis demonstrated abnormal progression of maturation of epidermal cells. In some of these, the cells of the basal and lower malpighian layers were tall, compressed and cylindrical, extending to the upper malpighian layers. In other areas, the cells were arranged more disorderly as in early solar keratoses. These features are consistent with those of XDP.

The proband's mother was 49 years of age (Fig. 1, I–2). She stated that she had had "dry skin" since age 16, which she cared for with lotions and salves. She had had symptoms suggestive of tension headache intermittently since age 18. She developed a peptic ulcer at age 49 which responded well to medical management. Hypertension of unknown etiology had been controlled medically for the past several years. Details of the hypertension management were not available. She had ten pregnancies, two of which terminated in abortion at less than three months' gestation. Two female children died at 3 days (Fig. 1, II–6 and II–7). Details on the cause of these deaths are lacking. The remainder of the medical history was unremarkable.

Physical examination revealed a healthy appearing, slightly obese, white woman. Her blood pressure was 160/90 mm mercury (Hg). Examination of the head, neck, breasts, heart, lungs, abdomen, and neurologic system was normal. The skin was universally dry, especially in the pretibial areas and the extensor surfaces of the arms. There was no evidence of XDP. She was not related to her husband.

A skin biopsy from the inner surface of the right upper arm revealed a normal granular cell layer with an overlying normal layer of keratin. There was suggestion of plugging of the eccrine sweat pores and hair follicles, but this was of minimal degree. The epidermis was of uniform thickness. Melanin pigment was evenly distributed through the basal layers of the epidermis, and there was normal progression of maturation of epidermal cells. Diagnostic evidence of either ichthyosis or XDP was lacking, though the slight poral and follicular plugging could possibly be of significance.

The father of the proband was 49 years old (Fig. 1, I–1). His growth and development were normal. There was no history of skin disease. He contracted malaria during World War II, but had had no recurrence of this disease. He had a perforated duodenal ulcer at age 20 which responded to limited surgical repair. At age 48, he had a venous thrombosis of the right leg, subsequently diagnosed as polycythemia. He underwent a splenectomy in 1966, but we have been unable to establish the reasons for splenectomy.

On physical examination, the patient appeared to be healthy, though mildly overweight. There were no external manifestations of polycythemia. Examination of the skin revealed no evidence of either ichthyosis or XDP. Approximately 30 moles were present on his body. Most were intradermal nevi but two were pigmented macular junctional nevi on the left sole.

A biopsy of the skin of the left arm showed no significant histopathological changes. There was normal progression of maturation of epidermal cells and normal granular cell and keratin layers. Melanin pigment was evenly distributed through the basal layers.

The oldest sister of the proband was 24 years of age (Fig. 1, II–1 and Fig. 3). She was born prematurely at 7 months. Development was normal though her growth rate was slightly retarded. She had had recurrent sinusitis beginning at age 12. Menarche occurred at age 15. She had mild dysmenorrhea through age 22. A diagnosis of XDP was established at age 14. Since then, approximately 20 basal and squamous cell carcinomas have been removed from exposed areas of her body. An active atypical junction nevus was removed in 1957 from an unstated skin site. She has been continually protected from ultraviolet ray exposure since age 14. The remainder of the history was noncontributory.

The physical examination revealed a woman of small stature (5 feet tall) and generally underdeveloped. Vital signs were normal. Complete physical examination results, except for the integument, were normal. Slowly progressive XDP of only a moderate degree of severity was found. There was relatively little difference in the degree of hyperpigmentation and freckling between exposed and unexposed areas of the skin. A striking feature was the presence of giant–sized freckles or lentigines of the face. These were not observed in other affected family members. A careful search was required to detect a slight amount of facial telan-

giectasia. The surfaces of the extremities were slightly dry without evidence of ichthyosis. Two small non–pigmented papules were detected in the right inner canthus. Clinically these appeared to be keratoses or early basal cell carcinomas. Telangiectasia was present on the lateral portion of the bulbar conjunctivae. A small pigmented macule was observed at the junction of the cornea and temporal portion of the left bulbar conjunctiva. The hyperpigmentation in this patient interfered with the detection of moles, but a careful search revealed that nevus cell nevi were scarce.

Biopsy of a small skin lesion on the nose revealed basal cell carcinoma. Of equal interest was the epidermis in the same specimen lateral to this tumor. It demonstrated marked dyskeratosis, accompanied in foci by acantholysis, as observed in some solar keratoses. Melanin pigment was irregularly distributed in areas associated with lentigo. The granular cell layer was present. No changes were present which suggested ichthyosis. A second biopsy from the skin of the leg was also free of ichthyosis, possessing normal granular cell and normal keratin layers. A feature of note was the irregular distribution of melanin pigment in areas associated with a lentigo pattern. Dyskeratosis, while suggested, was not as noticeable as in the exposed skin of the nose. In summary, histologic features consistent with XDP were present, while those of ichthyosis were lacking.

The next oldest sister of the proband was 22 years old (Fig. 1, II–2 and Fig. 4). Gestation, birth, growth, and development were normal. At age 12, this girl was the first member of the family to receive a diagnosis of XDP. However, freckling and areas of pigmentation had been present over her body since infancy.

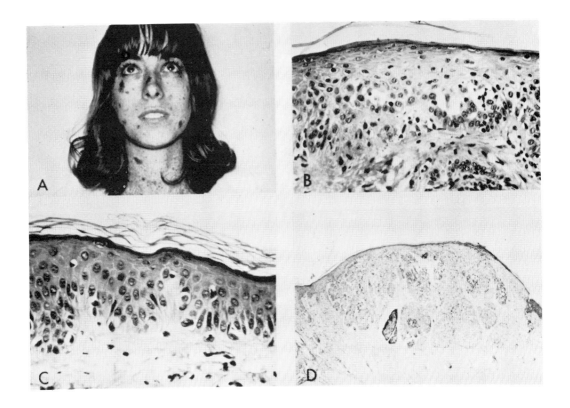

Figure 3. A. Front–face view of the proband's 24–year–old sister. Note numerous lentigines of varying size.

　　B. Epidermis showing dyskeratosis with suprabasalar acantholysis (specimen from area adjacent to lesion on nose.)

　　C. Epidermis showing increased numbers of melanocytes which was associated with irregular melanin pigmentation.

　　D. Basal cell carcinoma from nose.

At least 25 basal and squamous cell carcinomas, including a malignant melanoma excised from the integument, have been excised since the patient was 12 years old. Menarche occured at age 13. She had had recent dysmenorrhea. The remainder of the history was unremarkable.

Physical examination of the patient revealed normal vital signs. She was apprehensive and anxious, with emotional lability. Pigmentation was present over the entire body with relatively little difference between exposed and unexposed areas. The upper eyelids were pigmented and freckled. Mild telangiectasia was present over the center of the face. Prominent lentigines were noted over the head and neck, and the lips were freckled. Several small pigmented hyperkeratotic papules were observed over the malar areas and canthi. A scar caused by irradiation of the right lower lip was noted.

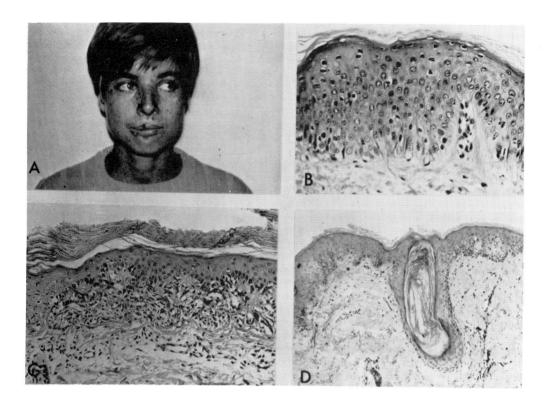

Figure 4. **A.** Front–face view of the proband's 22–year–old sister. Note the numerous lentigines and scars on her lips from removal of previous cancers.
  B. Epidermis shows dyskeratosis, an absent granular cell layer and slight to moderate hyperkeratosis.
  C. Active junction nevus associated with an absent granular cell layer and hyperkeratosis.
  D. Keratin plugging of a hair follicle.

The lateral portion of the bulbar conjunctiva had numerous telangiectatic vessels bilaterally. Some atrophy and thinning of the tissues of the nose were present, probably accentuated by prior management of tumors of both alae. The appearance of the facial skin suggested a moderately severe, slowly progressive XDP, with a number of cancer scars and precancerous lesions over the central fa-

cial areas. A moderate degree of ichthyosis, characterized by generalized dryness and scaly fish–like skin, was found on the legs and the extensor surfaces of the arms. The palms were dry, thickened, and hyperkeratotic.

A representative area of the skin of the leg was biopsied. The granular cell layer proved to be absent and the overlying keratin layer was less flaky and more dense than normal, similar to that observed in the skin of the proband. Keratin plugging of eccrine sweat pores and hair follicles was prominent. The epidermis was irregular, partly as a result of widespread lentigo and cellular nests of junction nevus cells. Melanin pigment distribution was irregular and patchy. Dyskeratotic changes, slight to moderate in degree, were present in the nonpigmented epidermis. These changes illustrate remarkably well the co-existing features of both ichthyosis and XDP.

A 19 year-old brother of the proband (Fig. 1, II-3) was delivered at 7 months' gestation without complications. Growth and development were normal. He has never manifested any freckling, increased pigmentation, or dryness of the skin. The remainder of the medical history was unremarkable.

Physical examination revealed a normally developed white boy. Results of the entire physical examination, including the skin, were normal, except for the finding of several nevus cell nevi. A skin biopsy was not performed.

A 14 year-old brother of the proband (Fig. 1, II-5 and Fig. 5) was delivered normally, despite the fact that his mother had possible eclampsia at 8½ months' gestation. Growth and development were normal. However, he had a lifelong history of dryness and scaliness of the skin, accentuated in the winter months. The remainder of the medical history was unremarkable.

Physical findings were entirely normal except for the skin. Generalized dryness of the skin was found, including the scalp and face. The palms and soles were slightly thickened and keratosis pilaris of the extensor surfaces of the extremities was present. The skin over the elbows, knees, and Achilles tendons was dry and hyperkeratotic with veruccous folds. Fish-skin appearance so characteristic of ichthyosis was prominent over the pretibial sites.

The exposed skin was similar to the unexposed skin and showed no evidence of abnormal sunlight damage. Approximately 12 pigmented nevi were present over the body with a predominance of the junctional type. The only clinical diagnosis in this patient was moderately severe ichthyosis.

Skin biopsies from an arm and a leg presented similar histologic features. In each, the granular cell layer of the epidermis was absent, and the overlying keratin layer, while not noticeably thickened, was more dense and homogeneous than normal. Plugging of eccrine sweat pores and follicles was prominent. Though clinically the patient did not present changes of XDP, slight irregularity and patchiness of melanin pigmentation was noted. This finding, together with the slight focal disorderly arrangement of cells, raises the question of a subclinical degree of XDP.

Eight-year-old identical twin brothers of the proband, (Fig. 1, II-8, II-9, and Fig. 6) were born prematurely at 7 months' gestation. Subsequent blood type studies proved them to be identical for 17 antisera. Deliveries were uncomplicated though the mother had considerable spotting throughout the pregnancy. Growth and development were normal for both children. Both showed freckling and pigmentation of the entire integument shortly after birth. Both had been protected from sunlight exposure since birth. To date, no skin cancers have developed. The remainder of the history was non-contributory.

Physical examination showed these boys to be virtually identical in appear-

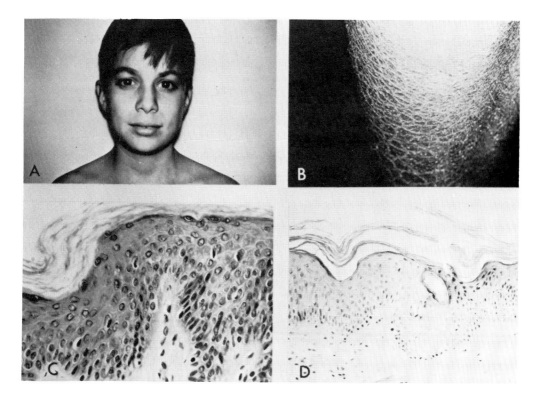

Figure 5. **A.** Front–face view of the 14–year–old brother of the proband. Note the absence of pigmentation.
    B. Gross evidence of congenital ichthyosis.
    C. Epidermis showing an absent granular cell layer with overlying slight to moderate hyperkeratosis. Early dyskeratotic changes are noted.
    D. Epidermis showing keratin plugging of an eccrine sweat pore.

ance. Both were above average intelligence. Except for the findings in the skin, physical findings were normal. A mild, slowly progressive XDP was readily recognizable in each child. It was characterized by freckling and hyperpigmentation, particularly on exposed sites. If the pigmentation follows the pattern of the older brother and sisters, the difference between exposed and unexposed sites will probably diminish with time. Slight telangiectasis of the bulbar conjunctiva was present. Both manifested generalized dryness of the skin with a mild ichthyosis of the extensor surfaces of the arms, which was most noticeable on the pretibial areas. One twin (Fig. 1, II–8) (Fig. 6) had keratosis pilaris of the arms and legs. Relatively few nevus cell nevi were present. The second twin (Fig. 1, II–9) (Fig. 6) had a hard subcutaneous iceberg–shaped mass of the left malar area which had been present, although asymptomatic, for approximately one year.

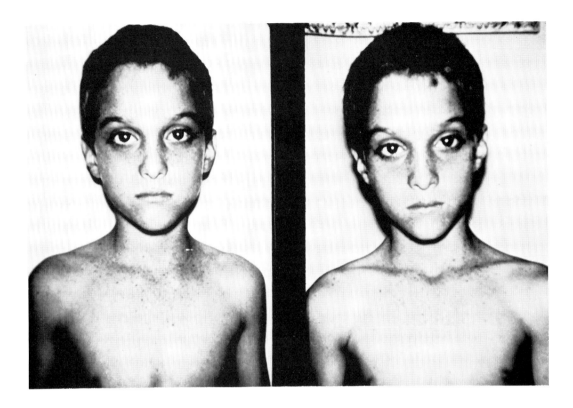

Figure 6. Eight–year–old identical twin brothers of the proband. Note numerous lentigines of the face and anterior thorax.

Representative skin from the legs of each of the 8–year–old twins was biopsied. Histologically, the features in each were virtually identical to those of the preceding patients, although they differed with regard to ichthyosis. The more pronounced changes were those related to XDP and consisted of irregular melanin pigmentation of the epidermis in areas in the form of lentigo and focal disorderly arrangement of the deeper epidermal cells. These changes coincided with the clinical observations and diagnosis of XDP. The histological difference from the preceding patients with ichthyosis was the presence of a granular cell layer, though focally diminished, and an overlying essentially normal flaky keratin layer in both twins. However, keratin which plugged hair follicles was relatively prominent. Some plugging of eccrine sweat pores was also present. These findings coincide with the clinical description of each having "mild ichthyosis" and one clinically having keratosis pilaris of the arms and legs. Thus, histologically, features of both diseases were present, though those of ichthyosis were less clear.

Discussion

The family presented here is interesting from the standpoint of the occurrence of XDP in five of seven siblings. In addition, four of these five also showed congenital ichthyosis, and two of these had a further and more grave complication, namely, malignant melanoma. One sibling manifested XDP and no ichthyosis and another sibling, while completely free of XDP, clinically presented with a classical and moderately severe form of congenital ichthyosis. This patient histologically, however, had changes which though minimal were albeit consistent with early changes of XDP. Thus, it appears that in this family we are dealing with two inherited diseases, XDP and congenital ichthyosis. The XDP appears to be behaving as an autosomal recessive factor, while the inheritance of congenital ichthyosis is not clear. A dominant factor with reduced penetrance of the gene cannot be excluded. Note that the mother had dryness of her skin, though histologic evidence for ichthyosis was lacking.

Congenital ichthyosis in association with XDP, so far as we can determine, is rare. A literature review has revealed only one authenticated report of this association, namely that of Couillaud[7] in 1898. In addition, a survey of dermatologists from several large institutions revealed that none had ever observed this association. Thus, the association in this family can be most reasonably explained in terms of fortuitous association of two hereditary diseases. It is suggested that other investigators search carefully for this occurrence in both affected as well as unaffected relatives of probands with XDP.

Congenital ichthyosis has been described previously in association with other genetic disorders. Lynch, et al[8] described congenital ichthyosis in association with secondary male hypogonadism in a family in which this combination was present in three members (and two additional members by history) through three generations. A sex-linked mode of inheritance was advanced for this. Congenital ichthyosis is also an essential component in the syndrome of Rüd[9]. However, the etiologic significance of these associations remains unclear.

The occurrence of malignant melanoma in two of the individuals in this family prompted us to make an extensive review of the association of this lesion with XDP (Table 1). Note the large number of reports documenting this association. [7,10-27] Moore and Iverson [25] summarized 360 cases of XDP which had been reported up to 1959 and estimated that melanoma was an associated finding in 3% of these. The present family, with two instances of malignant melanoma among five patients with XDP, provides additional support that these two cutaneous conditions may be associated more frequently than has heretofore been suspected. We emphasize this point because malignant melanoma is rarely considered to be a threat to patients with XDP in which generally, basal and squamous cell carcinomas are most frequently found. From the available data on XDP, malignant melanoma appears to be another manifestation of this severe recessively inherited skin cancer diathesis. When malignant melanoma occurs in families it usually behaves as an autosomal dominant.[28, 29] (See Chapter 6).

Finally there is an additional syndrome involving XDP, with associated neurological complications, known as the de Sanctis–Cacchione syndrome. The cardinal features of this syndrome include xeroderma pigmentosum, microcephaly, mental deficiency, dwarfism, and gonadal hypoplasia. This clinical entity was described by de Sanctis and Cacchione in

1932[30] when they reported three brothers with XDP and mental deficiency. Recently Reed and associates found 18 additional patients reported in the literature with confirmed XDP associated with clear–cut neurological complications.[3] In addition, these investigators have added 4 new cases of their own with the de Santis–Cacchione syndrome. The authors conclude that they do not consider that there are two separate forms of xeroderma pigmentosum, one with and one without neurological changes. Rather they postulate that the classical form without neurological changes is a less severe manifestation of the disorder resulting from incomplete penetrance of the gene for this disorder.

TABLE 1

XERODERMA PIGMENTOSUM, MELANOMA, AND ICTHYOSIS

Literature Review of Combined Xeroderma Pigmentosum and Malignant Melanoma

Author	Date	No. of Cases	Age at Onset of Malignant Melanoma	Sex	Others in Family With XDP	Comments
Pick[10]	1884	2	19 17	F F	2 Siblings 2 Siblings	– – – – – –
Mendes da Costa[11]	1889	1	21	M	1 sister	– – –
Eisenberg[12]	1890	3	5 12 15	M F F	1 sister	– – –
Benziger and Heuss[13]	1897	1	14	F	– – –	– – –
Couillaud[7]	1898	1	29	F	Paternal aunt	Both had ichthyosis (by history)
Wesolowski[14]	1899	2	4 7	M M	– – – – – –	– – – – – –
Havas[15]	1908	1	–	–	– – –	– – –
Stout[16]	1908	1	2	M	1 brother (by history)	– – –
Rouviere[17]	1910	1	21	F	2 sisters	– – –
Nakagawa[18]	1916	1	–	–	– – –	– – –
Nicolas et al[19]	1927	1	30	F	1 brother	– – –
Foldvari[20]	1934	1	7	F	– – –	– – –
Flarer[21]	1937	1	3	M	– – –	– – –
Merenlender and Ginzburgowa[22]	1938	1	15	F	– – –	– – –

Ronchese[23]	1953	1	24	F	older sister	Same patient followed for 25 years; intracranial metastases with "about 20 melanotic tumors."
Van Patter and Drummond[24]	1954	1	29	F	Brother, sister, paternal great aunt (by history)	– – –
Moore and Iverson[25]	1954	1	47	M	– – –	Estimated that of 360 cases of XDP 3% had malignant melanoma
Iijima et al[26]	1957	1	8	F	Brother	10 cases from Japan, 14 from other countries reported; frequency of malignant melanoma associated with XDP approximately 3%
Lemaire and Gaumond[27]	1965	1	14	M	Brother	– – –

References

1. Lynch, H.T.: Hereditary Factors in Carcinoma, in *Recent Results in Cancer Research,* monograph series, New York: Springer–Verlag, vol 12, 1967, pp. 1–186.

2. Attie, J.L., and Khafif, R.A.: *Melanotic Tumors: Biology, Pathology, and Clinical Features,* Springfield, Ill: Charles C. Thomas, Publisher, 1964, pp. 160–183.

3. Reed, W.B.; May, S.B.; and Nickel, W.R.: Xeroderma Pigmentosum With Neurological Complications, *Arch Derm 91*: 224–226, 1965.

4. El–Hefnawi, H., and Mortada, A.: Ocular Manifestations of Xeroderma Pigmentosum, *Brit J Derm 77*: 261–276, 1965.

5. Moss, H.V., Jr.: Xeroderma Pigmentosum: Report of Two Cases with Metabolic Studies, *Arch Derm 92*: 638–642, 1965.

6. Butterworth, T., and Strean, L.P.: *Clinical Genodermatology,* Baltimore: The Williams & Wilkins Company, 1962.

7. Couillaud, M.P.: Xeroderma Pigmentosum de Kaposi, *Ann Derm Syph 9*: 443–448, 1898.

8. Lynch, H.T., et al: Secondary Male Hypogonadism and Congenital Ichthyosis: Association of Two Rare Genetic Diseases, *Amer J Hum Genet 12*: 440–447, 1960.

9. MacGillivary, R.C.: The Syndrome of Rud, *Amer J Ment Defic 59*: 62–72, 1954.

10. Pick, F.J.: Ueber Melanosis lenticularis progressiva *Vschr Derm Syph 16*: 3, 1884.

11. Mendes da Costa, S.: Xeroderma Pigmentosum, *Nederl T Geneesk 1*: 1117–1118, 1900.

12. Elsenberg, A.: Xeroderm Pigmentosum (Kaposi): Progressive Lenticular Melanosis, *Arch Derm Syph 22*: 49–70, 1890.

13. Benziger, K., and Heuss: *Paracelsus,* Zurich, Switzerland, 1897.

14. Wesolowski, W.: Beitrag zur pathologischen Anatomie des Xeroderma pigmentosum, *Centralbl Allg Path 10*: 990–997, 1899.

15. Havas, cited by Nicolas, J.; Favre, M.; and Dupasiquier, D.: Du cancer melanique dans le xeroderma pigmentosum, *Ann Derm Syph 8*: 457–472, 1927.

16. Stout: A Case of Xeroderma Pigmentosum, *J Cutan Dis 26*: 380–381, 1908.

17. Rouviere, M.G.: Deux nonveaux cas de xeroderma pigmentosum, *Ann Derm Syph 1*: 34–37, 1910.

18. Nakagawa, cited by Nicolas, J.; Favre, M.; and Dupasquier, D.: Du cancer melanique dans le xeroderma pigmentosum, *Ann Derm Syph 8*: 457–472, 1927.

19. Nicolas, J.; Favre, M.; and Dupasquier, D.: Du cancer melanique dans le xeroderma pigmentosum, *Ann Derm Syph 8*: 457–472, 1927.

20. Foldvari, F.: Metastase sarcomateuse hepatique de xeroderma pigmentosum, *Acta Derm Syph 15*: 253–263, 1934.

21. Flarer, F.: Disceratosi: epiteliomi multipli e melanosarcoma in bambino di tre anni con xeroderma pigmentoso, *Riforma Med 53*: 635–638, 1937.

22. Merenlender, I.J., and Ginzburgowa, B.: Xeroderma Pigmentosum (Melanoneurinoma Consecutivum), *Acta Dermatovener 19*: 75–87, 1938.

23. Ronchese, F.: Spontaneous Bleaching of Melanotic Freckles, *Arch Derm 94*: 739–741, 1966.

24. Van Patter, H.T., and Drummond, J.A.: Malignant Melanoma Occurring in Xeroderma Pigmentosum: Report of a Case, *Cancer 6*: 942–947, 1954.

25. Moore, C., and Iverson, P.C.: Xeroderma Showing Common Skin Cancer Plus Melanocarcinoma Controlled by Surgery, *Cancer 7*: 377–382, 1954.

26. Iijima, S.; Watanabe, S.; and Shimoda, C.: A Case of Xeroderma Pigmentosum With Melanoma: Report of a Case With Review of Literature, *Acta Derm 52*: 163–167, 1957.

27. Lemaire, M., and Gaumond, E.: Xeroderma Pigmentosum, Huit cas d' evolution differente dans deux familles, *Canad Med Ass J 92*: 406–412, 1965.

28. Anderson, D.E.; Smith, J.L.; and McBride, C.M.: Hereditary Aspects of Malignant Melanoma, *J A M A 200*: 741–746 (May 29) 1967.

29. Lynch, H.T. and Krush, A.J.: Hereditary and Malignant Melanoma: Implications for Early Cancer Detection, *Canad Med Ass J 99*: 17–21, 1968.

30. de Sanctis, C. and Cacchione, A.: L'idiozia xerodermica, *Riv. Sper Fernita 56*: 269, 1932.

Chapter 6

MALIGNANT MELANOMA*

by Henry T. Lynch, M.D.

INTRODUCTION

Malignant melanoma is the most serious histologic variety of skin cancer affecting man, accounting for the greatest number of "dermatologic" deaths. For example, in the United States in 1965, approximately 2,687 individuals died from malignant melanoma. This figure accounted for approximately 27% of all patients who expired with a dermatologic diagnosis.[1] It is therefore, not surprising that heavily pigmented or black lesions of the skin cause concern and consternation in physicians and frequently give rise to anxiety in patients. In fact, notwithstanding the gravity of this disease, only about 2% of all black lesions of the skin are actually malignant melanomas; thus 98%, or the overwhelming majority of black lesions of the skin are not malignant melanomas and are therefore *not* a threat to the patient's life and well-being. A difficulty both to patients and their physicians is that of differentiating between those lesions which are benign and those which are either frank melanomas or are destined to become melanomas. Unfortunately, the establishment of a diagnosis of a benign skin lesion versus melanoma by inspection of the skin may be extremely difficult and indeed is often impossible. Competent dermatologists who have had experience and considerable interest in the diagnosis of malignant melanoma may have similar difficulties with the differential diagnosis and may err in 35% to 40% of the cases seen clinically. This fact of course dictates the absolute necessity for histopathologic confirmation in order to make a correct diagnosis of black cutaneous growths on the skin.

While occasionally malignant melanomas may arise *de novo* in the absence of preceding discernible skin changes, the characteristic presentation of melanoma is one which arises from a so–called junctional nevus. This growth is often flat, blue–black or black and may appear as a shiny macule or nodule; occasionally it may be brown in color with central or speckled blackening. The lesion may mimic a so–called blue nevus. Other lesions may mimic melanoma, including a capillary aneurysm which may show rapid growth in the form of a small, flat black nodule rapidly enlarging. However in the end analysis, the tissue must be examined by a competent pathologist in order to assure the diagnosis. The clinician must then be prepared to resort promptly to more radical surgical therapy should the histological diagnosis confirm his clinical impression of malignant melanoma.

*Portions of this paper are reprinted by permission of *Canadian Medical Association Journal*, from Lynch, H.T., and Krush, A.J., *Canad. Med. Ass. J. 99*: 17–21, 1968.

It is important to realize that many physicians have taken a pessimistic view concerning the prognosis of malignant melanoma. However, with *early* diagnosis and the benefit of skillfully directed therapy, patients with localized disease in the absence of metastatic spread to the lymph nodes, will have a five–year survival rate of 70 percent and a ten–year survival rate as high as 60%. Hence, we should not adopt a hopeless attitude once the diagnosis of malignant melanoma has been established. This not only discourages an attempt at successful therapy but also adds to the already severely fatalistic impression about cancer held by many patients.

Genetics and Malignant Melanoma

Malignant melanoma is ideally suitable for genetically oriented cancer control and research. Specifically, a hereditary etiology has recently been ascribed to this disease in several families.[2] The relative frequency of this disease, the fact that it almost invariably arises from a visible cutaneous lesion (pigmented nevus), and its grave prognosis when detected late in its course, make its study and control of major importance.

The following material is based on families originally under our investigation; it includes two families with cutaneous malignant melanoma (CMM) and two families wherein CMM and intraocular melanoma (IMM) occurred independently. Attention will be focused upon the practical aspects of family history and medical genetic knowledge as aids to early cancer diagnosis.

Methods

Four families with malignant melanoma were referred to us by physicians who were aware of our interest in cancer genetics. In the first two families medical genetic information was obtained from probands and their relatives, physicians, hospitals, and department of vital statistics. Verification of the histological diagnosis of malignant neoplasm was obtained whenever possible. The latter two families were referred by an ophthalmologist. Unfortunately, cooperation from these latter two families was restricted to the patients described below.

Results

Family 1

In the first family (Fig. 1 and Table I) CMM was histologically confirmed in the proband (Fig. 1, II–4), her sister (Fig. 1, II–2) and her son (Fig. 1, III–1). Thus, this disease was confirmed in three members of the family in two generations. One patient (Fig. 1, III–1) had five primary CMM's histologically verified during a period of six years. Excision of his most recent lesion followed as a result of his concern about the disease in his family and his desire to cooperate with us in our study of its genetic aspects. Of interest is the incidence of other histologic varieties of malignant neoplasms in this family (Table 1), and particularly the occurrence of histologically verified adenocarcinoma of the pancreas in the proband's father and the father's sister (Table I and Fig. 1, I–2, and I–1).

Family 2

In the second family (Fig. 2 and Table 2) CMM was histologically confirmed in the proband (Fig. 2, III–5), her paternal aunt (Fig. 2, II–10) and a paternal first cousin (Fig. 2, III–1). It was present by history in the proband's paternal grandfather (Fig. 2, I–6) and two paternal

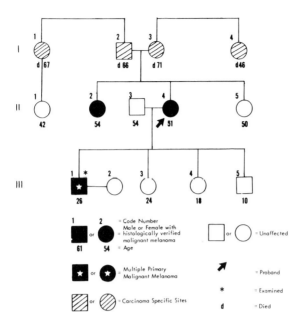

Figure 1. Pedigree of Family 1 with cutaneous malignant melanoma and cancer of other histologic types.

TABLE 1

Pedigree Number (Fig. 1)	Sex	Age	Malignant Melanoma	Cancer of Other Sites
I-1	F	d 67	—	Pancreas
I-2	M	d 66		Pancreas
I-3	F	d 71		Cervix
I-4	F	d 46		Breast Sarcoma right ilium
II-1	F	42		
II-2	F	54	+	
II-4	F	51	+	
II-5	F	50		
III-1	M	26	+*	
III-3	F	24		
III-4	F	18		
III-5	M	10		

Legend

    ➚ = Proband
    + = Histologically confirmed
    - = Medical history only
    * = 5 primary melanomas

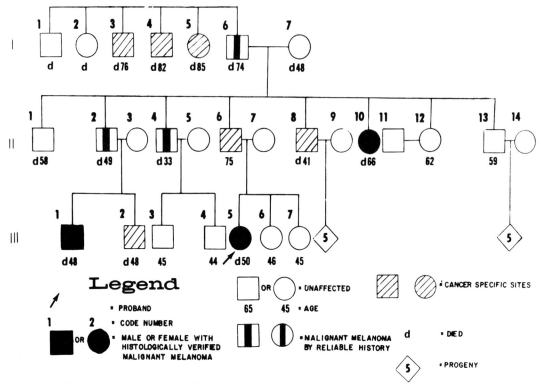

Figure 2. Pedigree of Family 2 with cutaneous malignant melanoma and cancer of other histologic types.

TABLE 2

Pedigree Number (Fig. 2)	Sex	Age	Malignant Melanoma	Cancer of Other Sites
I–3	M	d 76		Unknown site
I–4	M	d 82		"throat cancer"
I–5	F	d 85		Unknown site
II–2	M	d 46	−	
II–4	M	d 33	−	
II–6	M	75		larynx
II–8	M	d 41		lung
II–10	F	d 66	+	breast (age of 60)
III–1	M	d 48	+	
III–2	M	d 48		lung
III–5	F	d 50	+	

Legend
= proband
− = by medical history
+ = histologically verified

uncles (Fig. 2, II–2 and II–4). Thus CMM was histologically confirmed in three members in two generations and present by history in a third generation. An increased incidence of cancer of the respiratory tract occurred in other relatives. In addition, a paternal aunt of the proband (Fig. 2, II–10), had adenocarcinoma of the breast six years before diagnosis of CMM; thus there were two distinct primary cancers in this patient.

Family 3

In the third family a 61–year–old woman (Fig. 3A, II–1) had a diagnosis of IMM (histologically confirmed) while her sister, aged 51 (Fig. 3A, II–1) had a diagnosis of CMM (histologically confirmed).

Family 4

In the fourth family a 74–year–old man (Fig. 3B, I–1 had a diagnosis of IMM (histologically confirmed) and his son, aged 44 (Fig. 3B, II–1) had a diagnosis of CMM (histologically confirmed).

There was no evidence of consanguinity in these four families.

DISCUSSION

The hereditary aspects of malignant melanoma have only recently received attention in the medical literature. Familial CMM was first reported by Cawley[3] in 1952, when he described the disease in a father and two of his three children. Since this report, other investigators have confirmed the existence of a hereditary etiology for this disease in certain families.[4-14] Perhaps the most dramatic example of the role of hereditary factors in malignant melanoma was evidenced in the study by St-Arneault and associates.[13, 14] These investigators described the occurrence of cutaneous malignant

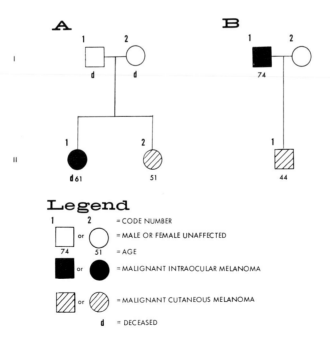

Figure 3. Pedigrees of Families 3 and 4 wherein cutaneous malignant melanoma and intraocular melanoma occurred independently.

melanoma in 53–year–old identical twins, children of one of a set of triplets. Each twin had a pre–existing mole nearly identically placed on the left chest each of which began to increase in size within a space of 2 months. Homozygosity of the twins was established with an extremely high degree of probability through use of blood typing, dermatoglyphics, lymphocyte culture, lymphocyte transfer and skin grafting. Thus in this particular genetic setting, we have concordance for cutaneous malignant melanoma as well as congruence for the anatomic site of the development of melanoma with an identical age of onset, or as the authors denote this remarkable occurrence, "congruent contemporaneous concordance." Approximately four and one half years following surgery, one of the twins had metastatic malignant melanoma while the co–twin was apparently free of tumor. This provided an opportunity to study tumor specific mechanisms in these twins. Findings showed that blastoid transformation of lymphocytes and cytoxicity of lymphocytes for melanoma cells in mixed lymphocyte–tumor subcultures were both substantially greater in lymphocytes from the tumor–free twin. Since the brothers were monozygous, it was believed that this phenomenon could not be attributed to transplantation–antigeneric differences. This data is believed to further existing evidence for immunity against tumor in man.[14]

Onset at an early age and multiple primary malignant melanomas have characterized the hereditary variety of this disease.[2] The frequency of the hereditary form of malignant melanoma in the general population is unknown. The estimate of approximately 3% given by Anderson, Smith, and McBride[4] was con-

sidered to be an underestimation of its true incidence. In their search of the medical records of approximately 1,000 patients with melanoma on file at the M.D. Anderson Hospital and Tumor Institute, they found 28 patients with a family history of malignant melanoma. However, they failed to verify the family histories of the remaining patients, since they relied solely upon statistics supplied by the Department of Epidemiology at that institution.[15] These statistics were based upon family histories from the medical records, which in our experience are often notoriously incomplete. We therefore, believe that in order to obtain a valid estimate of the frequency of any genetic disease, it is mandatory that hearsay family history be verified.[2]

In analyzing the pedigrees of families with CMM, autosomal dominance is apparent but it is complex, one explanation being reduced penetrance of the gene.[2] It is also possible that more than one gene is involved.[4] It is of interest that none of the reported genetic studies of CMM included patients with IMM.

IMM has shown a hereditary etiology in some families.[16-22] Lynch, Anderson, and Krush[23] have recently reviewed this work and have presented two families wherein the lesion was histologically confirmed in a brother and sister in one, and in the second family it was histologically confirmed in an uncle and his *niece,* present by history in a father, and histologically confirmed in his son and in his granddaughter. The frequency of the hereditary variety of IMM could not be estimated from these studies. However, the rarity of such cases in a review of medical reports and the world literature indicated that its familial occurrence is, in fact, infrequent. Overall genetic findings from these families and from those in the literature suggest autosomal dominant inheritance with reduced penetrance of the gene. No occurrence of CMM was found in families with IMM. Finally, Figure 4 illustrates in pedigree fashion the findings from four families reported in the literature showing intraocular melanoma on a site specific basis. Particular attention will be focused upon pedigree "C" which shows intraocular melanoma present in three and possibly four generations. The historical aspects of the pedigree are of interest and warrant detailed description. Specifically, the pedigree was compiled by Lynch and associates[23] based upon studies of the family by Silcock in 1892,[21] Parsons in 1905,[19] and Davenport in 1927.[17] Silcock and Parsons described the tumor in two generations and Davenport described it in three generations; however, these reports refer to the same family. We have taken the liberty of consolidating the information in the three reports to construct this pedigree. In summary, the proband was a 38–year–old woman whose left eye was enucleated for a spindle cell pigmented melanoma. Her father also had an eye removed but the reason for this enucleation was not given; however, it was stated

that it was "not from an injury." Her twin sister also had an eye removed, again for reasons other than an injury. Another sister had a tumor removed from the breast at age 40. The proband had seven children, two of whom were affected. The youngest child had her left eye enucleated at age 19 for a pigmented mixed round cell sarcoma of the choroid. She died 5 years later from metastatic melanoma. An older daughter had her left eye removed at about age thirty and her right eye was removed at about age thirty–eight because of melanotic sarcoma of the ciliary body and choroid. She apparently had disseminated melanoma at her last operation and died the following year. She had two daughters, each of whom had had the right eye removed for sarcoma of the choroid. The elder daughter had her eye removed at age 29 and died of metastatic melanoma 4 years later; the younger daughter had her eye removed at age 19 and, though having freely moveable, sharply defined, painless, subcutaneous "lumps," she was still alive 10 years after her enucleation. The average age of the five authenticated cases in this family was 28.6 years, according to Davenport, and all died from metasta-

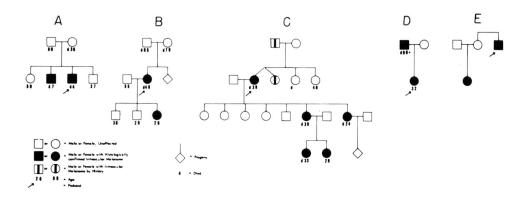

Figure 4. Abbreviated pedigrees of four families from the literature with intraocular melanoma histologically confirmed.

tic melanoma except one, who is known to have survived at least 10 years.

Malignant melanoma may also occur in association with other hereditary diseases. For example, Lynch *et al,*[24] recently described CMM and xeroderma pigmentosum (xdp) in two siblings (for further detail, refer to Chapter 5) and in a review of the world literature they provided a listing of 23 cases of cutaneous malignant melanoma associated with xdp. In addition, this review also showed that CMM may occasionally be associated with von Recklinghausen's neurofibromatosis, an autosomal dominantly inherited disorder.[25]

The findings of CMM in Families 1 and 2 reported here are consistent with autosomal dominant inheritance. An interesting observation among other family members in both families was the prevalence of malignant neoplasms of differing anatomic sites. Of particular interest was the finding of adenocarcinoma of the pancreas histologically confirmed in siblings (brother and sister) in Family 1 and an increased incidence of carcinoma of the respiratory tract in Family 2. Heretofore, investigations of the familial form of malignant melanoma have failed to record data on other malignant neoplasms occurring in the families.[2] Insight into the inheritance of cancer in man will be increased only by meticulous reporting of all varieties of cancer in the particular families under study. In the case of hereditary malignant melanoma, we may ultimately find that there is a specific predilection for this disease, possibly associated with a predisposition to other histologic varieties of cancer. This could be of practical importance in genetic counseling and cancer detection.

A unique finding in the present investigation was the independent occurrence of IMM and CMM in two sisters in Family 3 and in a father and son in Family 4. These families were not related to each other. Additional observations could increase our understanding of inheritance factors in malignant melanoma since CMM and IMM were previously thought to be inherited independently of each other.[10] It is, of course, possible that the occurrence of both CMM and IMM in these two families was fortuitous.

IMPLICATIONS FOR CANCER DETECTION

When malignant melanoma is found in a patient, its possible development in his relatives should be considered. All nevi in relatives at risk should be examined periodically and lesions showing suspicious changes should be biopsied. However, this must be achieved without unduly alarming the family, since provoking apprehension and anxiety could paradoxically cause them to repress the entire issue. This may be one of the most difficult problems encountered in the management of individuals at high genetic risk for cancer.[2]

An unusual opportunity is at hand for cancer control in families with CMM, since this lesion will often be apparent to the patient early in its clinical course. One obvious dilemma, however, concerns how many and which nevi should be biopsied in an individual at high genetic risk for CMM. Unfortunately, no single all-inclusive rule can be stated. At the present time clinical judgment must prevail. An example of such a problem appeared in the first family when the son of the proband advised us that his sister (Fig. 1, III–3) had a skin lesion which appeared to be similar to a malignant melanoma which he had recently had excised. She was reticent about seeing her physician and strongly repressed the issue of CMM in her family. When she finally consented to see a physician, biopsy of the lesion revealed a compound pigmented nevus with active junctional activity. Her physician wrote us as follows: "this is certainly a worrisome situation in view of the strong familial tendency for melanoma (in her family) and the fact that she has so many scattered nevi in areas of which we are generally suspicious. I think she should be watched closely and I have instructed her in the usual change to be looked for in moles . . . it is really a problem to determine which lesion to remove." Obviously all nevi on her body could not be removed. However, this physician took the opportunity to establish rapport with his patient and to provide her with a sound educational experience, carefully advising her of characteristic changes in nevi which might indicate malignancy, and urging periodic follow-up.

While some patients in a high cancer-risk category may elect to repress and deny early signs and symptoms of cancer,[26] others may overreact to the increased incidence of cancer in their family. For example, a patient in Family 2 was alarmed about a swift and fulminant course of CMM in his first cousin, a 49-year-old single woman who died from metastatic melanoma three months after excision of a lesion. He explained that many members of the family had moles of varying sizes and shapes. He himself undergoes yearly medical examinations and has been told by his physician that he should see a doctor only if he discovers an alteration in a nevus. He wrote, "In my opinion, however, I suspect that this would already be too late, since the family members who had these spots removed all died within three months." How can such a patient be alerted to the necessity for a wholesome concern about nevi without promoting undue or unrealistic concern or even a hypochondriacal reaction? We do not have the answer to the question, but we believe that such reactions may be avoided through frank and candid discussions between patient and physician. We have been impressed with the intense and crippling fear engendered in patients by their erroneous impressions about cancer. The patient's knowledge of his increased genetic risk for cancer will not necessarily compel him to seek medical attention early for signs and symptoms of cancer. He may react with fear, guilt and anxiety to the point of becoming fatalistic. Such a reaction may be effectively counteracted through a positive philosophy about the cancer problem instilled by the physician early in the patient's life and by emphasizing the cure potential through early diagnosis. On the other hand, a patient who is overly concerned about the cancer risk in his family may also harbor misconceptions and misinterpret signs and symptoms of cancer in his anxiety and fear of its development. This can lead to too frequent visits to the physician for minor symptoms.

In all instances the physician must accept his patient's attitude toward cancer in a sympathetic manner and be willing to take the necessary time not only to explain the significance of early signs and symptoms of malignant disease but also to help the patient gain insight into his feelings and attitudes about the cancer issue.

In summary, cutaneous malignant melanoma shows a hereditary etiology in about 3% of cases and in these it is consistent with autosomal dominant inheritance. The fact that the condition usually arises from a pre–existing mole which is often clearly visible emphasizes the need for education of patients about the risk for this disease, particularly when it has appeared in other members of the family.

References

1. Joint Committee on Planning for Dermatology: National Program for Dermatology, p.69 The Academy of Dermatology, 1964.

2. Lynch, H.T.: *Hereditary Factors in Carcinoma in Recent Results in Cancer Research,* Vol. 12, Springer–Verlag, New York, pp. 58–60, 1967.

3. Cawley, E.P.: Genetic Aspects of Malignant Melanoma, *Arch. Derm. Syph.,* 65, 440, 1952.

4. Anderson, D.E., Smith, J.L., Jr., and McBride, C.M.: Hereditary Aspects of Malignant Melanoma, *J A M A* 200, 741, 1967.

5. Katzenellenbogen, I., and Sandbank, M.: Malignant Melanoma in Twins, *Arch. Derm.* 94, 331, 1966.

6. Miller, T.R., and Pack, G.T.: The Familial Aspect of Malignant Melanoma, *Arch. Derm.,* 86, 35, 1962.

7. Salamon, T., Schnyder, V.W., and Storck, H.A.: A Contribution to the Question of Heredity and Malignant Melanomas, *Dermatologica,* 126, 65, 1963.

8. Schoch, E.P., Jr.: Familial Malignant Melanoma: A Pedigree and Cytogenetic Study, *Arch. Derm.,* 88, 445, 1963.

9. Smith, F.E., Henry, W.S., Knox, J.M., and Lane, M.: Familial Melanoma, *Arch. Intern. Med.* 117, 820, 1966.

10. Turkington, R.W.: Familial Factors in Malignant Melanoma, *JAMA,* 192, 77, 1965.

11. von Greifelt, A.: Malignes Melanom: Beziehungen zu Schwangerschaft, Pubertat, Kindheit: Familiare Maligne Melanome, *Arztliche Wocherschrift,* 7, 676, 1952.

12. Andrews, J.C.: Malignant Melanoma in Siblings, *Arch. Derm. 98:* 282–283, 1968.

13. St–Arneault, G., Nagel, G., Kirkpatrick, D., Kirkpatrick, R., and Holland, J.: Melanoma in Twins: Cutaneous Malignant Melanoma in Identical Twins from a Set of Triplets, *Cancer 25:* 672–677, 1970.

14. Nagel, G.A., St–Arneault, G., Holland, J.F., Kirkpatrick, D., Kirkpatrick, R.: Cell Meditated Immunity Against Malignant Melanoma in Monozygous Twins, *Cancer Res. 30:* 1828–1832, 1970.

15. Anderson, D.E.: Personal Communication, 1967.

16. Bowen, S.F., Brady, H., and Jones, V.L.: Malignant Melanoma of the Eye Occurring in Two Successive Generations, *Arch. Ophthal.* (Chicago) 71, 805, 1964.

17. Davenport, R.C.: Family History of Choroidal Sarcoma, *Brit. J. Ophthal.* 11, 443, 1927.

18. Gutmann, G.: Casuistischer Beitrag zur Lehre von den Geschwulsten des Augapfels, *Arch. Augenheilkunde* 31, 158, 1895.

19. Parsons, J.H.: The Pathology of the Eye, Vol. II, Histology, Part II, G.P. Putnam's Sons, 1905, pp. 496–497.

20. Pfingst, A.O., and Graves, S.: Melanosarcoma of Choroid Occurring in Brothers, *Arch. Ophthal.* 50, 431, 1921.

21. Silcock, A.Q.: Hereditary Sarcoma of Eyeball in Three Generations, *Brit. Med. J.,* 1, 1079, 1892.

22. Tucker, D.P., Steinberg, A.G., and Cogan, D.G.: Frequency of Genetic Transmission of Sporadic Retinoblastoma, *Arch. Ophthal.*, 57, 532, 1957.

23. Lynch, H.T., Anderson, D.E., and Krush, A.J.: Heredity and Intraocular Malignant Melanoma: Study of Two Families and Review of 45 Cases, *Cancer,* 21, 119, 1968.

24. Lynch, H.T., Anderson, D.E., Smith, J.L., Jr., Howell, J.B., and Krush, A.J.: Xeroderma Pigmentosum, Malignant Melanoma, and Congenital Ichthyosis: A Family Study, *Arch. Derm.,* 96, 625, 1967.

25. Gartner, S.: Malignant Melanoma of the Choroid and von Recklinghausen's Disease, *Amer. J. Ophthal.* 23, pp. 73–78, 1940.

26. Krush, A.J., Lynch, H.T., and Magnuson, C.W.: Attitudes toward Cancer in a "Cancer Family": Implications for Cancer Detection, *Amer. J. Med. Sci.* 249, 432, 1965.

Chapter 7

ATAXIA TELANGIECTASIA

by John F. Jackson, M.D.

Since Louis–Bar's original description in 1941 of a patient with progressive cerebellar ataxia and oculocutaneous telangiectasia,[1] a rather well–defined disease syndrome termed ataxia–telangiectasia has become established. Boder and Sedgwick proposed the name ataxia–telangiectasia (AT), added the additional manifestation of recurrent severe sino–pulmonary infection,[2] suggested the familial etiology of the disorder[3] and collected data on extensive numbers of cases.[4]

Cerebellar ataxia is usually the first sign of the disease, and may be noted at the time an affected child begins to walk. In addition to progressive cerebellar signs, choreic and athetoid movements,[5] a pseudopalsy of the eyes resembling oculomotor apraxia is typical.[6] Telangiectasia of the bulbar conjunctivae usually is manifest by age five or six, with extension later to the eyelids, ears, the butterfly area of the face and bridge of the nose, and periorbitally.[7] IgA immunoglobulin is often absent or severely deficient.[8] The absence of IgA, which is the predominant immunoglobulin secreted in nasal and bronchial secretions, may be the underlying cause for susceptibility to repeated sino–pulmonary infection. Autopsy routinely reveals thymic aplasia or dysplasia, with deficiencies of lymphocytes and Hassall's corpuscles.[9-11] The lymph nodes are usually abnormal with poorly developed lymphoid cuffs about the germinal centers. Some cases show reticulum cell hyperplasia, or lymphopenia. Since Peterson, Kelly and Good[8] called attention to the frequency of malignant tumors of lymphoid tissue in AT, other tumors have also been noted to occur in association with this disorder. Endocrine abnormalities including ovarian dysgenesis,[12] or follicular agenesis,[13] male hypogonadism[2] and anterior pituitary pathology[12] have been noted.

Inheritance Pattern

Ataxia–telangiectasia is now recognized to be inherited in a simple autosomal recessive fashion. A review of 64 families by Tadjoedin and Fraser[14] revealed no affected parents of affected children, an equal sex ratio, and a proportion of affected individuals among sibs of index cases consistent with the 25% expectation for autosomal recessive disorders. A higher than usual consanguinity rate also supported the hypothesis of recessive inheritance. Thus in most families in which AT appears, there are one or more affected sibs, with neither parent being affected, and usually no other affected relatives. In autosomal recessive inheritance, both unaffected parents of affected children must of necessity be heterozygous carriers, having one normal gene and one abnormal gene.

Neurologic Manifestations

Children with AT often are noted to be "unsteady" when learning to walk or "clumsy" as the first sign of the disorder. As the disease progresses, pronounced ataxia with weakness of the extremities develops. There may be cerebellar dysarthria, dyssynergia, dysmetria, and intention tremor. The limbs eventually become hypotonic and deep tendon reflexes diminished to absent. Nystagmus develops and voluntary eye movement becomes defective.[11] (Fig. 1)

The ocular features have been summarized by Smith and Cogan[6] to include normal vision, normal pupils, normal fundi, poor convergence, nystagmus that is worse in eccentric fixation than in primary position, poorly sustained conjugate gaze resembling partial ophthalmoplegia, conjunctival telangiectasia, essentially absent optokinetic responses, and involuntary maintained deviation of the eyes during rotation of the body. The ocular abnormality has been described as a halting extraocular movement and irregular conjugate gaze but with preservation of full range of excursion. The conjugate gaze disturbance has been called "oculomotor apraxia," "dysconjugate eye movements" or "pseudo–ophthalmoplegia".[15]

The neurological manifestations suggest that the cerebellar and extrapyra-

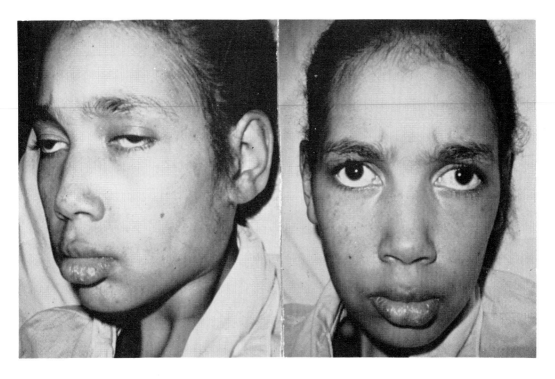

Figure 1. Oculomotor apraxia in Ataxia Telangiectasia demonstrating (a) intermittent ptosis and (b) divergent strabismus.

midal systems are the most severely affected,[15] and that there is no pyramidal or sensory involvement. Other than mental subnormality, there is no gross cerebral cortical disorder and seizures are rare. Autopsy findings correlate well with clinical findings.[16] The loss of Purkinje cells and losses of basket cell and granular layer of the cerebellar cortex account for the ataxia.[15]

Frequencies of clinical features are summarized in Table 1 below, based on Boder and Sedgwick's review of 101 cases of AT.[4]

Dermatologic Manifestations

Reed et al[7] have reviewed the cutaneous manifestations of ataxia–telangiectasia. Telangiectasia first appears on the exposed bulbar conjunctivae (Fig. 2).

The cutaneous telangiectasia is first noted on the ears, across the butterfly area

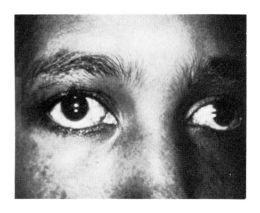

Figure 2. Telangiectasia of bulbar conjunctivae in Ataxia Telangiectasia.

TABLE 1
FREQUENCY OF CLINICAL FEATURES IN 101 CASES OF ATAXIA–TELANGIECTASIA
(After Boder and Sedgwick[4])

Feature

Neurological features
Feature	Frequency
Cerebellar ataxia, onset in infancy or childhood	100
Intact deep and superficial sensation	98
Flexor or equivocal plantar response	98
Diminished or absent deep reflexes	89
Negative Romberg's sign	78
Dysarthric speech	100
Characteristic facies and postural attitudes	98
Choreoathetosis	91
Drooling	88
Oculomotor signs	
Peculiarity of eye movements	84
Fixation or gaze nystagmus	83
Strabismus	47
Telangiectasia, oculocutaneous	100
Equable disposition	100
Changes of hair and skin	88
Frequent sinopulmonary infection	83
Retardation of statural growth	72
Familial occurrence	45
Mental deficiency	33

of the face, the bridge of the nose, and periorbitally, but with increasing age involves the neck, the dorsum of the hands and feet, and the antecubital and popliteal flexures. The areas of greatest sun exposure are most affected, with the ears becoming inelastic and the facial skin hidebound, similar to scleroderma. Telangiectases may also appear on the hard and soft palate, sometimes in association with repeated trauma of mucous membranes or radiation to the tonsils. The damaged skin areas may show mottled hyperpigmentation and hypopigmentation with cutaneous atrophy similar to the poikiloderma of advanced actinodermatitis or radiodermatitis. The "café au lait" spots described by Louis–Bar[1] and other investigators, are perhaps better described as ephelides (freckles) occurring with actinic damage.[7] Partial albinism (congenital absence of pigment in local areas) is frequent. Senile keratoses have appeared in a 23 year–old woman with AT. An effected man only 21 years old had multiple basal cell carcinomas.[7]

Cutaneous infections occur commonly in patients with ataxia–telangiectasia. But despite the immunoglobulin deficiency, nearly all of Reed's series[7] of patients were vaccinated, with none developing generalized vaccinia. Most had a successful vaccination scar. In addition, the childhood exanthemata (chicken pox, measles and mumps) caused no particular difficulty. Seborrheic dermatitis is common. Typical atopic dermatitis and nummular eczema also have occurred. Follicular keratosis, dry skin, and hirsutism of extremities in young affected females are almost always present.

Differential Diagnosis

The differential diagnosis should include other disorders that produce skin telangiectasia. The telangiectases in AT (Fig. 2) consist of linear diffuse vascular dilatations, unlike the discrete punctate lesions of hereditary hemorrhagic telangiectasia (Rendu–Osler–Weber Disease) in which the distribution is primarily over the lower face, lips, oral mucosa, and fingers (Fig. 3). The latter disorder also

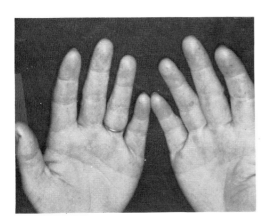
(a)

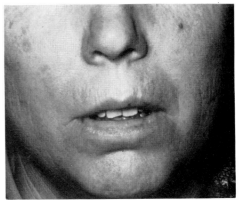
(b)

Figure 3. Punctate lesions of hereditary Hemorrhagic Telangiectasia involving (a) fingertips and (b) lips.

has associated hemorrhagic symptoms, especially epistaxis, whereas hemorrhage is not a feature of AT. Spider angiomata with typical central arteriolar filling and associated liver disease should likewise provide no serious problem. Bloom's syndrome[17] in addition to telangiectases from sunlight sensitivity, also includes dwarfism of the low–birth–weight type, and as in the previously mentioned disorders, has no prominent neurologic manifestations.

Disorders with neurologic manifestation, or mental retardation, may be more difficult to distinguish. The xerodermic idiocy of De Sanctis and Cacchione[18] has additional features including microcephaly, mental deficiency, dwarfism, gonadal hypoplasia and choreo–athetoid neurologic signs. Cockayne's syndrome[19] of premature aging, dwarfism, sunlight sensitivity, retinal degeneration, optic atrophy, and facial lipodystrophy, is also associated with mental deficiency. Cerebellar ataxia has also been noted with Hartnup disease, in which pellagra–like skin changes may appear.[20] The basic defect in Hartnup disease is an abnormal tryptophan metabolism producing amino–aciduria involving certain neutral alpha–amino acids. Werner's syndrome[21] includes sclerodermoid premature changes of the skin, cataract, subcutaneous calcification, premature arteriosclerosis, diabetes mellitus, and affected individuals may sometimes also be mentally defective. The Rothmund–Thomson syndrome of skin poikiloderma, scalp alopecia, dwarfism, hypogonadism, cataracts, and bony abnormalities should also be considered.[22]

Intense violaceous, telangiectatic facial flushing has been noted in homocystinuria.[23] Homocystinuria is characterized by autosomal recessive inheritance, osteoporosis with fractures, occasional ara-

chnodactyly, and ectopia lentis. Its resemblance to the Marfan syndrome is distinguishable by the osteoporosis, frequent venous and arterial thrombosis, mental retardation, cutaneous flushing, and excessive urinary excretion of homocystine, none of which are usual in the Marfan syndrome.

Immunologic Disorder

The aplasia or dysplasia of the thymus gland and other lymphoid tissue abnormalities produce in addition to deficient IgA immunoglobulins, abnormal cellular immunity, such as deficient delayed hypersensitivity to naturally occurring substances or to sensitization with contact vesicants, and lack of acute inflammatory response accompanying graft rejection. Failures of passive transfer of delayed hypersensitivity with sensitized cells indicate an effector–mechanism defect as well as the presumed defect in development of delayed allergy.[24] Other laboratory investigations have revealed lymphopenia,[10] reduced blastic transformation of lymphocytes stimulated in culture[25, 26] and increased chromosome breakage[25, 27, 28] in cultured lymphocytes from patients with ataxia telangiectasia (Fig. 4). The chromosomal breakage

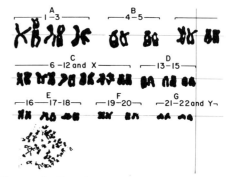

Figure 4. Isochromatid break in chromosome 1 in mitosis from cultured lymphocytes of patient with AT.

may produce translocations resulting in the appearance of dicentric chromosomes and large acrocentric chromosomes[28] resembling the chromosomal findings which occur spontaneously in malignant tumors.[29]

The exact pathogenesis of these diverse manifestations from a single gene defect through what appears to be basically abnormal lymphocyte function remains obscure. The absence of IgA in association with the chromosome loss in the formation of a ring–18 chromosome[30] has not shown a consistent association.[31] Thus chromosome breakage and IgA deficiency in ataxia telangiectasia can not yet be demonstrated to have a cause and effect relationship in the loss of part of chromosome 18. Pfeiffer[28] has recently confirmed the presence of chromosomal abnormalities in AT, but cautions that not all AT patients have chromosomal abnormalities. He also found no strong relationship of IgA deficiency to reduction in mitotic rate or chromosomal abnormality in lymphocyte cultures.

Sibships including AT and Swiss type agammaglobulinemia (SAG) have been found in a genetic isolate. Clinical similarities of the two disorders appearing under such conditions has prompted the suggestion that AT and SAG may even be expressions of the same gene.[32]

Other Observations

Untoward responses have been reported to radio–therapy in patients with ataxia telangiectaisa, resulting in severe dysphagia, skin pigmentation and desquamation, and a friable, oozing granulating skin surface,[33] or even deep tissue necrosis.[34]

Schalch et al[35] have found 10 of 17 AT patients studied to have an unusual form of diabetes mellitus, characterized by marked hyperglycemia, ketosis resistance, absent glycosuria and increased plasma insulin levels after glucose or tolbutamide administration. A decreased blood glucose response to insulin suggested that there was insulin resistance similar to that found in pregnancy, acromegaly and obesity. There was also evidence of liver disease.

Predisposition to Malignancy

Peterson, Kelly and Good[8] reported a case of lymphosarcoma and another with reticuloendotheliosis. They pointed out that six other cases of ataxia–telangiectasia had associated malignant tumors. Three had unspecified malignant tumors of lymphoid tissue, one had generalized reticulum cell sarcoma, one Hodgkin's disease, and another undifferentiated round–cell sarcoma. Hecht, *et al*[27] reported a family with one confirmed and two probable cases of leukemia associated with AT. Although most of the malignancies associated with AT have involved cells of the lymphoid system, there have been other tumors such as a cerebellar medulloblastoma,[36] a frontal lobe glioma,[37] bilateral ovarian dysgerminomas,[9] and multiple basal cell carcinomas.[7] These tumors arose in tissues known to be affected by the basic disease process. Our recent report[11] of two sibs with AT who both developed mucinous adenocarcinoma of the stomach in the second decade of life indicates that tumors may involve organs other than those primarily abnormal by virtue of the clinical manifestation of AT (Fig. 5). Thus the accepted predisposition to the development of lymphoreticular neo-

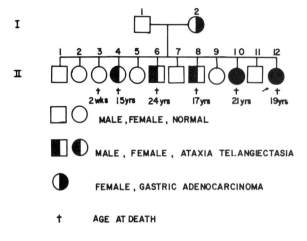

Figure 5. Pedigree of family with AT and gastric adenocarcinoma. (After Haerer, et al[11]).

plasms should be extended to include neoplasms in general.

Increased frequency of chromosome breakage has also been found in Fanconi's anemia[38, 39] and Bloom's syndrome,[17, 40] both of which appear to be associated with an increased risk of leukemia. Primary squamous cell carcinoma has also appeared in patients with Fanconi's anemia.[38] The predisposition for chromosomal breakage in these disorders has been suggested to be the basic mechanism for the associated neoplasia.[38] Such suggestion is supported by the association of chromosome breakage and neoplasia in post–irradiation leukemia.[41] Chromosomal abnormalities, though not always present, are now well–recognized features of malignant tumors in general,[42, 43]. In addition to radiation,[44] viruses[45, 46] and many chemicals[47] can break chromosomes. Thus it may be that individuals with these single gene inherited disorders share a propensity for the development of neoplasia mediated through chromosomal abnormalities.

Swift[48] has recently found that heterozygous carriers for Fanconi's anemia have a greater predisposition to malignancy than the general population. With this information, the need for extension of similar investigations to AT and Bloom's syndrome becomes obvious, since all three disorders share an increased susceptibility to chromosome breakage and neoplasia. Even in such rare disorders, the heterozygous carrier rate in the general population is relatively common. For example, at genetic equilibrium according to the Hardy–Weinberg equation, for a rare recessive disorder affecting only one in 100,000 individuals in the general population, there are about 1 in 160 of this population who are asymptomatic heterozygous carriers. Thus heterozygotes for a number of such disorders could be part of a polygenic predisposition to malignant tumors in general. In this regard, it is very interesting that the mother of the two sibs with AT and gastric adenocarcinoma[11] has developed gastric carcinoma also.[49] Her tumor appeared at the age of 62, rather than 19. She is, of course, an obligate heterozygote for the AT gene by reason of having affected children. Epstein et al[50] noted a high frequency of malignancy of all types in certain AT families. Tumors occurred mainly in older individuals, such as grandparents of probands. It is interesting that five of their 21 reported family members with malignancy had carcinoma of the stomach. This specific tumor exceeded in frequency all other specific tumor types including lymphoma. Additional studies of single gene inherited disorders which predispose to malignancy will undoubtedly contribute to our overall understanding of the basic mechanisms in the development of cancer.

References

1. Louis–Bar D: Sur un syndrome progressif comprenant des telangiectasies capillairescutanées et conjonctivae symetriques, a disposition naevoide et des trobles cerebelleux. *Confin Neurol 4*: 32, 1941.

2. Boder E, Sedgwick RP: Ataxia–Telangiectasia–A Familial Syndrome of Progressive Cerebellar Ataxia, Oculocutaneous Telangiectasia and Frequent Pulmonary Infection. *Pediatrics* 21: 526, 1958.

3. Boder E, Sedgwick RP: A Familial Syndrome of Progressive Cerebellar Ataxia, Oculocutaneous Telangiectasia, and Frequent Pulmonary Infection. *Arch. Derm 78*: 402, 1958.

4. Boder E, Sedgwick RP: Ataxia–Telangiectasia. A Review of 101 Cases. Little Club Clin Develop Med 8: 110, 1963.

5. Wells CE, Shy GM: Progressive Familial Choreoathetosis with Oculocutaneous Telangiectasia. *J Neurol Neurosurg Psychiat 20*: 98, 1957.

6. Smith J., Cogan DG: Ataxia–Telangiectasia. *Arch Opthal 62*: 364, 1959.

7. Reed WB, Epstein WL, Boder E, Sedgwick R: Cutaneous Manifestations of Ataxia–Telangiectasia. *J A M A 195*: 126, 1966.

8. Peterson RD, Kelly WD, Good RA: Ataxia–Telangiectasia. Its association with a defective thymus, immunological-deficiency disease, and malignancy. *Lancet* 1: 1189, 1964.

9. Dunn HG, Meuwissen H. Livingstone CS, Pump KK: Ataxia–Telangiectasia. *J. Canad Med Ass. 91*: 1106, 1964.

10. Peterson RD, Cooper MD, Good RA: Lymphoid Tissue Abnormalities associated with Ataxia–Telangiectasia. *Amer J Med 41*: 342, 1966.

11. Haerer AF, Jackson JF, Evers CG: Ataxia–Telangiectasia with Gastric Adenocarcinoma. *J A M A 210*: 1884, 1969.

12. Bowden DH, Davis PG, Sommers SC: Ataxia–Telangiectasia: A Case with Lesions of Ovaries and Adenohypophysis. J Neuropath Exp Neurol 22: 549, 1963

13. Miller ME, Chatten J: Ovarian Changes in Ataxia Telangiectasia. *Acta Paediat Scand 56*: 559, 1967.

14. Tajoedin MK, Fraser FC: Heredity of Ataxia–Telangiectasia (Louis–Bar Syndrome). *Amer J. Dis Child* 110: 64, 1965.

15. Karpati G, Eisen AH, Andermann F, Bacal HL, Robb P: Ataxia–Telangiectasia. Amer. J. Dis Child 110: 51, 1965.

16. Itatsu Y, Uno Y: An Autopsy Case of Ataxia–Telangiectasia. *Acta Path Jap* 19: 229, 1969.

17. Bloom D: The Syndrome of Congenital Telangiectatic Erythema and Stunted Growth. J *Pediat 68*: 103,

18. Reed WB, May SB, Nickel WR: Xeroderma Pigmentosum with Neurological Complications. *Arch Derm* 91: 224, 1965.

19. Paddison RM, Moossy J, Derbes VJ, Kloepfer W: Cockayne's Syndrome. A report of five new cases with biochemical, chromosomal, dermatologic, genetic, and neuropathologic observations. *Derm Trop* 2: 195, 1963.

20. Jepson JB: Hartnup Disease. in: The Metabolic Basis of Inherited Disease. 2nd Ed. Stanbury JB, Wyngaarden JB, Fredrickson DS (ed) McGraw–Hill New York, p 1283.

21. Epstein, CJ, Martin GM, Schultz AL, Motulsky AG: Werner's Syndrome. A review of its symptomatology, natural history, pathologic features, genetics, and relationship to the natural aging process.

Medicine 45: 177, 1966.

22. Blinstrub RS, Lehman R, Sternberg TH: Poikiloderma Congenitale. *Arch Derm* 89: 659, 1964.

23. Schimke RN, McKusick VA, Huang T, Pollack AD: Homocystinuria. Studies of 20 families with 38 affected members. *J A M A* 193: 711, 1965.

24. Peterson, RDA, Good RA: Ataxia-Telangiectasia. Birth Defects Original Article Series, Immunologic Deficiency Diseases in Man. IV. Bergsma D (ed) p 370, 1968.

25. Gropp A, Flatz G: Chromosome Breakage and Blastic Transformation of Lymphocytes in Ataxia-Telangiectasia. *Humangenetik* 5: 77, 1967.

26. Hayakawa H, Kobayashi N: Blasts in Ataxia-Telangiectasia. *Lancet* 1: 1279, 1967.

27. Hecht F, Koler RD, Rigas DA, Dahnke GS, Case MP, Tisdale V: Leukaemia and Lymphocytes in Ataxia-Telangiectasia. *Lancet* 2: 1193, 1966.

28. Pfeiffer RA: Chromosomal Abnormalities in Ataxia-Telangiectasia (Louis-Bar's Syndrome) *Humangenetik* 8: 302, 1970.

29. Jackson JF: Chromosome Analysis of Cells in Effusions from Cancer Patients. *Cancer* 20: 537, 1967.

30. Finley SC, Finley WH, Noto TA, Uchida IA, Roddam RF: IgA Absence Associated with A Ring 18 Chromosome. *Lancet* 1: 1095, 1968.

31. Stewart J, Go S, Ellis E, Robinson A: IgA and Partial Deletions of Chromosome 18. *Lancet* 2: 779, 1968.

32. McKusick VA, Cross HE: Ataxia-Tel angiectasia and Swiss-Type Agammaglobulinemia. *J A M A 195*: 119, 1966.

33. Morgan JL, Holcomb TM, Morrissey RW: Radiation Reaction in Ataxia Telangiectasia. *Amer J Dis Child 116*: 557, 1968.

34. Gotoff SP, Amirmokri E, Liebner EJ: Ataxia Telangiectasia. Neoplasia, Untoward Response to X-Irradiation, and Tuberous Sclerosis. *Amer J Dis Child 114*: 617, 1967.

35. Schalch DS, McFarlin DE, Barlow MH: An Unusual Form of Diabetes Mellitus in Ataxia Telangiectasia. *New Eng J Med 282*: 1396, 1970.

36. Shuster J, Hart Z, Stimson CW, Brough AJ, Poulik MD: Ataxia Telangiectasia with Cerebellar Tumor. *Pediatrics 37*: 776, 1966.

37. Young RR, Austen KF, Moser HW: Ataxia-Telangiectasia and the Thymus. *Trans Amer Neurol Ass 89*: 28, 1964.

38. Swift MR, Hirschhorn K: Fanconi's Anemia. Inherited Susceptibility to Chromosome Breakage in Various Tissues. *Ann Intern Med 65*: 496, 1966.

39. Zaizov R, Matoth Y, Mamon Z: Familial Aplastic Anaemia Without Congenital Malformations. *Acta Paediat Scand 58*: 151, 1969.

40. German J, Archibald R, Bloom D: Chromosomal Breakage in a rare and Probably, Genetically Determined Syndrome of Man. *Science 148*: 506, 1965.

41. Buckton KE, Jacobs PA, Brown WMC, Doll R: A Study of the Chromosome Damage Persisting After X-Ray Therapy for Ankylosing Spondylitis. *Lancet 2*: 676, 1962.

42. Sandberg AA: The Chromosomes and Causation of Human Cancer and Leukemia. *Cancer Res 26*: 2064, 1966.

43. Gottlieb SK: Chromosomal Abnormalities in Certain Human Malignancies. *J A M A 209*: 1063, 1969.

44. Langlands AO, Smith PG, Buckton KE, Woodcock GE, McLelland J: Chromosome Damage Induced by Radiation. *Nature 218*: 1133, 1968.

45. Nichols WW: Relationships of Virus-

es, Chromosomes and Carcinogenesis. *Hereditas 50*: 53, 1963.

46. Nichols WW: Studies on the Role of Viruses in Somatic Mutation. *Hereditas 55*: 1, 1966.

47. Kihlman B: Actions of Chemicals on Dividing Cells, Prentice–Hall, Englewood Cliffs, New Jersey, 1966.

48. Swift MR: Franconi's Anemia in the genetics of Neoplasia. Program and Abstracts the Amer Soc Human Genetics, San Francisco, Calif., Oct. 1–4, 1969.

49. Meena AL: Personal Communication, 1970.

50. Epstein WL, Fudenberg HH, Reed WB, Boder E, Sedgwick RP: Immunologic Studies in Ataxia–Telangiectasia. I. Delayed Hypersensitivity and Serum Immune Globulin Levels in Probands and First–Degree Relatives. *Int Arch Allerg* 30: 15, 1966.

Chapter 8

NEUROCUTANEOUS DISEASES

by William L. Harlan, M.D. and
Haruo Okazaki, M.D.

Since brain and skin are of a common ectodermal derivation it is not surprising that there are a group of conditions characterized by neurologic disorder and associated skin manifestations. Several of these conditions are easily recognized and were first reported during the golden age of descriptive clinical medicine before the turn of the century.

In 1879 Sturge described a case of Epilepsy in a young girl who demonstrated an angioma of the face with congenital glaucoma and postulated a similar angioma of the brain.[1] The following year, Tuberous Sclerosis was described by Bournville. His patient was a two and a half year-old retarded girl who presented with convulsions, and a "rosaceous pustular acne of the face." The patient died in status epilepticus and at autopsy "hypertrophic sclerosis of various portions of the cerebral convultions"[2] was noted. Von Recklinghausen first described Multiple Neurofibromatosis in 1882.[3] Thus began the documentation of the Neurocutaneous diseases; (Sturge–Weber–Dimitri Disease, Tuberous Sclerosis, and Multiple Neurofibromatosis). To these three we may add Ataxia-Telangiectasia described by Madame Louis Bar in 1941[4] and a pathologic entity, Melanosis Cerebri, which should be included in our discussion of Neurocutaneous diseases because of its relationship to Giant Pigmented Nevi and Malignant Melanoma. We might also include a sixth condition, the Multiple Nevoid Basal Cell Carcinoma Syndrome, because of its frequent association with Medulloblastoma and Pheochromocytoma, both of which are tumors of neural origin. A recent addition to the group is the Multiple Mucosal Neuromata Syndrome which is described in detail in Chapter 13. Finally, the Nevus Sebaceum of Jadassohn which was first described in 1895 is associated with neurologic symptoms which have heretofore received little attention. There are other skin conditions, e.g. xeroderma pigmentosum, in which there may be associated neurologic symptoms. As some of these conditions become more widely known and more thoroughly investigated it seems likely that the list of neurocutaneous diseases will increase well beyond those entities included in this chapter.

Multiple Neurofibromatosis

Clinical Manifestations:

Clinically, Multiple Neurofibromatosis is a disease associated with a wide variety of skin, neurologic, endocrine, skeletal, ocular, as well as other visceral manifestations. The diagnosis is easily established when the skin findings are severe, though this is not always the case. Neurofibromas involving skin are usually multiple, flesh colored nodules which are sessile or pedunculated and which show a "buttonholing" phenomenon in that they can be pushed back through a defect in the underlying dermis into the subcutaneum. Such lesions are illustrated in Figure 1. Yet another type is the Plexiformneurofibroma, which is a mass of subcutaneous cords "like a bag of worms." Even in cases where such skin lesions do not exist, café au lait spots, usually more than six[5] are often found. These are brown pigmented macules of varying shape and size and these have been shown to differ histologically where associated with Neurofibromatosis from those are not associated with the disease.[6] Occasionally large bathing trunk nevi or angiomatous lesions may also be seen in Multiple Neurofibromatosis.

The neurologic manifestations of multiple neurofibromatosis are many and varied. Any of the cranial nerves may be affected but most commonly it is the eighth nerve that is involved with tumor producing deafness, loss of corneal reflex, facial palsy and cerebellar signs. Frequently such tumors are bilateral, 87% being so in one reported series. Nerve tumors may also involve spinal nerves growing through the intervertebral foramen, enlarging it and at the same time producing paraplegia as a result of pressure against the spinal cord. Of equal importance is the occurrence of a high incidence of other central nervous system tumors (meningiomas and gliomas) in association with the disease.[7] Unilateral proptosis as a result of neurofibroma of

the orbit may occur and glioma of the optic nerve is common in children.[8] It has been noted that some families showing only minimal skin findings have an extremely high incidence of brain tumor.[9] Similarly superficial neurofibromata seldom undergo malignant change, but neurogenic sarcoma or fibrosarcoma may arise from deeply situated tumors. Even in the absence of any demonstrable tumor epilepsy may be present and many patients, perhaps as many as 50% have a mild degree of mental subnormality.

Skeletal changes in Multiple Neurofibromatosis include scoliosis, hypertrophy of bone, underdevelopment of bone and congenital pseudoarthrosis. Pressure necrosis may occur due to the presence of adjacent tumor. Intraosseous cystic lesions are also described.[5] It has been argued that Fibrous Dyplasia is a manifestation of neurofibromatosis and it has been reported in a family in which nine members had Neurofibromatosis.[10] Albright's syndrome, which consists of bone changes, endocrinopathy and café au lait spots may be differentiated on the basis of the histology of the melanotic macules which differ in the two conditions.[6] Saville and his co-workers[11] have demonstrated osteomalacia in neurofibromatosis associated with congenital renal tubular defect similar to that of resistant rickets and Daly et al[12] have reported hyperparathyroidism associated with neurofibromatosis in two cases.

Retardation of sexual maturation and somatic underdevelopment which is sometimes clinically suggestive of panhypopituitarism has been described,[5] but the laboratory results were equivocal. A high incidence of pheochromocytoma associated with neurofibromatosis has been found and Humble points out the danger of a misdiagnosis of eclampsia

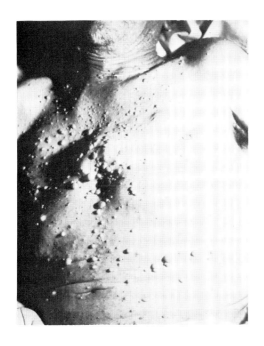

Figure 1A. Patient with neurofibromatosis.

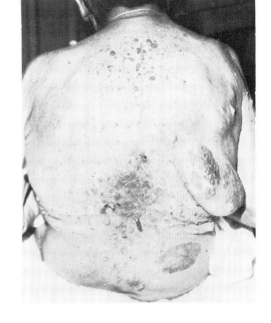

Figure 1B. Patient with neurofibromatosis.

when pheochromocytoma is present during pregnancy.[13] Yet another mechanism for the production of hypertension is the involvement of the renal arteries by an adjacent neurofibroma with resultant renal ischemia.[14] Pancreatic duct obstruction with steatorrhea due to neurofibromatosis has also been reported, and so has aneurysm of the Vena Cava.[15] Involvement of the intestine by neurofibromata may produce obstruction, intussuseption, or melena and these lesions may occur without cutaneous manifestations of the disease.[16] Cystic lesions of the lung producing exertional dyspnea, cough, fever and hemoptysis also occur.[17]

Pathology

The basic lesions of neurofibromatosis may be looked upon as multiple, localized hyperplasia and neoplasia of various ectodermal and mesodermal protective, supportive elements in the skin, peripheral nerves, central nervous system and other organs. Added to these is a vascular component, either independently as vascular lesions or as vascularized supportive lesions. Rarely, parenchymatous elements may participate in the process (Lichtenstein, 1949).[18]

The most important are of course the tumors of the peripheral nerve and cerebrospinal nerve roots, known variously as neurinoma, neurilemmoma, neurofibroma, perineurial fibroblastoma, and schwannoma to name a few reflecting a long history of uncertainty and controversy regarding the basic type of cells responsible. There have been two polar groups recognized: schwannomas and neurofibromas. Most recently it appears to be generally agreed that both of them share Schwann's cells as their predominant neoplastic cells. By electron microscopy, the Schwann's cells are noted to have cellular basement membranes with insertions of collagen fibers into its matrix. The difference in the appearance of schwannomas and the neurofibromas may be related to the varying degree of collagenization encountered in these neoplasms and does not detract from the identification of their schwannian nature. It is not evident whether variations in collagen production represent distinct differences in the activity of the Schwann cells which have been observed in the tissue cultures to produce such fibers or reflect different kinds of fibroblastic responses in these tumor types.[19]

While recognizing the probable basic identity of these two tumors, it may still be convenient to discuss them separately because of different histology and gross appearance in typical cases, and fundamental dissimilarity in their relationships to the surroundings.[20]

The predominant peipheral nerve tumors in von Recklinghausen's disease are neurofibromas whereas infinitely more schwannomas involve multiple sites of cranial and spinal roots, most commonly the eighth nerve, often bilaterally, and the sensory roots of the spinal cord. Schwannomas seen in the peripheral nerves in von Recklinghausen's disease are generally limited to one or more of the large nerve trunks. It is to be noted in this connection that solitary forms of nerve tumors are almost exlcusively schwannoma in type when they involve cranial and spinal roots and both schwannomas and less frequently, neurofibromas may be seen as solitary lesions in peripheral nerves, unassociated with any other evidence of von Recklinghausen's disease.

Neurofibroma

The neurofibroma involves a peripheral nerve in a more diffuse fashion resulting in, at least initially, a fusiform enlargement of the nerve. Its texture is soft and elastic, white, devoid of cystic change or hemorrhages.[21] Only occasionally a most circumscribed mass similar to schwannomas may be seen. It is by definition an irregular overgrowth of the Schwann's cells, associated with an increase of reticulin and collagen and intimately penetrated by nerve fibers. Occasionally, areas closely resembling those of schwannoma are incorporated. Neurofibromas can be seen in almost every conceivable locality, including skin, nerve trunks, and sympathetic nervous system. The entire G.I. tract from the mouth to rectum can be involved; the urinary bladder, adrenals, and the pituitary and other endocrine organs, bones and the periostium can be involved. The retina and iris may also be involved. The *skin lesions* can assume various nodular forms of varying size such as flattened, sessile, pedunculated, spherical, conical and lobulated, etc. (Fig. 2). Characteristically, they are soft to touch as is the old term "fibroma molluscum" suggests, although they can be harder at times. Neurofibromas in the terminal distribution of the nerve fibers ("plexiform neuroma") may be accom-

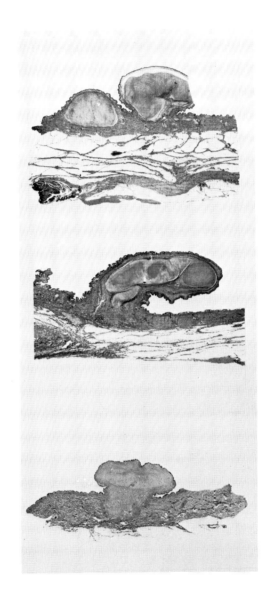

Figure 2. Histologic sections of 3 examples of superficial dermal neurofibromas, all from the same patient. Hematoxylin and Eosin stain original magnification X 3.

panied by a diffuse fibrous thickening of the skin and subcutaneous tissue in which cords of involved enlarged nerves can be palpable. (Fig. 3). When it hangs down in folds, it is referred to as pachyderma-tocele. When it is more voluminous, particularly in the extremities, with or without associated hyperostosis, it is referred to as elephantiasis neuromatosa.

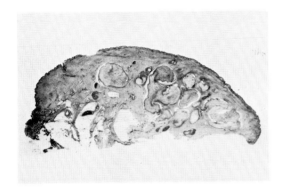

Figure 3. von Recklinghausen's disease: section of surgically resected plexiform neurofibroma of the labia in a patient with von Recklinghausen's disease.There is a diffuse thickening of the dermal tissue in addition to the presence of tortuous, irregulary swollen nerve bundles. H & E stain, original magnification × 2.

Similar hyperplasia may occur in one–half of the tongue and in the gum on one side. The face may show hermihypertrophy. Hypertrophy of the viscera has been reported in association with the plexiform neurofibroma of the autonomic nervous system. When seen at birth, neurofibromas are in the form of a diffuse regional overgrowth whereas later in adolescence, or in early adulthood, they appear as more localized nodules.

Neurofibromas of *nerve trunks* are generally firmer and more discrete (Fig. 4). At the beginning, they may be in spindle shape but may bulge spherically on one side and sometimes loosely attached to nerve sheaths. They may eventually become confluent forming uniformly or irregularly thickened nerves (plexoform neurofibroma). The microscopic features are illustrated in Fig. 5. These larger growths may arise in the neck, mediastinum, and in the retroperitoneal tissue or on a major peripheral nerve but the massive growth of von Recklinghausen's disease may as already noted be a schwannoma on occasion.

It may be said that although usually associated with von Recklinghausen's disease, neurofibromas are sometimes solitary and then usually superficial and localized. More extensive neurofibromas, whether superficial or deep are rarely truly solitary. A discrete tumor on a deep nerve in the absence of other evidence of von Recklinghausen's disease is likely to be a schwannoma.[20]

Schwannomas

There is a remarkable tendency for sensory nerve roots, both cranial and spinal, to be selectively affected. In general, these tumors are firm, circumscribed and encapsulated. Small examples tend to be spheroidal, eccentrically bulging out from a parent nerve, compressing with the remaining portion. The larger tumors are often irregularly lobulated. Many of the latter contain hemorrhages and opaque, creamy–yellow areas but otherwise the texture is firm, rubbery, and somewhat slimy with some indication of whirling.

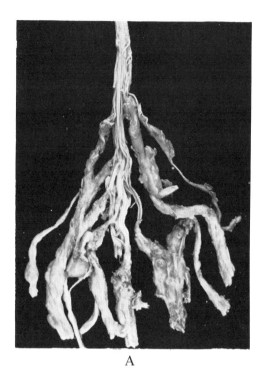

A

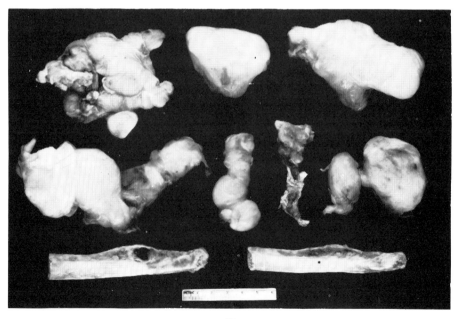

B

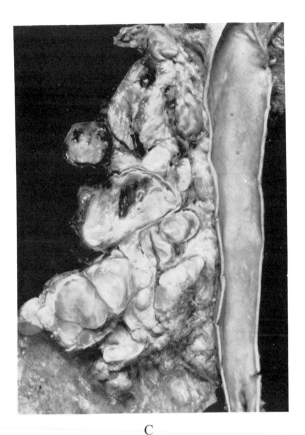

C

Figure 4. von Recklinghausen's disease.
   A. diffuse enlargement of the nerves of the lumbar plexuses.
   B. Surgical specimen of multiple neurofibromas in the posterior mediastin-
       um and midthoracic spinal roots compressing on the spinal cord. On the
       bottom row are the ribs removed.
   C. Residual tumors in the mediastinum along the thoracic aorta in the same
       patient as Figure 4 B. Areas of hemorrhages are due to surgery and the
       typical cross–sectional appearance of neurofibromas is seen in the lower
       portion of the mass.

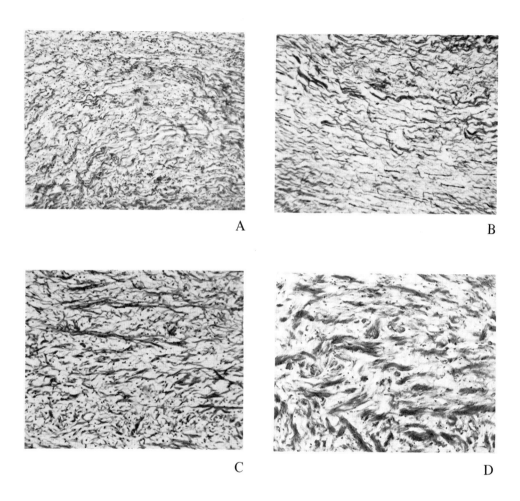

Figure 5. von Recklinghausen's disease

    A. Photomicrograph of neurofibroma involving the right lumbar plexus. This area represents a portion of the nerve trunk which began to show diffuse fusiform enlargement involving its entire circumference. There is a diffuse proliferation of Schwann cells and collagen fibers which retain the orientation of nerve fibers. H & E stain, original magnification X 110.

    B. Same area as in Figure 5A showing dark staining axons spread apart but still recognizable. Bodian stain, original magnification X 110.

    C. Early mucoid degeneration of neurofibroma with relatively poor cellularity and decreased density of collagen fibers. H & E stain, original magnification X 110.

    D. An area of intense collagenization within neurofibroma. H & E stain, original magnification X 110.

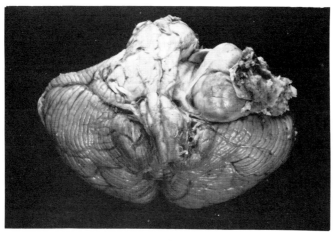

A

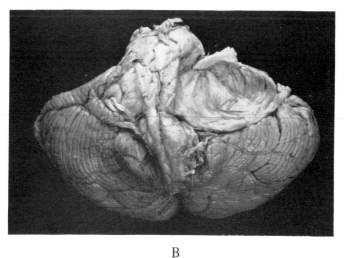

B

Figure 6. Unilateral (lt.) schwannoma of the 8th cranial nerve.

    A. The tumor in situ with the lt. 7th nerve seen running over the medial aspect of the tumor. This 60 year–old man had an additional small schwannoma involving one of the cauda equina roots, but no other stigmata of von Recklinghausen's disease.

    B. View of the same brain stem and cerebellum after removal of the tumor, demonstrating a marked indentation and deformity of these structures.

1. Cranial nerve roots.

The most common acoustic nerve tumors occupy the cerebellar pontine angle (Fig. 6) and when fully developed, produce great deformation of the brainstem and adjacent cerebellum which accounts for various long–tract and nuclear signs and symptoms, aside from the loss of functions of the eighth nerve. It may obstruct the fourth ventricle and result in hydrocephalus above which may explain some of the mental symptoms that are not infrequent in this condition. The parent nerve fibers and the neighboring nerve roots are stretched over the surface of the mass resulting in loss of function of these nerves. They are often bilateral (Fig. 7) and may be seen in the relative absence of other stigmata of the disease.[22]

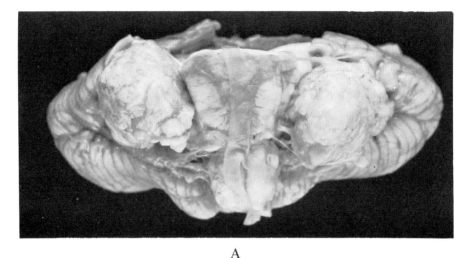

A

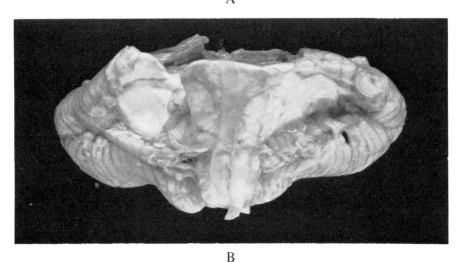

B

Figure 7. von Recklinghausen's disease.
    A. Bilateral acoustic schwannomas in a patient with von Recklinghausen's disease.
    B. View with the tumors removed.

Association of multiple meningiomas in this situation constitutes one of the frequent forms of a so-called central type of von Recklinghausen's disease. As indicated by small and clinically silent examples, the point of origin is the vestibular portion of the nerve at the mouth of the internal auditory meatus which becomes invariably enlarged as the tumors grow (Fig. 8). By comparison, the trigeminal tumors are rare. It appears that most are confined to the middle fossa, where they arise from the gasserian ganglion. In sightly fewer cases, the tumor occupies the cerebellar pontine angle. In a few cases, it is of hour glass

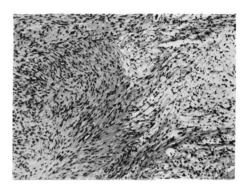

Figure 9. von Recklinghausen's disease: typical histologic appearance of schwannoma of the 8th nerve with the compact cellular Antoni type A tissue on the left and the loose type B tissue on the right. H & E stain, original magnification X 90.

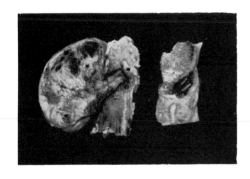

Figure 8. Acoustic schwannoma: cross section of the acoustic tumor shown in Fig. 6 through the internal auditory meatus which is enlarged by the tumor.

form, involving both locations.[23] Microscopically, (Fig. 9) more compact areas (Antoni's type A) is composed of interwoven bundles of long spindle cells (Schwann's cells). They are associated with numerous, fine, hair–like argyrophilic fibers which accompany the cells and are parallel to their long axis. In places, the cell bundles form formations of varying size and complexness. Palisading of the nuclei is infrequent in the acoustic tumors and is more characteristic of the spinal examples. Other areas, Antoni's type B, show loose texture with pleomorphism of the tumor cells. They are responsible for macroscopic yellowish zones and eventually show the presence of foam cells containing sudanophilic lipid. While it is often assumed that Type B tissue is a result of the degeneration of Type A tissue, Murry and Stout, 1940,[24] found a distinct type of Schwann cells in a tissue culture. Other secondary changes are referrable to vascular thrombosis. Other cranial nerves such as vagus, glossopharyngeal, and the motor roots in general are known to be involved in von Recklinghausen's disease, but are extremely rarely the sites for solitary tumors.

2. Spinal nerve roots.

The solitary schwannoma is a common, intrathecal growth approximating in the frequency to the meningiomas of this region (Fig. 10). The posterior roots are selectively involved though occasional examples of involvement of motor roots has been recorded; except in cauda equina, tumor deforms the adjacent spinal cord because of the limitation of the space within the spinal canal. It is characteristically a smooth, encapsulated,

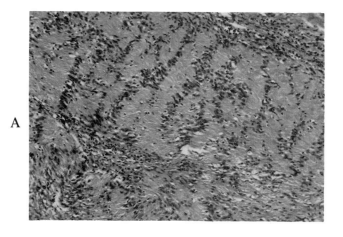

A

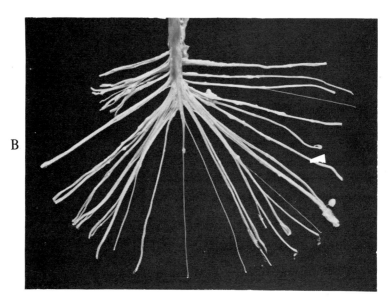

B

Figure 10. A. Schwannoma of a thoracic spinal root: a typical palisading pattern of Schwann cell nuclei is evident.
B. von Recklinghausen's disease: an example of multiple schwannomas along the cauda equina roots.

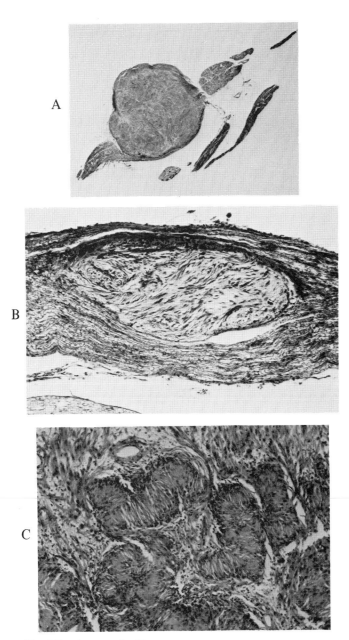

Figure 11. von Recklinghausen's disease.
    A. Histologic section of a small discrete schwannoma growing out in a typically eccentric fashion out of a cauda equina root. The attenuated portion of the parent nerve is seen along the inferior border of the tumor. H & E stain, original magnification X 12.
    B. One of the multiple schwannomas found in the cauda equina roots with the characteristic focal expansive growth pattern displacing adjacent nerve fibers. H & E stain, original magnification X 110.
    C. Schwannoma of the ulnar nerve showing Verocay bodies. H & E stain, original magnification X 110.

ovoid, or sausage–shaped mass of elastic consistency. It may extend out through an intervertebral foramen to form a dumb–bell shaped mass. Cysts are frequently found on section and the tissue is usually devoid of xanthomatous areas. The nerve roots of the cauda equina are frequently involved in multiplicity. Microscopically, they resemble the intracranial examples, except that the palisading of Antoni's A area seem to be more pronounced (Fig. 11). Small clumps of these cells are often to be likened to Wagner–Meissner tactile corpuscles (Verocay bodies).

3. Peripheral nerve.

The solitary tumors of this type in von Recklinghausen's disease are exceptional, on the course of the peripheral nerves (Fig. 12).

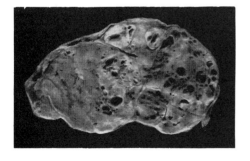

Figure 12. Solitary schwannoma: characteristic cross–sectional appearance of a schwannoma resected from the postero-lateral chest wall between the 7th and 8th ribs on the right. The tumor was 4cm. in diameter.

Malignant transformation

1. Neurofibromas.

Large neurofibromas of the peripheral nerves occasionally become malignant (Fig. 13). True incidence of malignant transformation in von Recklinghausen's disease is difficult to assess. The widely quoted figure of 13% by Hosoi[25] who in 1931 calculated this incidence from the literature is regarded by most pathologists too excessive, since, as pointed out by Stout,[26] many mild cases of the disease are unrecorded and indeed unrecognized. D'Agostino et al[27] found, among 678 patients with a clinical diagnosis of multiple neurofibromatosis seen at the Mayo Clinic, 21 patients who had associated malignant neoplasms of the peripheral nerves and somatic tissue. They were unable to arrive at any satisfactory estimation of the incidence of malignant transformation since no attempt was made to follow the subsequent course of these patients. Uniform spindle cell sarcomas ("malignant neurilemmomas") adjacent to neurofibromatous tissue were seen in 12 patients. Nine other patients had pleomorphic sarcomas (rhabdomyosarcoma, liposarcoma and unclassified) but the authors were of the opinion that they are further expressions of the biologic capacities of the neurilemmal (i.e. Schwann) cell.

2. Schwannoma.

Whether a schwannoma ever acquires malignant attributes is seriously questioned, since strict histological criteria[28] have been seldom observed in those reported in the literature. Stout[29] rejected all previously reported cases of this transformation on the ground that it was not stated whether the benign tumor was a schwannoma or a neurofibroma. Only recently,

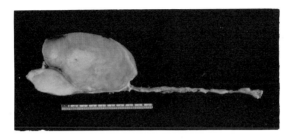

A

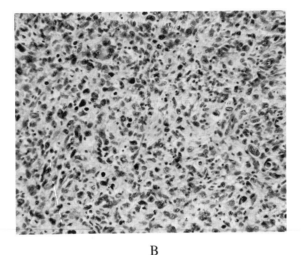

B

Figure 13. von Recklinghausen's disease
    A. Surgical specimen of neurofibromas in the cervical portion of the left vagus nerve with malignant transformation in a 17 year–old girl with von Recklinghausen's disease.
    B. Microscopic appearance of the sarcomatous portion of the tumor showing cellular pleomorphism and atypical mitoses. H & E stain, original magnification X 50.

as case report is made of a schwannoma with malignant transformation of a benign tumor of the thumb in a 93–year–old female.[30] This woman had no evidence of von Recklinghausen's disease. The few reported malignant schwannomas appear to have been malignant from the onset (ab initio). They are often microscopically similar to fibrosarcoma and usually show many local recurrences before distant metastases, commonly to the lungs, occur.

Pheochromocytoma may be regarded as an example of ectodermal parenchymatous involvement. Spinal ganglioneuroma has also been reported.[31]

The involvement of the central nervous system and its meningeal covering is not infrequent in von Recklinghausen's disease. All integumentary and peripheral nervous system lesions observed in neurofibromatosis may occur as isolated hyperplasias or tumors and one is probably not justified in making a diagnosis of von Recklinghausen's disease from the observation of an isolated lesion. The nervous system, in such cases, however, may show multiple intracranial and intraspinal foci of hyperplasia and neoplasia. In this central form, bilateral acoustic neurilemmomas generally associated with meningiomas of the dura mater occur.

Hyperplasia and neoplasia of the neu-

roglia are constant features of the so-called central type of neurofibromatosis. They are usually in the form of gliomas of astrocytic series, often termed as spongioblastomas. Astrocytoma of the optic nerves, chiasm and the tracts with associated involvement of the hypothalamus are classical examples of the former type (Fig. 14). According to Davis,[32] 10% of the optic gliomas show some evidence of neurofibromatosis. The other parts of the cerebral hemispheres, the brainstem and the cerebellum are also involved. More malignant forms of astrocytomas (Glioblastoma multiforme) have been reported.[7] Since many of these astrocytic neoplasms have bipolar cells with spindle-shaped nuclei, they were in the past given the designation of central neurinoma. Ependymomas are commonly found in the spinal cord and may involve

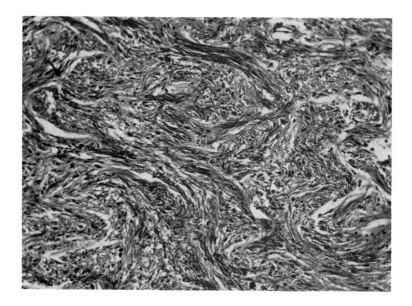

Figure 14. Photomicrograph of astrocytoma of the optic nerve, composed of relatively mature astrocytes with bipolar fibrillary processes which form interwoven bundles.

several segments independently (Fig. 15). Some of these lesions are associated with syringomyelia.[33]

Hyperplasia of neuroglial cells in the form of nests of atypical cells are seen in almost all instances of central neuro-

fibromatosis (Fig. 16). They occur primarily in the cerebral cortex[34] but may be seen elsewhere, such as internal capsule and the spinal cord white matter. Proliferation of marginal (subpial) glial cells (marginal gliosis) may occur in the cere-

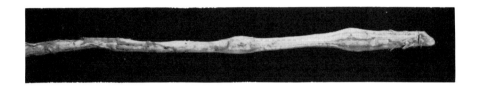

A

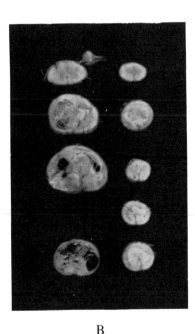

B

Figure 15. von Recklinghausen's disease.

    A. Dorsal view of the spinal cord with cervical and thoracic ependymomas in a patient with von Recklinghausen's disease.

    B. Cross sections of the cervical (the left row) thoracic (the right row) spinal cord with ependymomas. There is a small schwannoma arising from a posterior root of an upper cervical segment (the tip piece on the left).

bral cortex and spinal cord. This may lead to gliomatosis of these subarachnoid spaces as was reported in the cerebellum by Walker[35] as astrocytosis arachnoidea cerebelli. Double diagnosis of central neurofibromatosis and tuberous sclerosis has sometimes been made on the basis of nonspecific changes common to both diseases such as glial proliferation and fibrous dermal tumors.

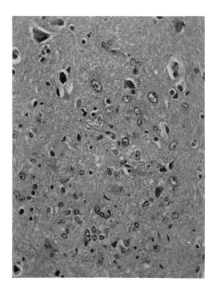

Figure 16. von Recklinghausen's disease: one of the multiple foci of atypical astrocytic proliferation seen in the cerebral cortex. H & E stain, original magnification × 280.

Participation of the extrinsic supporting structures of the CNS (leptomeninges) is mostly in the form of *meningiomas,* which are often multiple (Fig. 17). They can also be seen in the choroid plexus. Focal hyperplasia in the cerebrospinal arachnoid and fibroma of the pia mater are also reported. Optic astrocytomas may be associated with reactive proliferation of meningothelial cells or true neoplasia of these cells (meningiomas).[32] Proliferation of the capsule cells of the spinal ganglia reported by Kernohan and Parker[36] and fibrosis of the capsule of the same structures reported by Henneberg and Kock[37] can be regarded as evidence of the participation of intrinsic and extrinsic supporting cells in these structures respectively. The choroid and ciliary bodies of the eye, comparable to the leptomeninges, may show diffuse thickening due to proliferation of elongated cells of probable Schwann cell origin mixed with ganglion cells and nerve fibers. Melanin pigment in varying amount is often present in some of these cells.[38]

Vascular components participate in the form of vascular nevi of the skin, frequently associated with pigmented nevi, and of the oral and nasal mucosa. Similar lesions may be found in the choroid of the eye and the leptomeninges, the last two forming the link of this disorder and Sturge–Weber disease, at least morphologically.

Associated developmental anomalies of the nervous system seen in von Recklinghausen's disease include meningomyelocele or meningocele, hydrocephalus, aqueductal stenosis, microscopic or gross neuronal heterotopia, glial heterotopia, and cortical dysgenesis. Syringomyelia has already been mentioned.

Multiple neurofibromatosis behaves genetically as an autosomal dominant condition with fairly complete penetrance of the gene, but with highly variable phenotypic expression. Since the cutaneous manifestations of the disease are usually present from an early age[39] early recognition of the disease in the children of affected individuals is often possible. In the absence of skin manifestations or an adequate family history the disease can be quite cryptic, however. Because of its association with so many serious medical and surgical problems, the importance of a positive family history regarding multiple neurofibromatosis deserves emphasis.

Tuberous Sclerosis

Clinical Findings

Like multiple neurofibromatosis, tu- berous sclerosis is characterized by multiple organ system involvement. The skin manifestations are even more varied than those of von Recklinghausen's neurofibromatosis. These two conditions share café au lait spots as a common manifestation though they tend to be less numerous in Tuberous Sclerosis than in Neurofibromatosis and whether or not they differ histologically is yet to be determined. The most constant skin finding however is adenoma sebaceum which according to some investigators[40] is present in 100% of affected individuals over 35 years old and in at least 50% of cases under age 5. In milder cases these lesions are small (1–7mm.) nodules the

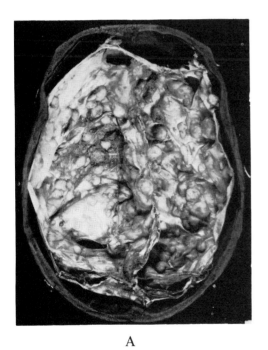

A

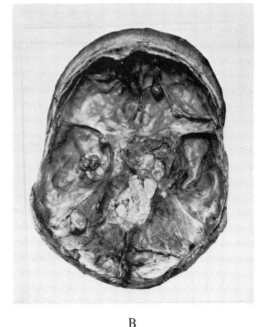

B

Figure 17. von Recklinghausen's disease
  A. Multiple meningiomas along the inner surface of the calvarial dura and along the falx.
  B. Multiple meningiomas at the base of the skull.

color of normal skin and sparsely distributed over the nose, cheeks and forehead as in Figure 18. Occasionally, however, the lesions are red, seed–like, and quite vascular. It has been noted that they tend to have this appearance in the earlier stages of their development.[41] In later stages, they may become confluent or undergo ulceration. In rare instances they may become quite large and disfiguring, resembling a cavernous hemangioma or plexiform neuroma.[42]

Another skin finding which may be of great diagnostic importance in early life before the appearance of adenoma sebaceum is the white leaf–shaped macule. These lesions differ from vitiligo in that the depigmentation is less complete and the patches tend to be oval or lancet-shaped rather than irregular. In one study[43] these white macules were found in 78% of 23 children with tuberous sclerosis. These macules are often present at birth and in many cases are the only demonstrable skin finding to suggest the etiology of convulsions in an affected infant. Examination with a Woods light may facilitate recognition of these lesions. Yet another finding characteristic of Tuberous Sclerosis is the

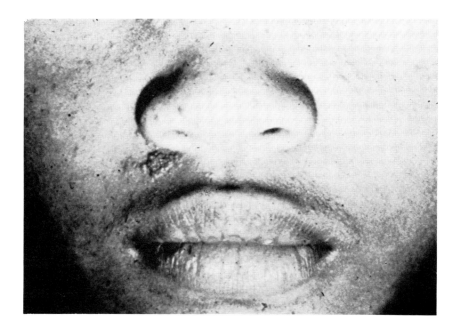

Figure 18. Patient with Adenoma Sebaceum

shagreen plaque. These are rough, slightly elevated lesions showing transverse wrinkling suggesting the skin of a shark and hence the appelation. Such a lesion is demonstrated in Figure 19.

A subungual fibroma is illustrated in Figure 20. These are flesh colored tumors arising beneath or at the margin of the nail. These lesions seem to appear later in the course of the disease and are probably present in less than 20% of patients. Even more rare are small fibromas involving the mouth and gums.

While the skin manifestations may be diagnostic it is, as a rule, the neurologic symptoms that bring the patient to medical attention. The commonest presenting complaint is that of convulsions, which in a series reviewed at the Mayo Clinic were present in 70% of cases, usually with the onset before the age of 5 years. Various investigators have found nothing particularly characteristic about the siezures, which seem to vary greatly in all parameters, that is frequency, form and severity. In the Mayo Clinic series it is of interest that of the 62% of patients demonstrating mental retardation all (100%) had siezures whereas siezures were present in only 44% of the group with normal intelligence.[44] Contrary to some reports in the literature, these authors stress the point that many patients (38% in their series), do have normal intelligence. At the other extreme of the spectrum the disease may appear very early in life and be lethal. Thibault and Manuelidis reviewed 13 cases documenting the presence of brain lesions during the first week of life.[45]

One need only examine a brain of one patient with tuberous sclerosis to understand how diverse other neurologic manifestations of the disease may be. An

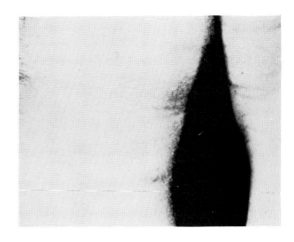

Figure 19. Shagreen Plaque

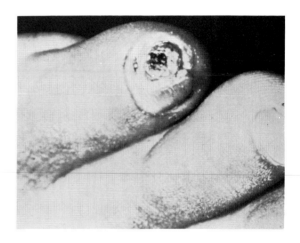

Figure 20. Ulcerated Subungual fibroma.

intraventricular lesion may produce obstructive hydrocephalus, or the multiple potato–like nodules may increase in size producing increased intracranial pressure or neurologic deficit according to their anatomic distribution. Of 48 cases reviewed at Duke University, 7 (15%) had brain tumor confirmed by surgery, ventriculography or autopsy.

Funduscopic findings (in addition to optic atrophy or papilledema which may occur as a result of the brain lesions) include two types of phakomata. One type is a small, flat, yellowish nodule which may be seen in any part of the retina. The other is a large, mulberry like nodule projecting from the surface of the disc. The latter type is illustrated in Figure 21 and may as in this case resemble drussen of the disc. Small grey nodules on the tarsal conjunctiva are also described. Ocular lesions are probably more common than is generally believed if the fundi are examined adequately; having been found in 49% of the eyes examined in the Mayo Clinic series.[44] Ordinarily however, vision is not impaired and the diagnosis is made as a result of a routine screening examination rather than from investigation of a specific eye complaint.

Pulmonary cystic lesions similar to those of neurofibromatosis may cause progressive exertional dyspnea. Pleural effusion has also been described.[46] In addition, multiple angiomata and adenomata have also been described. The majority of the reported cases have been in affected adult females.[47]

Angiomyolipomata of the kidney (Fig. 22) are estimated to occur in 50 to 80% of cases. They are usually small and multiple and often produce no symptoms. A large solitary angiomyolipoma may present with flank pain, hematuria, or abdominal mass. They have been known to rupture, producing retroperitoneal hemorrhage and shock.[48] Renal failure is surprisingly rare but when it occurs the differential diagnosis with congenital polycystic kidney disease can be difficult.[49] These tumors are said to seldom undergo malignant change but eight cases of metastasis of the lesions are noted in the literature.[50] Hamartomas of the spleen[51] and of the liver[50] are rare, but have been reported.

In a review of primary tumors of the heart Griffith states that over half the patients having rhabdomyomas of the heart have demonstrable tuberous sclerosis. Of 13 cases developing within the first week of life cited by Thibault and Manuelidis eleven had rhabdomyomata of the heart. In addition, four cases of fibroelastosis have been cited by Crome.[52]

Cardiac arrhythimas[53] (multifocal ventricular extra systoles and intraventicular conduction defects) have been reported both in Caucasians and in the Zulu.[54]

Pathology

1. *Tubera* (or tubers)

There are two basic characteristic lesions in the brain tuber and subependymal nodules. Some reduction of the brain weight is not uncommon in patients with mental subnormality. However, the convolutional pattern is generally within normal limits except for local abnormalities due to the presence of tubera. Frank microcephaly or very heavy brain is ex-

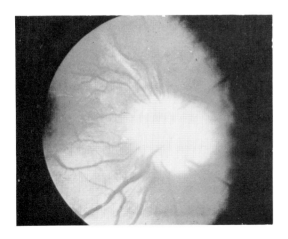

Figure 21. Phakoma of the optic disc.

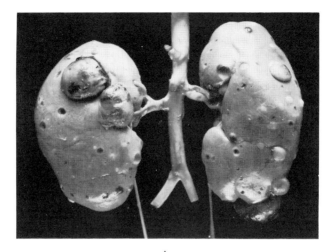

A

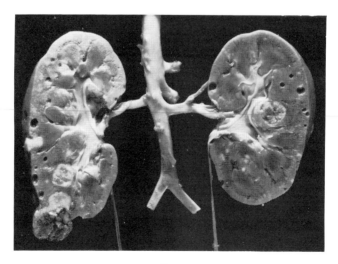

B

Figure 22. Tuberous sclerosis: multiple angiomyolipomas of both kidneys.
      A. External view.
      B. Cross–sectional view.

ceptional. These pathognomonic sclerotic lesions are most commonly seen in the cerebral gyri but are rarely recorded in the cerebellum, brainstem, basal ganglia and spinal cord. The affected gyri show widening, pallor and increase in consis-

tency with flattened and smooth crests (Fig. 23). The change is focal but is poorly defined. On cross section, there is an obscuration of the cortical medullary junction of the involved convolution. Microscopically, there is a considerable

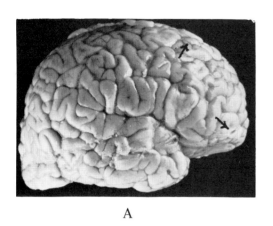

A

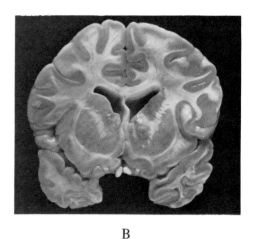

B

C

Figure 23. Tuberous Sclerosis

    A. External view of the right cerebral hemisphere with arrows pointing to two of the cortical tubera.

    B. Cross section through the frontal lobes and basal ganglia. Cortical tubera are best seen in the right superior frontal gyrus and left middle frontal gyrus. Two subependymal nodules are seen at the lower angle of the lateral ventricles on both sides.

    C. Cross section through the parietal lobes. Multiple "gutterings of a candle" are seen along the ventricular walls bilaterally.

distortion of the cortical pattern with decreased numbers of nerve cells, and increased numbers of fibrous astrocytes which contribute to an increase in glial fibers in the rather nonvascular background stroma (Fig. 24). There are many, large, bizarre–shaped cells, many of which can be recognized as astrocytic in nature while others are found to be neurons with Nissl bodies and neurofibrils, by appropriate histologic stains. Monster glial cells constitute the majority while the atypical ganglion cells are in the minority. In the molecular layer, there is usually proliferation of fibrous astrocytes. This marginal gliosis may be found focally elsewhere without obvious tuber formation. The underlying white matter appears somewhat loose in texture and contains fewer myelinated fibers and shows an increase in astrocytes, some of which are large and bizarre–shaped.

A minor form of these dysplastic changes may take the form of localized, convolutional hypertrophy with relatively well retained cortical striata, with or without the features of macro or micropolygyria and islets of glial sclerosis in the white matter with proliferation of astrocytes. Fibrillary gliosis may be more diffuse throughout the white matter and is often associated with an atypical astrocyte.

Recently, Hirano (1968), noted occurrence of Alzheimer's neurofibrillary tangles, Simchowiz's granulovacuolar degeneration and argentophilic globules in giant neurons in the affected area in a 13–year-old.[55] These changes are seen, although not exclusively in senile and presenile dementias and among certain numbers of "normally" aged individuals. One is thus reminded of vascular fibrosis and a tendency to form senile plaques reported in young patients with tuberous sclerosis.[56]

A

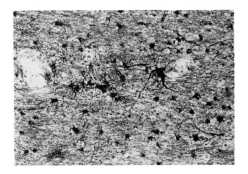

B

Figure 24. Tuberous Sclerosis

A. Microscopic appearance of a cortical tuber showing general disorganization of the cortical pattern and the presence of giant neurons and astrocytes against the background of diffuse fibrous gliosis. H & E stain, original magnification X 75.

B. Microscopic appearance of giant astrocytes in a cortical tuber as demonstrated by Cajal gold sublimate method. Original magnification X 160.

2. *Subependymal, periventricular nodules.*

These fairly well circumscribed nodules are commonly found along the terminal sulcus of the lateral ventricles and appear as sausage–shaped projections into the ventricular cavity, the deeper portion of which is imbedded within the substance of the caudate nucleus or thalamus (Fig. 23). They are likened to gutterings of a candle. They are occasionally found within the subcortical white matter, rarely in the cerebellum and brainstem. The nodules are composed of a large astrocytic cells in clusters separated by bands and whirls of fibrillary glial fibers (Fig. 25). Sometimes, fibrillary astrocytes predominate the picture. Iron–calcium deposits appear as small concretions or confluent masses interspersed among the abnormal astrocytic cells. Although bi- or multinucleated cells are not infrequ t, there is usually no evidence of active malignant growth, and these nodules are generally looked upon as hamartomatous, rather than neoplastic in nature, although they are at times referred to as astrocytomas.

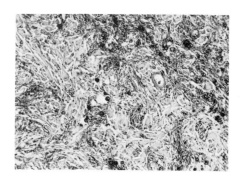

Figure 25. Tuberous Sclerosis: microscopic appearance of a subependymal nodule composed of large astrocytes with hyaline cytoplasm. Scattered mineral deposits are also seen. Mallory's phosphotungstic acid hematoxylin stain, original magnification X 100.

3. *Neoplasms*

Uncommonly, true neoplastic development may be seen in patients with tuberous sclerosis, presumable arising from the areas of dysplastic malformation. They may take the form of a malignant, giant–celled neoplasm, referred to as spongioblastoma or glioblastoma, a fibrillary astrocytoma of localized nature or a diffuse hemispheric gliomatosis. Occasionally, abnormal nerve cells are thought to be involved in the neoplastic process and these tumors are referred to as spongioneuroblastomas.[57]

4. *Retinal lesions (phakomas).*

The large nodular lesion usually lying at the edge of the nerve head and smaller, multiple, flattened forms present elsewhere in the fundus are recognized. Both are histologically similar and involve primarily the nerve fiber layer of the retina. While the precise nature of these lesions is not determined, they are thought to be composed of abnormal forms of retinal neuroglia, and glial fibers and sometimes of ganglion cells. The frequent whorling pattern of glial fibers, occasional calcification is reminiscent of the subependymal tumors described above. It is not certain if true malignant neoplasia develops in these lesions.

Genetic Considerations

Tuberous Sclerosis is considered to be inherited as an autosomal dominant trait and it has indeed been recorded in as many as five successive generations of a family. The incidence of sporadic cases however, is extremely high. Bundey and Evans[40] found an incidence of 87% sporadic cases in their series. Since Adenoma Sebaceum is present in nearly 100% of affected persons it serves as a convenient marker and makes it seem highly unlikely that these investigators were overlooking forme fruste cases in the parents; though Schnitzer[58] did describe an autopsy case of a 62–year–old woman with typical lesions of brain, kidneys, and lungs who had no cutaneous evidence of Tuberous Sclerosis.

The outlook for long life in patients seems quite poor. Of 18 autopsy cases reviewed by the Armed Forces Institute of Pathology, 78% were under age 25 at the time of death.[49]

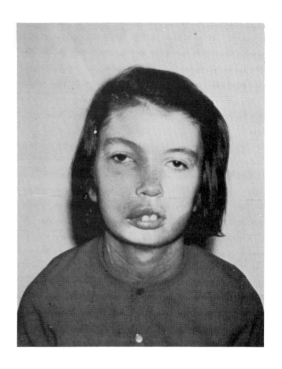

Figure 26. Sturge–Weber disease: note bilateral port wine nevus, predominant on the left with contralateral craniofacial assymetry.

Sturge–Weber Disease

Clinical Findings

Sturge–Weber disease is characterized by a port wine mark (a telangiectatic hemangioma) in the distribution of the trigeminal nerve with an associated angiomatosis of the meninges, which is present usually from birth. The typical appearance of such a patient is demonstrated in Figure 26. In addition to the angiomatous malformation involving the meninges there is often associated cerebral cortical calcifications. These follow the contour of the convolutions and present radiographically as a characteristic double curvilinear calcification as illustrated in Figure 27. Clinically, patients with Sturge-Weber disease frequently present with

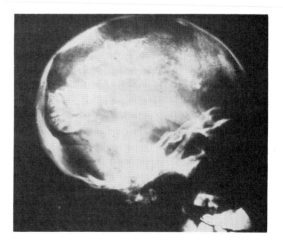

Figure 27. Skull x–ray in Sturge Weber disease; note characteristic double curve linear calcifications.

mental retardation, focal convulsions and sometimes hemianopsia and hemiparesis. Since the first division of the trigeminal distribution is almost invariably involved, telangiectasis of the bulbar conjunctiva, buphthalmos or microphthalmos, and glaucoma frequently occur. In rare cases, the facial nevus may be absent[59] and at times the facial nevus does not conform precisely to the distribution of the trigeminal nerve.[60] Occasionally the hemangioma may be cavernous rather than telangiectatic, such forms being contiguous with Klippel–Trenaunay syndrome which consists of extensive cavernous hemangiomatosis involving one side of the body as well as the face, and associated with hemihypertrophy of that side. Rarely Sturge–Weber disease may be associated with angiomata of other organs,[61] such forms merging with Osler–Weber Rendu disease which is an autosomal dominant condition in which one finds hemangiomas scattered throughout many organs including the brain, and telangiectatic lesions of the face, ears, and hands. Clinically this condition presents with episodes of bleeding from these hemangiomas. Frequent bouts of epistaxis are most common but bleeding from the lung, kidney, bowel, and occasionally cerebral hemorrhage have been described.

In 1936, Greenwald and Koota[62] reviewed all the cases of Sturge–Weber Dimitri disease reported in the literature. Of 82 cases angiomata of the brain had been confirmed by surgery or autopsy in 24. In the remaining 58, neurologic findings or x–rays suggested the diagnosis. In three cases nevi were found in organs other than in the brain. Convulsions were the most frequent neurologic symptom occurring in 68 (82%) of cases. Paralysis occurred in 51 (62%) and in two cases paralysis was ipsilateral to the facial nevus suggesting that the brain lesion was either bilateral or on the side opposite the facial telangiectasis. Mental retardation occurred in 50 (61%) of the series and varied from mild to severe. Ocular symptoms were present in 29 cases (36%) and included exophthalmos, glaucoma and ocular palsies. Headache was a prominent symptom in only four cases. Many patients died in the second or third decades of life indicating that the disease has a poor prognosis.

Pathology

The basic neuropathologic lesion of Sturge–Weber disease[61] consists of leptomeningeal vascular malformations ("angiomatosis"), involving the portions of the cerebral hemisphere usually ipsilateral to the facial angiomatosis, mostly in the occipital or parieto–occipital region (Fig. 28). There is a general correspondence of the facial cerebral lesions. When the ophthalmic division of the trigeminal the ophthalmic division of the trigeminal nerve, the meningeal lesion is found in the occipital region; the involvement of the maxillary division is usually associated with a comparable lesion in the parietal convexity, while the meningeal angiomatosis involving the entire hemispheric convexity, inclusive of the frontal lobe, as a rule, occurs in conjunction with nevus involvement of all three divisions of the trigeminal nerve. The leptomeningeal angiomatosis is seen to extend into the depths of the sulci, but not directly into the brain substance (Fig. 29). Microscopically, most of these vessels are thin–walled, dilated venous or capillary structures which show the persistence of sinusoidal embryonal character. This apparently reflects the lack of structural

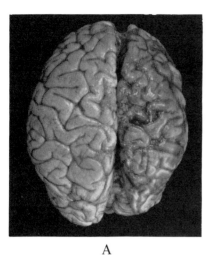
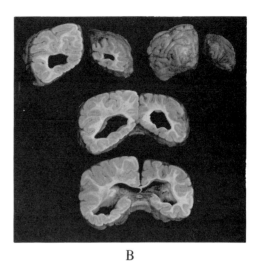

A   B

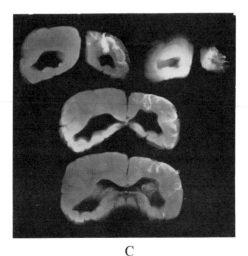

C

Figure 28. Sturge–Weber Syndrome

    A. Dorsal view of the cerebral hemispheres of a patient with Sturge–Weber syndrome. The affected right hemisphere is atrophic and shows a darker surface due to leptomeningeal hemangiomatosis.

    B. Cross sections of the posterior half of the cerebral hemispheres.

    C. Roentgenograph of (B) showing lines of calcification along the cortical ribbons particularly in right occipitoparietal region.

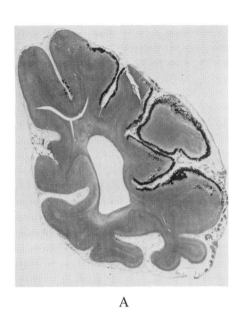

A

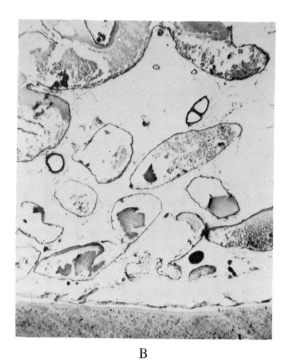

B

Figure 29. Sturge–Weber Syndrome

    A. Photomicrograph of a section through the right posterior parietal region showing a generalized increase in vascularity in the leptomeninges and laminar calcification within the cortex over the dorsolateral aspect. H & E stain, original magnification.

    B. Photomicrograph of leptomeningeal hemangiomatosis in which thin–walled and dilated blood vessels constitute the majority.

differentiation of the vascular wall. However, secondary degenerative changes such as hyalin collagenous thickening of the walls and thrombosis may occur. The changes within the brain substance notably in the underlying cerebral cortex appear to be largely secondary in nature. While penetration of these abnormal vessels into the cortex is rare, increase of intracortical capillaries and the presence of anomalous convoluted large vessels have been reported.[63] Some large vessels are occasionally seen in the convolutional white matter. The most characteristic change here consists of the presence of mineral deposits, initially, as fine concretions along the capillaries. They become enlarged and confluent causing apparently secondary damage to neurons and reactive gliosis. When large, they apparently lie free in the tissue without any relationship to the vasculature. However, some of the larger vessels may show circumferential mineral deposits in their walls. While generally referred to as "calcification," the chemical composition of these concrements is disputed. It is apparently variable but calcium and phosphorous are the major constituents with or without the addition or iron. Some of the cortical changes in the way of neuronal loss may be related to circulatory and metabolic disturbances related to the repeated episodes of epileptic seizures. Changes frequently seen in the cerebellum consisting of Purkinje cells and later, granular cell loss and associated gliosis are more probably attributable to this mode of damage.

Occasionally, anomalies in the gasserian ganglia and sensory nerve roots consisting of proliferation of capsule cells and ectopic ganglion cells[61] are recorded. Other cerebral malformations reported include disturbance of neuroblastic migration towards the cerebral cortex from the subependymal germinal matrix resulting in neuronal heterotopia in the white matter.

To complete the discussion of diseases associated with angiomatosis mention must be made of Von Hippel Lindau disease, though in a strict sense it is not a neurocutaneous disorder in that no characteristic skin lesions are described. Angiomatous cystic lesions of the retina were first described by Von Hippel in 1904.[64] The association of these eye lesions with hemangioblastoma of the cerebellum was made by Lindau in 1926. The retinal lesions are raised orange colored masses located in the periphery of the fundus and often fed by aberrant vessels. These lesions ultimately produce retinal detachment with resultant blindness.[65] The cerebellar vascular tumors (commonly referred to as hemangioblastoma or Hemangioendothelioma) produce signs of posterior fossa tumor and sometimes subarachnoid hemorrhage (Fig. 30). There may be associated polycythemia and hypertension. Pheochromocytoma has also been reported. Both autosomal dominant and autosomal recessive modes of inheritance have been described.[66]

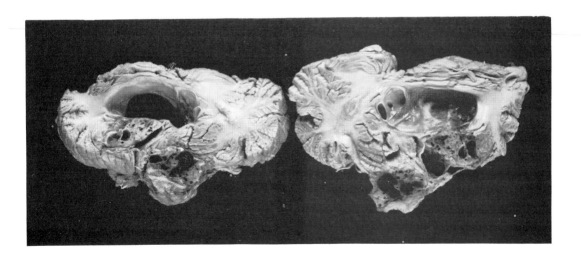

Figure 30. von Hippel–Lindau's disease: multiple hemangioblastomas of the cerebellum in a patient with von Hippel–Lindau's disease.

Ataxia Telangiectasia

Ataxia telangiectasia is described in detail in Chapter 7. This disease begins with ataxia in early life due to cerebellar degeneration. Later telangiectasis of the conjunctiva and butterfly area of the face appears. The disease is associated with immune globulin deficiency, upper respiratory infections and a high incidence of lymphosarcoma. On the skin, white macules, basal cell carcinomas and early appearance of senile keratosis have been reported.[67] A Negro family in which five of 12 members were affected and two of which had gastric carcinoma has also been reported.[68] The condition has also been linked with medulloblastoma and gliomas. Of particular interest is a case of ataxia telangiectasia with lymphosarcoma and coexisting tuberous sclerosis.[69]

Pathology

The atrophy of the cerebellum, the predominant feature in this disorder, consists of loss of Purkinje cells and to a lesser extent, granular cells and many of the remaining Purkinje cells show degenerative changes. The atrophy involves the entire cerebellar cortex but the vermis or lateral lobes may be preferentially affected. While there are not telangiectatic lesions comparable with the ocular lesion in the central nervous system, the presence of abnormally large veins in the leptomeninges of the cerebellum and cerebrum has been described in some cases. These vessels were held responsible by some for the cerebellar neuronal loss due to venous stasis but this view is challenged by others since there are cases documented without such vascular abnormalities. Clinically, the development of the ocular telangiectasia is preceded by cerebellar ataxia. Therefore, at the present time, no established pathogenesis of the cerebellar degeneration is known in the human. It is of interest that Tedeschi produced a lesion in rats similar to the human condition by neonatal thymectomy, pointing to a relationship between thymic dysplasia and cerebellar degeneration. Some of the features of ataxia telangiectasia are compared with Sturge–Weber Dimitri disease and Osler–Weber Rendu disease in Table I.

Multiple Nevoid Basal Cell Carcinoma Syndrome

The Multiple Nevoid Basal Cell Carcinoma Syndrome will be reviewed at length in Chapter 9. The essential findings in this condition are multiple basal cell carcinomas, jaw cysts and skeletal anomalies. Other skin manifestations include café au lait spots and palmar plantar pits. Evidence of central nervous system involvement in the form of a high incidence of medulloblastoma, and congenital communicating hydrocephalus will suffice to justify classification of this syndrome with the neurocutaneous diseases. A high incidence of pheochromocytoma has been reported as has pseudohyperparathyroidism and ovarian fibromata. Fibrosarcoma has occurred. Eye findings include corneal opacity, cataract, glaucoma and congenital coloboma.

Melanosis Cerebri

Leptomeningeal Melanosis is a rare condition characterized by proliferation of melanocytes in the meninges causing them to be grossly black in appearance. The condition might go entirely unrecognized during life except for the frequent association with giant pigmented nevi

Table I. Differential Diagnosis of Cutaneous Telangiectasia

EPONYM	STURGE–WEBER	LOUIS–BAR	OSLER–WEBER–RENDU
Proper Name	Encephalo-Trigeminal Syndrome	Ataxia Telangiect-asia	Hereditary Hemorrhagic Telangiectasia
Age of Discovery	At Birth	Childhood	Adult
Skin Findings	Port wine mark of face, palate, neck-Rarely bilateral	Mild, Telangiect-asis of conjunctiva, nose & ears. Bilateral	Telangiectasis of face, sometimes hands and feet. Bilateral
CNS Findings	Hemangiomatosis of Meninges – calcification of Cortex	Degeneration of Cerebellar Cortex	usually none – may have Cerebral A–V anomalys
Outstanding CNS Symptoms	Convulsive disorder–mild mental retardation	Ataxia Retardation Choreo–Athetosis	Rarely convulsions or a Cerebral hemorrhage
Presenting Complaint	Skin lesion Convulsions	Ataxia Infections	Nosebleed Internal bleeding
Eye Findings	Microphthalmia Glaucoma	Telangiectasis of Conjunctiva Nystagmus–oculo Gyric crises	Telangiectasis of Conjunctiva which may bleed
Other Organ Involvement	None	Thymus Gonad	Hemangiomas of Liver, Lung, Gut
Genetics	Not Confirmed	Recessive	Dominant
Cytogenetics	Normal	Chromatid breaks and rearrangements and endoreduplica-tions	Normal
Cancer Association	Neurofibromatosis	Lymphoma Gastric Carcinoma	None
Corroborating Tests	Skull X–Ray EEG	Serum Globulin Electrophoresis	Arteriography Endoscopy

and with malignant melanoma. Reed and his associates report an incidence of 43% of patients with giant pigmented nevi as showing cerebral meanocytosis.[70] Cerebral melanocytosis was most often associated with occipital giant nevi. Of particular interest is a case reported by Slaughter et al which clearly demonstrated neurofibromatosis with giant pigmented nevus and malignant melanoma and melanosis cerebri.[71] This case clearly links Melanosis Cerebri with the other Neurocutaneous disorders. These authors point out a high incidence of malignant melanoma (13%) in children with neurocutaneous melanomatosis. It has been argued that Malignant Melanoma in the brain is always metastatic from a cryptic lesion elsewhere in the body, but Reed and his associates.[70] point out an age descrepancy with a peak incidence of meningeal melanomas in the fourth decade while cutaneous melanomas are most prevalent in patients over 60. It would seem reasonable to suppose that cerebral melanocytes could undergo malignant change as readily as cutaneous melanocytes. Seizures and hydrocephalus are associated with cerebral melanomatosis. Malignant melanoma involving the central nervous system frequently produces subarachnoid hemorrhage. Diffuse melanosis with melanuria and generalized darkening of the skin may also occur with Metastatic Malignant Melanoma.[72]

The Nevus of Ota is a diffuse dark blue–grey pigmentation about the eyes and sometimes involving the sclera. It is commonly seen in Oriental peoples and a review of a large series of Oriental patients demonstrating Nevus of Ota failed to demonstrate a single case of malignant transformation.[73] This however, has not been the case with Occidentals demonstrating Nevus of Ota where development of

malignant melanoma does occur.[74] Intraocular malignant melanoma has been reported in more than one member of a family in several instances[75] but by in large the condition is sporadic and a mode of inheritance has not been determined.

Differential Diagnosis of Neurocutaneous Disorders

While the neurocutaneous disorders can be clearly differentiated on the basis of the associated skin lesions and while each has its own distinctive clinical history and heredity, these conditions do share in many instances common symptoms, signs and relationships to a variety of clinical entities. These relationships are briefly outlined in Table II. It is noted that café au lait spots are common to neurofibromatosis, Tuberous Sclerosis, Sturge–Weber Dimitri disease and the multiple nevoid basal cell carcinoma syndrome. They are often more numerous in Multiple Neurofibromatosis than in the others and whether or not they differ histologically remains to be seen. It is also noted that an increased incidence of basal cell carcinoma is seen in both the Multiple basal cell carcinoma and in Ataxia telangiectasia. There is also a relationship between giant pigmented nevi and both Melanosis cerebri and multiple Neurofibromatosis. In this regard it is of interest that a melanotic schwannoma of the acoustic nerve has been reported.[74]

A high incidence of mental subnormality has been noted in multiple neurofibromatosis, tuberous sclerosis and in Sturge–Weber Dimitri disease. Mental deficiency is usually less severe in Neurofibromatosis though patients of normal intelligence may be seen in any of these conditions. There does seem to be an inverse relationship between intelligence and the incidence of seizures. Seizures are a more prominant feature of Tuberous Sclerosis and Sturge–Weber Dimitri disease than they are in Neurofibromatosis. Hemiparesis, hemianopsia and other evidence of a lateralized cerebral lesion are commonly seen in Sturge–Weber Dimitri disease, occur less frequently in Tuberous Sclerosis and are relatively uncommon in the other neurocutaneous disorders. Conversely parplegia or other evidence of spinal lesion is much more common in Neurofibromatosis. Congenital communicating hydrocephalus occurs in both Melanosis Cerebri and Multiple Nevoid Basal Cell Carcinoma Syndrome is common to Ataxia. Cerebellar Ataxia is common to Ataxia Telangiectasia and Von Hippel Lindau disease. Subarachnoid hemorrhage may occur with Cerebral Malignant Melanoma, Cerebellar Hemangioblastoma (Von Hippel Lindau), Osler-Weber Rendu disease, and Sturge–Weber Dimitri disease.

Ocular Telangiectasis occurs in Ataxia Telangiectasia, Osler–Weber Rendu disease and Sturge–Weber Dimitri disease, and Multiple Nevoid Basal Cell Carcinoma and Sturge–Weber disease Glaucoma may occur. In both Multiple Neurofibromatosis and Tuberous Sclerosis, Phakomata of the retina are to be found.

Cystic lesions of bone are found in Von Recklinghausen's disease and these are radiographically indistinguishable from bone cysts seen in Tuberous Sclerosis. Fibrous dysplasia of the skull similar to that seen in Albright's Syndrome may be seen in Multiple Neurofibromatosis and indeed it has been argued that these two conditions are one and the same disease. Lesser, but similar changes in the skull have been noted in Tuberous Sclerosis.[76] Pseudoarthrosis occurs in both diseases and Scoliosis is common to both

Multiple Nevoid Basal Cell Carcinoma Syndrome and Von Recklinghausen's neurofibromatosis. Hemihypertrophy or hemiatrophy of the skeleton may be seen in Multiple Neurofibromatosis, in Klippel–Trenaunay, and in Sturge–Weber Dimitri disease respectively. A very similar type of cystic lung disease is seen in both Multiple Neurofibromatosis and Tuberous Sclerosis.

Osteomalacia may result from either renal tubular defect with Vitamin D resistant Rickets or as a result of Hyperparathyroidism in Multiple Neurofibromatosis and also occurs in Multiple Nevoid Basal Cell Carcinoma Syndrome as a result of tubular hyposensitivity to parathormone. Pheochromocytoma is of unusually high incidence in both Multiple Neurofibromatosis, Multiple Nevoid Basal Cell Carcinoma Syndrome and in Von Hippel Lindau disease. Crowe emphasizes delayed physical and sexual maturation in Multiple Neurofibromatosis and gonadal dysgenesis is seen in Ataxia Telangiectasia.

In completing the investigation of a diagnosed case of any of the neurocutaneous syndromes it is well to bear in mind the high incidence of malignancy associated with this group of diseases. This is particularly true in Melanosis Cerebri in children, but an increased incidence of Melanoma is also noted in Multiple Neurofibromatosis in addition to the numbers of Neuroblastomas and Fibrosarcomas associated with the disease. The high incidence of Medulloblastoma found in multiple neurofibromatosis is shared with the Multiple nevoid basal cell carcinoma syndrome which in turn shares an increased incidence of basal cell carcinoma with Ataxia Telangiectasia. The latter condition has been associated with gastric carcinoma

Table II. Clinical Features of Neurocutaneous Diseases

	Skin	Brain	Skeletal	Endocrine
Neurofibro-matosis	1) Neurofi-bromas 2) Plexiform neuromas 3) Café–au–lait 4) Giant Nevi 5) Angiomas	1) Acoustic & spinal neuromata 2) Meningiomas 3) Gliomas	1) Fibrous Dysplasia 2) Cystic lesions 3) Scoliosis 4) Pseudo-arthrosis	1) Parathyroid adenomas 2) Vit. D Resis-tant osteo-malacia 3) Pheochromo-cytoma
Tuberous Sclerosis	1) Adenoma sebaceum 2) Shagreen spots 3) Subungual fibroma 4) Café–au lait 5) White macules	1) Gliomas 2) Ganglio-gliomas	1) Cystic lesions 2) Sclerotic lesions	
Sturge-Weber	1) Telangiec-tatic Heman-gioma 2) Café–au–lait 3) Cavernous Hemangiomas	1) Meningeal Hemangioma-tosis	1) Hemiatrophy 2) Hemihyper-trophy	
Ataxia Telangiec-tasis	1) Telangiec-tasis 2) White macules 3) Basal Cell Carcinoma 4) Senile Keratosis	1) Medullo-blastoma 2) Cerebellar degener-ation 3) Glioma	None	1) Immune globulin deficiency 2) Ovarian dysgenesis
Multiple Nevoid Basal Cell Carcinoma Syndrome	1) Basal Cell Carcinoma 2) Café–au–lait 3) Palmar-plantar pits	1) Medullo-blastoma 2) Congenital communicating hydroceph-alus	1) Hypertel-iorism 2) Short meta-carpals 3) Bifurcate ribs 4) Klippel-Feil Syndrome 5) Scoliosis 6) Platybasia	1) Pseudohyper-parathyroid-ism 2) Ovarian fibromata 3) Pheochromo-cytoma
Melanosis Cerebri	1) Giant Bath-ing Trunk nevus	1) Melanoma 2) Congenital communicating hydrocephalus 3) Subarachnoid Hemorrhage		

Lung	Kidney	Heart	Other Malignancy	Eye
1) Cystic lesions	1) Constriction or aneurysm of Renal artery 2) Polycystic Kidney disease		1) Melanoma 2) Neuroblastoma 3) Myeloma 4) Fibrocarcinoma	1) Glioma of Optic nerve 2) Retrobulbar Neurofibromatosis 3) Phakomata of the Retina
1) Cystic lesions 2) Adenomata 3) Angiomata	1) Angiomyolipomata	1) Rhabdomyomata 2) Fibroelastosis		1) Phakomata of Retina
				1) Glaucoma 2) Neurofibroma 3) Telangiectasis 4) Melanoma
			1) Lymphosarcoma 2) Gastric Carcinoma 3) Basal Cell Carcinoma 4) Ovarian Dysgerminoma	
			1) Fibrosarcoma	1) Corneal opacity 2) Cataract 3) Glaucoma 4) Coloboma
			1) Melanoma	1) Ocular Melanoma

and a high incidence of lymphosarcoma. To come full circle there has been at least one case of familial Multiple Neurofibromatosis associated with Multiple Myeloma.[77] The relationship of Medullary Carcinoma of the Thyroid to the Multiple Mucosal Neuromata Syndrome which is presented in detail in Chapter XIV is of interest, for in some cases of this condition Cutaneous Neurofibromatosis also occurs.

Sturge–Weber Dimitri disease and Tuberous Sclerosis, both deadly conditions in their own right, from which patients often expire at an early age show less association with malignancy, though Metastatic Sarcomas associated with the kidney lesions of Tuberous Sclerosis have been reported and the relationship to Astrocytoma in Tuberous Sclerosis is problematical in view of the histopathology of the brain lesions.

Table II illustrates clinical entities as they are associated with each individual Neurocutaneous Syndrome.

A summary, which compares the incidence of seven of the most commonly observed clinical signs among the neurocutaneous disorders is presented in Table III. Each + indicates an incidence of approximately 25% or less for the finding as it is observed at some time in the course of the disease.

TABLE III

RELATIVE FREQUENCY OF COMMONLY OBSERVED

MANIFESTATIONS OF NEUROCUTANEOUS DISEASES

	Mental Subnormality	Epilepsy	Localizing Neurologic Signs	Hydrocephalus	Skin Manifestations	Ocular Findings	Skeletal Deformity
Multiple Neurofibromatosis	++	+	+	—	+++	+	+++
Tuberous Sclerosis	+++	+++	++	+	++++	++	+
Sturge–Weber Dimitri Disease	++	+++	++	—	++++	++	+
Ataxia Telangiectasia	+	—	+++	—	+++	++++	—
Multiple Nevoid Basal Cell Carcinoma Syndrome	+	—	—	+	++	+	+++
Melanosis Cerebri	++	++	+	+	++	—	—

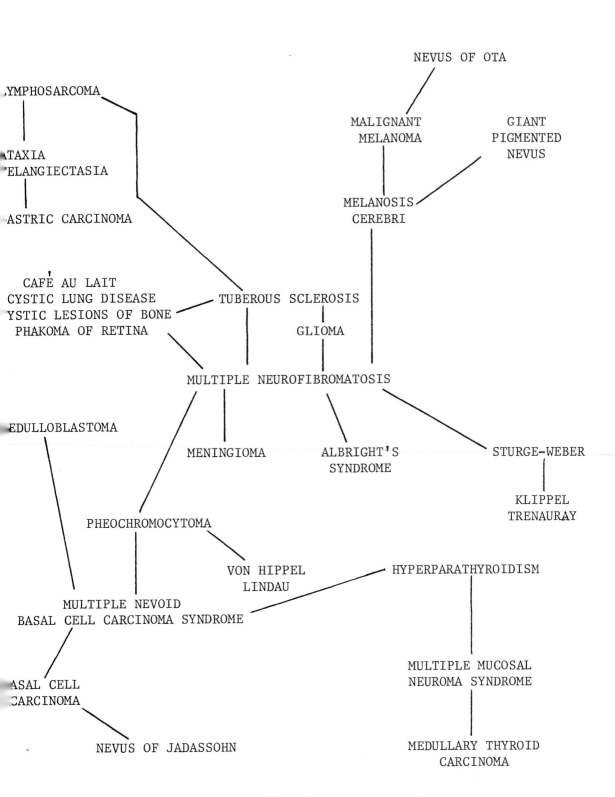

Figure 31. Interrelationships of neurocutaneous diseases.

Interrelationships Among Neurocutaneous Diseases

We have already observed that the neurocutaneous diseases are linked together indirectly with each other through a number of other clinical conditions which share a common association with two or more neurocutaneous diseases. These associations are illustrated in Figure 31. The numbers coincide with the appropriate reference from the bibliography. From the diagram it is noted that rarely but repeatedly the presence of lesions characteristic of two neurocutaneous diseases are noted in the same patient or within the same kindred. Both Crowe and Chao and their associates document the coexistence of Tuberous Sclerosis and Multiple Neurofibromatosis within the same kindred. The occurrence of Tuberous Sclerosis with Ataxia Telangiectasia, reported by Gotoff, et al has been cited earlier. Since Neurocutaneous diseases are rare,[5, 58] the probabilty of chance association of these conditions if they were unrelated is infinitely small. It would seem reasonable to suppose then that there is a hamartomatous diathesis which links at least four and possibly all of the Neurocutaneous diseases together developmentally.

BIBLIOGRAPHY

1. Sturge, W.A.: A case of partial epilepsy, apparently due to a lesion of one of the vasomotor centers of the brain. *Tr. Clin. Soc.* London, *12*: 162, 1879.

2. Bourneville, D.M.: Contribution à l'etude de l'idiotie. *Arch. Neurol. 1*: 69–91, 1880.

3. Von Recklinghausen F.: Über die multiplen Fibrome der Haut und ihre Beziehung zu den multiplen Neuromen, Berlin, A. Hirschwald, 1882; p. 138.

4. Louis–Bar, D.: Sur un syndrome progressif comprenant des telangiectasies capillaires cutanees et conjonctivae symetriques naevoide et des trables cerebelleux. *Confin. Neurol. 4*: 32, 1941.

5. Crowe, F.W., Schull, W.J., and Neel J.V.: Multiple Neurofibromatosis. Springfield, Illinois, Charles C. Thomas, 1956.

6. Benedict, P.H., Szabo, G., Fitzpatrick, T.B., and Sinesi, S.J.: Melanotic Macules in Albright's Syndrome and in Neurofibromatosis. *J.A.M.A. 205*: 618–618–626, (August) 1968.

7. Pearce, J.: The Central Nervous System Pathology in Multiple Neurofibromatosis. *Neurology. 17*: 691–97, (July) 1967.

8. Penfield, W., and Guthrie, R.R.: Congenital Ectodermosis (Neurocutaneous Syndrome) in Epileptic Patients. *Arch. Neurol & Psychiat. 26*: 1145, 1931.

9. Lee, D.K., and Abbott, M.L.: Familial Central Nervous System Neoplasia. *Arch. Neurol. 20.* 154–160, (February) 1969.

10. Rosenberg, R.N., Sassin, J., Zimmerman, E.A., and Carter, S.: The Interrelationship of Neurofibromatosis and Fibrous Dysplasia. *Arch. Neurol. 17*: 174–179, (August) 1967.

11. Saville, P.D., Nassim, J.R., Stevenson, F.H., Mulligan, L., and Carey, M.: Osteomalacia in Von Recklinghausen's Neurofibromatosis. *Brit. Med. J.* 1: 1311–13, (May) 1955.

12. Daly, D., Kaye, M., and Estrada, R.L.: Neurofibromatosis and Hyperparathyroidism – A New Syndrome? *Canad Med Ass J 103*: 258–59, (August) 1970.

13. Humble, Roy M.: Phaeochromocytoma, Neurofibromatosis and Pregnancy. *Anaesthesia 22*: 296–303, (April) 1967.

14. Halpern, M., Currarine, G.: Vascular Lesions Causing Hypertension in Neurofibromatosis. *New Eng J. Med. 273*: 248–51, (July) 1965.

15. Knight, J.A., and Cancilla, P.A.: Neurofibroma Involving the Superior Vena Cava With Formation of an Aneurysm. *Arch. Path. 86*: 427–430, (October) 1968.

16. Lipton, S., and Zuckerbrod, M: Familial Enteric Neurofibromatosis *Medical Times 94*: 544–548, (May) 1966.

17. Massaro, D., Katz, S., Matthews, M.J., and Higgins, G.: Von Recklinghausen's Neurofibromatosis Associated with Cystic Lung Disease. *Amer. J. Med. 38*: 233–240, (February) 1965.

18. Lichtenstein, B.W.: Neurofibromatosis (von Recklinghausen's Disease of the Nervous System). Analysis of the Total Pathologic Picture. *Arch. Neurol Psychiat. 62*: 822–839, 1949.

19. Fisher, E.R. and Vuzevski, V.D.: Cytogenesis of Schwannoma (Neurilemmoma), Neurofibroma, Dermatofibroma, and Dermatofibrosarcoma as Revealed by Electron Microscopy. *Amer J. Clin Path. 49*: 141–154, 1968.

20. Heard, G.: Nerve Sheath Tumours and von Recklinghausen's Disease of the Nervous System. *Ann. Roy. Coll. Surg. Eng 31*: 229–248, 1962.

21. Russell, D.S. and Rubinstein, L.J.: Pathology of Tumours of the Nervous System. pp. 31–33, Edward Arnold (publishers), Ltd., London, 1959.

22. Gardner, W.J. and Frasier, C.H.: Bilateral Acoustic Neurofibromas: A Clinical Study and Field Survey of a Family of Five Generations with Bilateral Deafness in the Thirty–Eight Members. *Arch. Neurol. Psychiat. 23*: 266–302, 1930.

23. Olive, I. Svien, H.J.: Neurofibroma of the Fifth Cranial Nerve. *J. Neurosurg. 14*: 484–505, 1957.

24. Murray, M.R. and Stout, A.P.: Schwann Cell versus Fibroblast as the Origin of the Specific Nerve Sheath Tumor: Observations Upon Normal Nerve Sheaths and Neurilemmomas in Vitro. *Amer J Path 16*: 41–60, 1940.

25. Hosoi, K.: Multiple Neurofibromatosis (von Recklinghausen's Disease) with Special Reference to Malignant Transformation. *Arch. Surg. 22*: 258–281, 1931.

26. Stout, A.P.: Atlas of Tumor Pathology Section II – Fascicle 6. Tumors of the Peripheral Nervous System. Washington, D.C., Armed Forces Institute Of Pathology, 1949.

27. D'Agostino, A.N., Soule, E.H., and Miller, R.H.: Sarcomas of the Peripheral Nerves and Somatic Soft Tissues Associated with Multiple Neurofibromatosis (von Recklinghausen's Disease). *Cancer 16*: 1015–1027, 1963.

28. Evans, R.W.: Histological Appearance of Tumours. pp. 374–381, 2nd Edition, Edinburgh and London, E. & S. Livingston, Ltd., 1966.

29. Stout, A.P.: The Peripheral Manifestations of the Specific Nerve Sheath Tumor (neurilemmoma). *Amer J Cancer 24*: 751–796, 1935.

30. Carstens, P.H.B. and Schrodt, G.R.: Malignant Transformation of a Benign Encapsulated Neurillemmoma. *Amer J Clin. Path. 51*: 144–149, 1969.

31. Canale, D., Bebin, J. and Knighton, R.S.: Neurologic Manifestations of von Recklinghausen's Disease of the Nervous System. *Confin. Neurol. 24*: 359–403, 1964.

32. Davis, F.A.: Primary Tumors of the

Optic Nerve (A Phenomenon of Recklinghausen's Disease): A Clinical and Pathologic Study with a Report of Five Cases and a Review of Literature. *Arch. Ophthal. 23:* 735–830 and 957–10022, 1940.

33. Poser, C.M.: The Relationship Between Syringomyelia and Neoplasm, Springfield, Illinois, C.C., Thomas, 1956.

34. Bielschowsky, M.: Über tuberose Sklerose und ihre Beziehungen zur Recklinghausenschen Krankheit. *Z. ges. Neurol Psychiat. 26:* 133–155, 1914.

35. Walker, A.E.: Astrocytosis Arachnoideae Cerebelli. A Rare Manifestation of von Recklinghausen's Neurofibromatosis. *Arch, Neurol. Psychiat. 45:* 520–532, 1941.

36. Kernohan, J.W. and Parker, H.L.: A Case of Recklinghausen's Disease with Observations on the Associated Formation of Tumors. *J. Nerv. Ment. Dis. 76:* 313–330, 1932.

37. Henneberg and Koch, M.: Über "centrale" Neurofibromatose und die Geschwulste des Kleinhirnbruckenwinkels (Acusticusneurome). *Arch. Psychiat. Nervenkss 36:* 251–304, 1903.

38. Hogan, M.J. and Zimmerman, L.E.: Opthhalmic Pathology. An Atlas and Textbook, 2nd Edition, pp. 443–449. W.B. Saunders Co., Philadelphia and London, 1966.

39. Chao, D.H.: Congenital Neurocutaneous Syndromes in Childhood: I, Neurofibromatosis. *J. Pediat 55:* 189–199, (August) 1959.

40. Bundey, S., and Evans, K.: Tuberous Sclerosis, a genetic study. *J. Neurol. Neurosurg. Psychiat. 32:* 591–603, 1969.

41. Chao, D.H.: Congenital Neurocutaneous Syndromes in Childhood: II, Tuberous Sclerosis. *J. Pediat 55:* 447–58, (October) 1959.

42. Alvarez, E.: Unusual Cutaneous Manifestations of Tuberous Sclerosis: Case Report. *Plast Reconstr Surg 40:* 153–56, (August) 1967.

43. Fitzpatrick, T.B., Szabo, G., Yoshiaki, H., Simone, A.A. Reed, W.B., and Greenberg, M.H.: White Leaf-Shaped Macules. *Arch. Derm. 98:* 1–6 (July) 1968.

44. Lagos, J.C., and Gomez, M.R.: Tuberous Sclerosis: Reappraisal of a Clinical Entity. *Mayo Clin. Proc. 42:* 25–49, (January) 1967.

45. Thibault, J.H., and Maneulidis, E.E.: Tuberous Sclerosis In A Premature Infant, *Neurology 20:* 139–146, (February) 1970.

46. Broughton, R.B.K.: Pulmonary Tuberous Sclerosis Presenting with Pleural Effusion. *Brit. Med. J. 1:* 477–478, 1970.

47. Harris, J.E., Waltuch, B.L., and Swenson, E.W.: The Pathophysiology of the Lungs in Tuberous Sclerosis, *Amer. Rev Resp Dis 100:* 379–387, 1969.

48. Seshanarayana, K.N., and Keats, T.E.: Angiomyolipoma of the Kidney: Diagnostic Roentgenographic Findings.

49. Anderson, D., and Tannen, R.L.: Tuberous Sclerosis and Chronic Renal Failure, *Amer. J. Med. 47:* 163–168, 1969.

50. Viamonte, M., Ravel, R., Politano, V., and Bridges, B.: Angiographic Findings In A Patient With Tuberous Sclerosis.

51. Van Heerden, J.A., Longo, M.D., Cardoza, F., and Farrow, G.M.: The Abdominal Mass in the Patient With Tuberous Sclerosis. *Arch. Surg. 95:* 317–319, 1967.

52. Crome, L.: The Structural Features of Epiloia with Special Reference to Endocardial Fibroelastosis. *J. Clin. Path. 7:* 137.

53. Taylor, T.R.: Tuberous Sclerosis Presenting as Cardiac Arrhythmia. *Brit. Heart J. 30*: 132–134, 1968.

54. Cosnett, J.E., and Gibb, B.H.: Tuberous Sclerosis and Cardiac Arrhythmia in Three Zulu Patients. *Brit. Med. J.* 30: 132–134, 1968.

55. Hirano, A., Tuazon, R., and Zimmerman, H.M.: Neurofibrillary Changes, Granulovacuolar Bodies and Argentophilic Globules Observed in Tuberous Sclerosis, *Acta Neuropath. 11*: 257–261, 1968.

56. Hallervorden, J. and Krucke, W.: Die Tuberose Hirnsklerose. Ein Handbuch der speziellen pathologischen Anatomie u. Histologie, Lubarsah, O., Henke, F.u. Rossie, R. (Ed.) XIII. 4th Part, pp. 602–663, 1956.

57. Jervis, G.A.: Spongioneuroblastoma and Tuberous Sclerosis. *J. Neuropath. Exp Neurol. 13*: 105–116, 1954.

58. Schnitzer, B.: Tuberous Sclerosis Complex. *Arch. Path. 76*: 626–632, 1963.

59. Lund, M.: On Epilepsy in Sturge–Weber Disease. *Acta. Psychiat. Neurol. 24*: 569, 1949.

60. Chao, D.H.: Congenital Neurocutaneous Syndromes of Childhood: III, Struge–Weber Disease. *J. Pediat 55*: 635–649, 1959.

61. Wohlwill, F.J., and Yakovlev, P.I.: Histopathology of Meningo–Facial Angiomatosis (Struge–Weber's Disease) Report of Four Cases. *J. Neuropath Exper. Neurol. 16*: 341–364, 1957.

62. Greenwald, H.M., and Koota, J.: Progress in Pediatrics: Associated Facial and Intracranial Hemangiomas. *American Journal of Diseases of Children* : 868–896.

63. Craig, J.M.: Encephalo–Trigeminal Angiomatosis. (Sturge–Weber's Disease) A Case Report, *J. Neuropath. Experim. Neurol. 8*: 305–318, 1949.

64. Von Hippel, E.: Uber eine sehr seltene Erkrankung der Netzhaut: Klinische Beobachtungen. *Arch Ophthal 59*: 83–106.

65. Melmon, K.L., and Rosen, S.W.: Lindau's Disease; Review of the literature and Study of a Large Kindred. *Amer. J. Med. 36*: 595–617.

66. Shokeir, M.H.K.: Von Hippel–Lindau Syndrome: A Report of Three Kindreds, *J. Med. Gen. 7*: 155–157 1970.

67. Reed, W.B., Epstein, W.L., Boder E., and Sedgewick, R.: Cutaneous Manifestations of Ataxia Telangiectasia, *J.A.M.A. 195*: 126, 1966.

68. Haerer, A.F., Jackson, J.F., and Evers, C.G.: Ataxia–Telangiectasia With Gastric Adenocarcinoma, *J.A.M.A. 210*: 1884–1887, 1969.

69. Gotoff, S.P. Amirmokri, E., and Liebner, E.J.: Ataxia Telangiectasia. *Amer. J. Dis. Child. 114*: 617–625, 1967.

70. Reed, W.B., Becker, (Jr.), S.W., Becker, (Sr.), S.W., and Nickel, W.R.: Giant Pigmented Nevi, Melanoma, and Leptomeningeal Melanocytosis. *Arch. Derm. 91*: 100–119, 1965.

71. Slaughter, J.C., Hardman, J.M., Kempe, L.G., and Earle, K.M.: Neurocutaneous Melanosis and Leptomeningeal Melanomatosis in Children. *Arch. Path. 88*: 298–304, 1969.

72. Silberberg, I., Kopf, A.W., and Gumport, S.L.: Diffuse Melanosis in Malignant Melanoma: Report of a Case and of Studies by Light and Electron Microscopy, *Arch. Derm. 97*: 671–77, 1968.

73. Hidano, A., Kajima, H, Ikeda, S. Mizutani, Miyasato, H., and Nimura, M.: Natural History of Nevus of Ota, *Arch. Derm. 95*: 187–195, 1967.

74. Dastur, D.K., Sinh, G., and Pandya, S.K.: Melanotic Tumor of the Acoustic

Nerve.

75. Lynch, H.T., Anderson, D.E., and Krush, A.J.: Heredity and Intraocular Malignant Melanoma: Study of Two Families and Review of Forty-five Cases, *Cancer 21*: 119–125, 1968.

76. Lagos, J.C., Holman, C.B., and Gomez, M.R.: Tuberous Sclerosis: Neuroroentgenologic Observations. *Amer. J. Roentgen 104*: 171–176, 1968.

77. Unpublished data, personal case.

Chapter 9

THE MULTIPLE NEVOID BASAL CELL CARCINOMA
SYNDROME REVISITED *

by Robert J. Gorlin, D.D.S., M.S. and
Heddie O. Sedano, D.D.S.

Over a decade has elapsed since the senior author became interested in the multiple nevoid basal cell carcinoma syndrome.[1] During the intervening years many facets of the syndrome have been examined and the evidence weighed concerning new findings. The original triad of signs: multiple nevoid basal cell carcinomas, jaw cysts and skeletal anomalies has been greatly expanded to include intracranial calcification, ovarian fibroma, hyporesponsiveness to parathormone, lymphomesenteric cysts, medulloblastoma and a whole host of minor and/or occasionally (but valid) associated anomalies. The present survey encompasses over 100 publications which have described over 250 individuals with the syndrome. In addition, the authors have personally examined at least 30 affected individuals in the United States and abroad and have been consulted in correspondence on numerous documented but unpublished cases. A tenth anniversary appears to us to be a rather convenient point in time for summing up what is known about this most intriguing syndrome.

Historical Review

Reliable evidence exists that the syndrome dates from early Egyptian times.[2] The first reported case of the syndrome was possibly that of Jarisch in 1894.[3] One cannot be certain, however, since he emphasized the cutaneous lesions. Nomland, in 1932,[4] distinguished the basal cell nevus as an entity. In 1939, Straith[5] described a family in which several members presented nevoid basal cell carcinoma of the skin and cysts of the jaws, but this report went largely unnoticed.

In 1951, Binkley and Johnson[6] reported a 31-year-old woman with multiple nevoid basal cell carcinomas and dental cysts. The jaw lesions were treated with roentgenotherapy over seven years. Subsequently, a fibrosarcoma arose in this area and metastasized to the lungs and bone, resulting in death. Ovarian fibroma, bifid rib, and absence of the corpus callosum were noted at autopsy. A daughter of this patient, 6 years of age, had skin cancers but no jaw cysts. Boyer and Martin (1958)[7] emphasized

*This study was made possible in part by U.S.P.H.S. Program Grant in Oral Pathology DE-1770.

the Marfanoid build in their patient but failed to identify the condition. Howell and Caro (1959)[8] presented four patients with the syndrome, defined the complex and first brought it to the general attention of the dermatologist.

Palmar–plantar pits were noted to be associated with the syndrome by Ward (1960),[9] although they were illustrated as early as 1905 by Pollitzer.[10] Gorlin and Goltz (1960)[1] and Gorlin, et al. (1963)[11] tabulating and analyzing all known cases thought that the combination of these clinical signs constituted a syndrome. They suggested that the condition was inherited as an autosomal dominant trait. Herzberg and Wiskemann (1963)[12] noted the association of medulloblastoma with the syndrome, and Block and Clendenning,[13] in the same year, suggested that ovarian fibromas and lymphomesenteric cysts were other components of the condition. Gorlin, et al, (1963)[11] surmised and Clendenning (1963)[14] demonstrated that affected individuals present a hyporesponsiveness to parathormone.

Systematic Survey

Facies

A characteristic facies appears to be part of the syndrome though it is not present in every case. Frontal and temporoparietal bossing is often marked, giving the skull a pagetoid appearance. This, combined with well–developed supraorbital ridges[1, 15, 16] imparts a sunken appearance to the eyes. Occasionally multiple Wormian bones are noted in the lambdoidal sutures.[17] Exotropia may also be present. Broad nasal root is extremely common and may be associated with true ocular hypertelorism (increased inter–inner canthal, interpupillary, and inter–outer canthal distances) or dystopia canthorum (increased distance between inner canthi only). Ocular hypertelorism was especially marked in a patient described by Kirsch (1956).[18] Mild mandibular prognathism has been present in most patients. Figure 1 clearly denotes several of these mentioned anatomic features. Table 1 shows the signs and symptoms with their relative frequency.

Skin

In this syndrome, the multiple nevoid basal cell carcinomas usually appear at puberty or during the second or third decade (usually 17–35 years), but may occur as early as the second year of life in both exposed and unexposed cutaneous areas. They may not appear throughout the life of the individual. It should be emphasized that in large kindreds carefully examined for all stigmata, only about half of affected individuals 20 years of age or older, manifest skin tumors.[19] They are usually numerous, appearing as tiny, flesh–colored to brownish dome-shaped papules, soft nodules or flat plaques varying in size from 1 mm to 1 cm in diameter. In order of decreasing frequency they occur on the face and neck, back and thorax, and abdomen and upper extremities. Some patients have had more than 1,000 individual lesions.

While the smaller lesions are usually flesh colored, the larger are usually pigmented. Ulceration is common. The midface is especially involved. The preiorbital areas, eyelids, nose, malar region, and upper lip have also been favored sites.

The nevoid basal cell carcinoma thus contrasts with the usual basal cell carcinoma which is usually single and occurs in areas of the skin exposed to increased amounts of sunlight. The patient is usually middle aged and of fair complexion. In his survey, Maddox (1962)[20] found the nevoid form to constitute about 0.4% of all cases of basal cell carcinoma and/or epithelioma adenoides cysticum. Summerly (1965)[21] found two cases of the syndrome among 125 patients with basal cell carcinoma. The basal cell nevus has been considered to differ from the basal cell carcinoma, largely in its appearance at a young age and its occurrence in cutaneous areas not especially exposed to sunlight.

Nevoid basal cell carcinomas exhibit a diversity in histopathological appearance, the spectrum ranging from that of a benign adnexal tumor to a typical, aggressive, ulcerating, basal cell carcinoma. They arise in the epidermis and in the upper part of the hair follicle.[22]

Maddox[20, 23] divided the skin tumors of the syndrome into 5 groups and estimated their frequency: solid (72%), adenoid (27%), cystic (19%), morphea-like (17%), and superficial (6%). About one-third of the patients exhibited two or more types. Mason, et al., (1965)[24] noted similar findings. When compared with a control series of basal cell carcinomas, the tumors seen in the syndrome appeared to be more often associated with an inflammatory infiltrate and with minute calcification but were otherwise indistinguishable. Graham, et al. (1965),[25] found bone or osteoid in about one-third of the nevoid basal cell lesions and an abundance of sulfated acid mucopolysaccharides. Mason, et al. (1965),[24] however, found bone or osteoid in only 11 of 370 tumors. Murphey (1969)[26] described

generalized subcutaneous calcification of the scalp.

Cysts of the skin vary in size from minute milia common to the face, to those 1 to 2 cm in size, more often found on the extremities. They are found in at least 20 per cent of the patients. [15, 19, 22, 24, 27–30] Gilhuus–Moe, et al., (1968)[19] noted chalazion in their patients.

Comedones have also been stated to be common[31, 32] and *café-au-lait* pigmentation is occasionally noted.[33, 34] In several patients, there has been hirsutism and/or multiple pigmented nevi.[35]

Palmar–plantar pits have been noted in several patients.[10, 22, 34, 36–42] These punctate lesions represent a localized retardation of the maturation process of the basal cells. These have been eminently well–illustrated microscopically by Pollitzer (1905)[10] and Zackheim, *et al.* (1966).[22] They may also occur on the dorsa and sides of the fingers and toes.

Electron microscopic studies have demonstrated an increased number of basal cells, a reduction of desmosomal attachments, formation of plasmalemmal microvilli and a disturbance in the maturation of keratohyaline granules and keratinosomes.[22] Basal cell carcinomas have occurred on the palms or soles in a few cases developing at the base of the pits.[9, 43]

Musculo–Skeletal Anomalies

Skeletal anomalies are common, being present in 60–75% of individuals affected with the syndrome. Among the more common anomalies are splayed and/or bifurcated rib. Bifurcation may involve several ribs and may be bilateral. Other costal anomalies include synostosis, partial agenesis, pseudoarthrosis and cervical rudimentary ribs.[44]

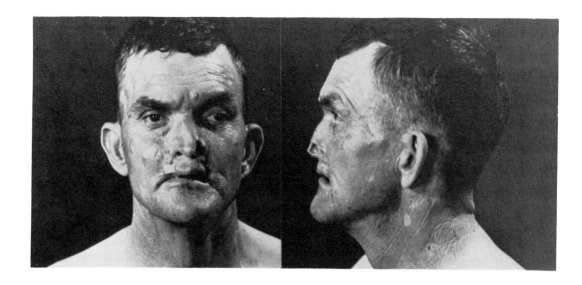

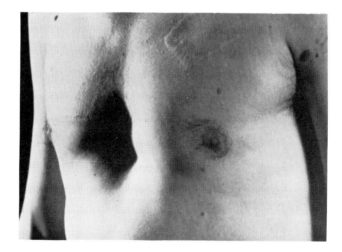

Figure 1. Patient showing several striking phenotypic characteristics of the multiple nevoid basal cell carcinoma syndrome. Note ophthalmoplegia, hypertelorism, prognathism, pectus excavatum, and evidence of excision of many basal cell cancers.

It should be pointed out that similar rib anomalies may occur in ostensibly normal people. However, their frequency is rather rare. Etter (1944)[45] found the prevalence of presumably isolated bifid rib, rudimentary rib and synostosis of ribs to be 6.2, 2.0 and 2.6., respectively, per 1000 live births. Ashbury, *et al.* (1942),[46] in examination of more than 22,000 United States Army inductees, noted a frequency of 3.0, 1.2, and 1.0 per 1000 men. These figures would make fortuitous association of the costal abnormalities in this syndrome highly unlikely. Skeletal anomalies such as these are often overlooked and only discovered when sought. Therefore, their incidence in the syndrome, although high, would probably be even higher if a thorough roentgenologic survey were given to each patient.

Kyphoscoliosis has been observed in at least 50 percent of affected individuals. Cervical and/or upper thoracic vertebral fusion or lack of segmentation has also been noted.[37, 42, 44, 47–50] Fusion between the occiput and first cervical vertebra was described by Pimenta, *et al.* (1965).[51] In the case of Eisenbud, *et al.* (1952),[47] there was incomplete segmentation of the 4th–6th cervical vertebral segments and six, rather than seven cervical vertebrae. Pollard and New (1964)[37] noted fusion of D2–D3 and D3 and D4 and Mills and Foulkes[48] observed lack of segmentation of the fourth and fifth cervical vertebrae. Van Erp (1968)[49] noted block vertebrae bodies. To use the term Klippel–Feil syndrome to describe this situation[47] only confuses the issue since this term has been used to refer to so many different entities. The brilliant article of Gunderson, *et al.* (1967)[52] clarifies this problem.

Spina bifida occulta also commonly (about 40 percent) involves these same vertebrae.[15, 19, 32, 37, 53–56]

Sprengel's deformity has been described by several authors.[21, 28, 39, 49, 50, 58–60] Medial hooking or dysplasia of the scapulae has been noted.[37, 60–63] Pectus excavatum and carinatum has also been described but possibly is the result of kyphoscoliosis which occurs in at least one–half of the affected.[37, 60, 64]

Shortened metacarpals (brachymetacarpalism), especially the fourth, were seen by Gorlin, et al. (1963),[11] Clendenning (1964),[33] Pollard and New (1964),[37] Berlin, et al., (1966),[65] Tobias (1967),[34] Becker, et al. (1967),[53] Gilhuus–Moe, et al., (1968),[19] Lile, *et al.* (1968)[55] and Cernea, et al. (1969).[66] It should be noted however, that about 10 percent of the normal population has a positive metacarpal sign.[67] Lausecker (1952),[68] Davidson and Kay (1964),[69] Mordecai (1966)[70] and Ziprkowski (1967)[40] noted polydactyly. Arachnodactyly was described by Boyer and Martin (1958),[7] Meerkotter and Shear (1964),[71] Maddox, et al., (1968).[23] Hallux valgus was seen in the cases of Clendenning, *et al.* (1964),[33] Anderson and Cook (1966),[39] Stevanovic (1967),[64] and Becker (1967).[53] Minor cortical defects of long bones were noted by Cairns (1965);[73] Cerena, *et al.* (1969)[66] and Bataille, *et al.* (1969).[74]

Bilateral syndactyly of the second and third fingers was described by Mordecai[70] of the same fingers in one of our patients. Polydactyly of both thumbs and the right hallux was noted by Kahn and Gordon (1967)[17] as well as an extra fused terminal phalanx in the left hallux. Lile, *et al.* (1968)[55] remarked on shortened distal phalanges in the thumbs of their patients. Mordecai (1966)[70] also described polydactyly in one patient but the digits involved were not mentioned.

An extra metatarsal was noted by Davidson (1962).[75]

Pes Planus has also been observed.[20, 33, 37, 39, 59, 60, 72, 75–79]

Frontal bossing has already been mentioned. It is usually combined with bi-parietal bossing, producing a head circumference in adults of approximately 60 cm or more. Broadened nasal root has been noted in at least one–fourth of these patients and may exist without increased distance between inner canthi or without increased distance between the pupils.

Bridging of the sella was noted to occur in about 60 percent by Mills and Foulkes (1967),[48] a far higher incidence than in the normal population. This observation has been made by other authors.[37, 66, 72] Mills and Foulkes (1967)[48] also described platybasia in four of nine patients.

Of considerable interest is the Marfanoid build or unusually great height attained by several of these patients.[7, 33, 53, 57, 70, 73, 74, 76, 80, 81] Syndactyly and/or oligodactyly has been seen in several cases.[20, 32, 39, 48, 53, 59, 60, 70, 75, 81, 82]

Central Nervous System

Mild mental retardation and schizophrenia have been described.[1, 3, 6, 13, 32, 35, 53, 54, 58, 64, 66, 73, 83]

The normal occurrence of lamellar calcification of the dura in the parietal region, falx and petroclinoid ligament have been extensively studied by many authors. Nicotra (1929)[84] carried out a most extensive study on 400 clinical cases and 200 cadavers. Roentgenograms were correlated with dissection. Calcification was found in 0.75% and osteoma formation in 1%. These combined findings of about 2% probably represent a truer value than the 6–7% noted by others[85, 86] since Nicotra's original estimate of 8%, obtained roentgenographically, was not substantiated on dissection. Calcifications occur with somewhat greater frequency in males, the peak incidence being in the fourth decade.[87]

Calcification of the petroclinoid ligament is normally present in about 12.5% of individuals. The incidence is higher (19.5%) in skulls in which there is calcification of the falx.[88] Familial occurrence of this change as an autosomal dominant trait has been reported by the same authors.

Normally, the calcified falx is manifested as a clearly visible vertical thread–like shadow between 0.5 and 2.0 mm in width in the median sagittal plane in the A.P. projection. The most extensive survey has been that of Bruyn (1969)[86] who studied 2,595 roentgenograms, finding 5% to have either calcification or osteoma of the falx. Males more often had calcification while females more frequently had ossification of the falx.

The roentgenographic appearance of the calcification found in the multiple nevoid basal cell carcinoma syndrome is quite different from that noted in the normal population. Its lamellar appearance with one or more flat sheets is quite distinctive and usually extends more widely than that in the normal individual. The lamellar form of calcification has also been seen in patients with profound disturbances of calcium and phosphorus metabolism.[37]

Congenital communicating hydrocephalus was noted by Gross (1953),[89] Schamberg, (1960),[27] Maddox (1962),[20] Cawson (1964),[90] Gorlin, et al., (1965),[59] Formas (1967),[91] Rater, et al., (1968)[92] Tamoney (1969)[93] and Bang (1970).[35] It has been established in all cases, however, that this did not simply represent an abnormality of head form. Kahn and Gordon (1967)[17] described cysts of the choroid plexus of the third and lateral ventricles and glial nodules projecting into the walls of the lateral ventricles. Taylor, *et al.* (1968)[61] also described cysts in the brain and Binkley and Johnson (1951)[6] noted partial agenesis of the corpus callosum.

One of the more fascinating facets of the syndrome is medulloblastoma.[12, 15, 39, 61, 71, 74, 90, 94, 96] The occurrence was first pointed out by Herzberg and Wiskemann (1963).[12] The medulloblastoma which has occurred in cases of the multiple nevoid basal cell carcinoma syndrome usually appears during the first two years of life. It would seem likely that medulloblastoma was not heretofore recognized as a manifestation of the syndrome, since the affected child usually died of the tumor prior to the development of the rest of the syndrome. It is conceivable that more cases might be uncovered if family pedigrees were more carefully analyzed for the cause of death of "unaffected siblings". The brain tumor described by Moynahan (1964)[95] as "astrocytoma" was examined by one of the authors (R.J.G.) and found to be desmoplastic medulloblastoma. A child of the patient described by Telle (1965)[97] was stated to have died of a "meningeal sarcoma." A daughter of the proband described by Kennedy and Abbott (1968)[41] died of a "brain stem tumor" at the age of 2 years but information concerning its pathologic nature is lacking.

Medulloblastoma normally comprises about 20–25 percent of childhood intracranial tumors spreading via the cerebrospinal fluid to the subarachnoid space from which area seeding may occur either along the spinal cord or intracranially. Its prognosis has been considered to be extremely grave.

The number of cases of multiple nevoid basal cell carcinoma having associated medulloblastoma is far too small from which to draw conclusions concerning comparative behavior of the brain tumor. However, the odds of 1 per 600,000 population for this brain tumor calculated by your authors would make its co–occurrence by chance highly unlikely and thus we must conclude that it too arises in some way from the effect of the pleiotropic gene.

Craniopharyngioma was noted by Tamoney (1969)[93] in his patient. This is not too surprising since this tumor is the counterpart of ameloblastoma. A meningioma was noted in the same patient.

Nerve deafness was seen in the cases of Nichols and Solomon (1967)[32] and Mordecai (1966).[70]

Eye

Congenital blindness due to corneal opacity, cataract, glaucoma, and/or coloboma of the choroid and optic nerve have been recorded by Hermans, *et al.* (1960),[15] Oliver (1960),[98] Gorlin, *et al.* (1963),[11] Rasmussen (1963),[28] Meerkotter and Shear (1964),[71] Cawson (1964),[90] Anderson and Cook (1966),[39] Mills and Foulkes (1967),[48] Kahn and Gordon (1967),[17] Shear and Wilton (1968),[78] van Erp (1968)[49] and Cernea, *et al.* (1969).[66]

Hermans, *et al.* (1960)[15] thought that the eye changes which they described as "dysgenesis neuroblastica gliomatosis" were so characteristic as to be classified as a fifth type of phakomatosis. Kedem, *et al.* (1970)[50] described melanoma of the iris.

Convergent or divergent strabismus was seen by Jablonska (1961);[16] Gorlin, *et al.* (1963);[11] Block and Clendenning (1963);[13] Pimenta, *et al.* (1965);[51] Anderson and Cook (1966);[39] Anderson *et al.* (1967);[99] Veltman and Adari (1967);[83] van Erp (1968);[49] Cerneá, *et al.* (1969);[66] Bang (1970).[35]

Endocrine System

Gorlin, *et al.* (1963)[11] suggested that the shortened metacarpals and calcifications in various parts of the body might signify abnormal calcium and/or phosphorus excretion. Block and Clendenning (1963)[13] almost simultaneously published findings that demonstrated an almost complete lack of end–organ response to parathormone, almost no phosphorus diuresis being experienced. This finding has been substantiated in other laboratories.[53, 65, 66] It may be present in about 80 percent of patients affected with the syndrome.

Shortening of one or more metacarpals occurs in several other conditions among them pseudohypoparathyroidism, where it is called the dimple or Albright's sign and in Turner's syndrome. A positive metacarpal sign is obtained if a line touching the distal–most portion of the fourth and fifth metacarpals, crosses the third metacarpal. Hyporesponsiveness to parathormone attributed to a renal tubular defect is seen in pseudohypoparathyroidism and in Turner's syndrome.

Ovarian fibromas and/or cysts with ovarian or uterine calcification have been noted by a number of authors.[6, 11, 13, 14, 19, 28, 37, 39, 49, 50, 61, 66, 79, 92, 100] Dijk and Sanderink (1967)[60] noted bicornuate uterus. Lile, et al. (1968)[55] found a theca–cell tumor in one of their patients. Furthermore, several authors[7, 20, 28, 34,] [38, 49, 59, 64, 68, 69, 72, 75] have reported that several male patients have manifested hypogonadism. They have had cryptorchidism, a missing testicle, female pubic–hair pattern, gyneocomastia and/or scanty facial hair. The female patient reported by Swanson and Jacks (1961)[57] had never menstruated.

Oral Anomalies

Jaw cysts appear to be one of the more constant features, being seen in 65–75 percent. They have been classified as primordial cysts or odontogenic keratocysts. Often appearing initially during the first decade of life, they have been the chief source of complaint in about one–half the cases due to swelling of the jaws, dull pain, or drainage of the cysts intraorally. They are scattered throughout both jaws but are more common in the mandible. They vary in size from microscopic to several centimeters in diameter, occasionally being so large as to produce a pathological fracture.

If the cysts arise during the stage at which tooth root formation is progressing, the pressure engendered may result in bending or dilaceration of the adjacent roots, and the adjacent teeth are often markedly displaced. As the cysts become larger they may contain a displaced tooth, may bulge the anterior wall of the maxilla, and cause elevation of the infra–orbital rim. Maxillary teeth may often be displaced immediately beneath the orbit.

Microscopically, the uninfected cyst is lined by a monotonously uniform layer of keratin. This type of cyst has been designated as "primordial" by Shear (1960)[101] and as "odontogenic keratocyst" by Philipsen (1956).[102] Some cysts exhibit budding, reminiscent of embryonal skin, and it is likely that some tendency exists for the transformation of these cysts to ameloblastoma, as may be seen from the cases of Thoma (1959),[103] Davidson (1962),[75] Maddox (1962),[20] Gorlin, et al (1963),[11] and Pollard and New (1964).[37]

Recurrence of the curetted cysts is common, possibly from adjacent micro-cysts. These were nicely illustrated by Thoma and Blumenthal (1946)[104] and resulted in the term "polycystoma".[103]

It should be pointed out that there are a large number of cases reported in the literature in which several members of a kindred had multiple dentigerous cysts. Gorlin, et al. (1965)[59] suggested that several of these cases probably rep-resented examples of the syndrome in which the cutaneous component was either missing or minimally expressed. The nature of the neurogenic–appearing jaw "cyst" reported by Laugier, et al. (1966)[105] needs further investigation.

Fibrosarcoma of the palate of maxi-llary antrum has been noted in the cases of Binkley and Johnson (1951),[6] Howell and Caro (1959),[8] Reed (1968)[79] and Tamoney(1969).[93]

Cleft of the lip and/or palate has been seen in the cases of Clarkson and Wilson (1960),[82] Summerly (1965),[21] Storck, et al. (1966),[38] Tobias (1967),[34] Becker, et al. (1967),[53] Formas (1967),[91] Dijk and Sanderink (1969),[60] Veltman and Adari (1967),[83] Rater, et al. (1968)[92] and Bopp, et al. (1968).[106] Since the incidence of cleft lip with or without cleft palate in the normal population is approximately 1 per 700 births and that of isolated cleft palate is 1 per 2,500 births, the association of clefting of the primary and/or secondary palates in this syndrome does not appear to be due to chance.

Other Findings

A variety of kidney malformations [24, 59, 61, 62, 91,] have been noted and adrenal cortical adenomas have been found on autopsy in two patients.[61]

Of interest is the finding of lymphatic cysts of the mesentery of the small in-testines.[14, 24, 73, 79, 107, 108] Mesenteric cysts are remarkably rare, their occur-rence being somewhere in the range of 1 per 100,000 population.[109] Congenital rhabdomyosarcoma of the anterior chest wall was described in a patient by Schweisguth, et al. (1968)[110] and the present authors have seen a similar example.

Multiple leiomyomata, 0.1–3.0 cm. in diameter, were distributed over the mes-entery of the bowel and beneath the diaphragm of an infant described by Kahn and Gordon (1967)[17] and leiomyo-mas of the esophagus were noted on post-mortem in a patient by Taylor, et al. (1968).[61]

Heredity

As originally suggested by Gorlin and Goltz (1960),[1] the genetic pedigrees of many families exhibiting the syndrome clearly demonstrate that it is inherited as an autosomal dominant trait.[23, 58, 59, 99, 111] Penetrance appears to be marked and expressivity variable. The syndrome occurs almost equally in both sexes and analysis of pooled data from thoroughly examined kindreds exhibits an almost 1 : 1 ratio of affected and normal after correction for ascertainment bias. Off-spring of affected males are as frequently affected and without sex predilection as children of affected mothers. Neither is there a birth order effect. Many case reports have indicated that the patient was an isolated example implying new mutation. However, we cannot be certain, since in many cases, a really thorough examination has not been conducted and the expressivity of the syndrome is so remarkably variable.

The contention that the syndrome is inherited as an X–linked dominant trait, as stated by Block and Clendenning (1963)[13] is certainly not valid. With such a pattern, the syndrome should be transmitted to all daughters but to no sons of an affected male, and this is clearly not the case.[59, 99]

Discussion

Many terms have been employed in designation of this syndrome. Analysis of the appended bibliography reveals: basal cell nevus syndrome; nevoid basal cell carcinoma syndrome; epitheliomatose multiple multiforme generalisee (type Ferrari); syndrome of jaw cysts, basal cell tumors and skeletal anomalies; polycystoma; Fünfte Phakomatose, hereditary cutaneomandibular polyoncosis; Ward's syndrome and Gorlin's syndrome.

It should be obvious that at this time there is no ideal designation. The term "multiple nevoid basal–cell carcinoma syndrome" signifies and selects out but a single facet of this symptom–complex that affects so many of the body's systems. While the adnexal tumors constitute perhaps the most obvious or striking aspect, are they really of more intrinsic importance than any other aspect? To string out several of the clinical findings into a compound descriptive term seems terribly unwieldy. Furthermore, the implication that this syndrome represents a phakomatosis, a term in itself often subject to many interpretations and erroneous uses, seems rather unjustified.

As to the use of eponyms to describe a syndrome, while we can assure you that it is flattering for an author to have a syndrome named for him, it is unfair to others who have made outstanding contributions. It often becomes nationalistic and it is confusing if the author has more than one syndrome named in his honor. Further, it does little for the neophyte entering the field other than to serve as a hurdle in the mental gymnastics of memorizing the manifold syndromes and diseases relevant to his special interests.

There appear to be striking analogies between the cutaneous and jaw lesions. For example, the jaw cysts correspond to the cutaneous milia, and the adnexal skin tumors have their analogue in the mural proliferations seen in some of the jaw cysts. Furthermore, the ameloblastoma and craniopharyngioma are counterparts of the cutaneous basal–cell carcinoma.

The reported failure of the kidneys to respond to administered parathormone, is a most interesting phenomenon and may eventually provide the key to the biochemical defect that is the basis of the syndrome. The gene defect acts over a considerable period of development—during the early embryologic period—to produce bizarre rib anomalies and extends into mature adult life with continued formation of skin tumors and jaw cysts. The abbreviation of the fourth metacarpal is also seen in pseudohypoparathyroidism and in Turner's syndrome, conditions which also manifest hyporesponsiveness to parathormone. One may conjecture about a shared metabolic pathway in these three conditions. It should also be of interest that a patient with the so–called basal ganglia syndrome had medulloblastoma.[65]

No one component of the syndrome

is present in all patients, i.e., there is variable expressivity of the several facets. Some are more common, e.g., skin tumors, jaw cysts, skeletal anomalies, intracranial calcifications, and hyporesponsiveness to parathormone while other aspects may be more subtle and have heretofore been overlooked.

BIBLIOGRAPHY

1. Gorlin, R.J. and R.W. Goltz: Multiple Nevoid Basal–cell Epithelioma, Jaw Cysts and Bifid Rib Syndrome. *New Eng. J. Med. 262*: 908–912, 1960.

2. Satinoff, M.I. and C. Wells: Multiple Basal Cell Naevus in Ancient Egypt. *Med. History 13*: 294–296, 1969.

3. Jarish, –: Zur Lebre von den Hautgeschwulsten. *Arch. Derm. Syph. 28*: 163–222, 1894.

4. Nomland, R.: Multiple Basal Cell Epitheliomas Originating From Congenital Pigmented Basal Cell Nevi. *Arch. Derm. Syph. 25*: 1002–1008, 1932.

5. Straith, F.E.: Hereditary Epidermoid Cyst of Jaws. *Am. J. Orthodont. 25*: 673–691, 1939.

6. Binkley, G.W. and H.H. Johnson, Fr., Epithelioma adenoides cysticum: Basal Cell Nevi, Agenesis of Corpus callosum and Dental Cysts. *Arch. Derm. Syph. 63*: 73–84, 1951.

7. Boyer, B.E. and M.M. Martin: Marfan's Syndrome: Report of Case Manifesting Giant Bone Cyst of Mandible and Multiple (110) Basal Cell Carcinomata. *Plast. Reconstruct. Surg. 22*: 257–263, 1958.

8. Howell, J.B. and M.R. Caro: Basal–Cell Nevus: Its Relationship to Multiple Cutaneous Cancers and Associated Anomalies of Development. *Arch. Derm. 79*: 67–80, 1959.

9. Ward, W.H.: Naevoid Basal Celled Carcinoma Associated with Dyskeratosis of Palms and Soles: New Entity. *Australian J. Derm. 5*: 204–208, 1960.

10. Pollitzer, J.: Eine eigentumliche Karzinose der Haut (Carcinoderma pigmentosum–Lang) Nebenher: Punkt–und strichformige Defekte im Hornstratum der Palmae und Plantae. *Arch. Derm. Syph. (Berlin). 76*: 323–345, 1905.

11. Gorlin, R.J. and J.J. Yunis and N. Tuna: Multiple Nevoid Basal–Cell Carcinoma, Odontogenic Keratocyts and Skeletal Anomalies Syndrome. *Acta Dermatovener. 43*: 39–55, 1963.

12. Herzberg, J.J. and A. Wiskemann: Die funfte Phakomatose, Basalzellnaevus mit familiarer Belastung and Medulloblastom. *Dermatologica 126*: 106–173, 1963.

13. Block, J.B. and W.E. Clendenning: Parathyroid Hormone Hyporesponsiveness in Patients with Basal–Cell Nevi and Bone Defects. *New Eng. J. Med. 268*: 1157–1162, 1963.

14. Clendenning, W.E., J.R. Herdt, and J.B. Block: Ovarian Fibromas and Mesenteric Cysts; Their Association with Hereditary Basal Cell Cancer of Skin. *Amer J Obstet Gynec 87*: 1008–1012, 1963.

15. Hermans, E.J., J.C.M. Grosfield, and L.E.M. Valk: Eine funfte Phakomatosis; Naevus epitheliomatodes multiplex. *Hautarzt 11*: 160–164, 1960.

16. Jablonska, S.: Basaliome naevoider Herkunft (Naevo–basaliome bzw. Basalzellnaevi). *Hautarzt 12*: 147–157, 1961.

17. Kahn, L.B. and W. Gordon, Basal Cell Naevus Syndrome. *S. Afr: Med. J. 41*: 832–835, 1967.

18. Kirsch, T: Pathogenetische Beziehungen zwischen Kieferzysten und Hautveranderungen unter besonderer Berucksichtigung der Hautkarzinomatose.

Schweiz. Monatsschr. Zahnkeilk. *66*: 687–701, 1956.

19. Gilhuus–Moe, O., L.K. Haugen and P.M. Dee: The Syndrome of Multiple Cysts of the Jaws, Basal Cell Carcinomata and Skeletal Anomalies. *Brit. J, Oral Surg. 6*: 211–222, 1968.

20. Maddox, W.D.: *Multiple Basal Cell Tumors, Jaw Cysts and Skeletal Defects. A Clinical Syndrome.* M.S. Thesis, University of Minnesota (1962).

21. Summerly, R.: Basal Cell Carcinoma. An Aetiologic Study of Patients Aged 45 and Under with Special Reference to Gorlin's syndrome. *Brit. J. Derm. 77*: 9–15, 1965.

22. Zackheim, H.S., J.B. Howell, and A.V. Loud: Basal Cell Carcinoma Syndrome. *Arch. Derm. 96*: 317–323, 1966.

23. Maddox, W.D., R.K. Winkelmann, E.G. Harrison, K.D. Devine and J.A. Gibilisco: Multiple Nevoid Basal Cell Epitheliomata, Jaw Cysts and Skeletal Defects. *JAMA 188*: 106–111, 1964. 111, 1964.

24. Mason, J.K., E.B. Helwig, and J.H. Graham: Pathology of the Nevoid Basal Cell Carcinoma Syndrome. *Arch. Path. 79*: 401–408, 1965.

25. Graham, J.H., J.K. Mason, H.R. Gray and E.B. Helwig: Differentiation of Nevoid Basal–Cell Carcinoma from Epithelioma Adenoides Cysticum. *J. Invest. Derm. 44*: 197–200, 1965.

26. Murphey, K.J.: Subcutaneous Calcification in the Naevoid Basal Cell Carcinoma Syndrome. Response to Parathyroid Hormone and Relationship to Pseudohypoparathyroidism. *Clin. Radiol. 20*: 287–293, 1969.

27. Schamberg, I.L.: Basal–cell Nevi. *Arch. Derm. 81*: 269, 1960.

28. Rasmussen, P.E.: Folikulaere Kaebecyster, basal–celle–tumorer og knogle-

anomalier som led i et hereditareret syndrom. *Nord. Med. 69*: 606–612, 1963.

29. Noury, J.Y.: *La naevonatose baso-cellulaire.* Thesis, Paris, 1967.

30. Howell, J.B., D.E. Anderson, and J.L. McClendon: Multiple Cutaneous Cancers in Children: The Nevoid Basal-Cell Carcinoma Syndrome. *J. Pediat. 69*: 97–103, 1966.

31. Carney, R.G., Linear Unilateral Basal–Cell Nevus with Comedones. Report of Case. *Arch. Derm. Syph. 65*: 471–476, 1952.

32. Nichols, L. and L.M. Solomon: Basal Cell Nevi Syndrome. *Arch. Derm. 91*: 188–189, 1965.

33. Clendenning, W.E., J.B. Block and I.C. Radde: Basal Cell Nevus Syndrome. *Arch. Derm. 90*: 38–53, 1964.

34. Tobias, C.: Zum Basalzellnaevus-Kieferzysten Syndrome (Ward Syndrom) mit familiarem Auftreten. *Schweiz. med. Wschr. 97*: 949–952, 1967.

35. Bang, G., Keratocysts, Skeletal Anomalies, Icthyosis and Defective Response to Parathyroid Hormone in a Patient with Basal Cell Carcinoma. *Oral Surg. 29*: 242–248, 1970.

36. Calnan, C.D.: Two Cases of Multiple Naevoid Basal Cell Epitheliomata? Porokeratosis of Mantoux. *Brit. J. Derm. 65*: 219–221, 1953.

37. Pollard, J.J. and P.F.J. New: Hereditary Cutaneomandibular Polyoncosis. A Syndrome of Myriad Basal Cell Nevi of the Skin, Mandibular Cysts, and Inconstant Skeletal Anomalies. *Radiology 82*: 840–849, 1964.

38. Storck, J., K. Schwarz and I. Cavegn: Naevoid Basaliome mit Kieferzysten (Ward Syndrome). Icthyosis vulgaris palmo–plantar keratose. Kryptorchismus. Gespaltene Uvula. *Dermatologica 133*: 145–150, 1966.

39. Anderson, D.E. and W.E. Cook:

Jaw Cysts and the Basal Cell Nevus Syndrome. *J. Oral Surg. 24*: 15–26, 1966.

40. Ziprowski, L., Exhibit on Genodermatoses. Basal Cell Nevus Syndrome. XII Internat. Congress Dermatology, Munich, 1967, Springer–Verlag, Berlin–Heidelberg – New York, p. 1419.

41. Kennedy, J.W. and P.L. Abbott: Nevoid Basal–Cell Carcinoma Syndrome. *Oral Surg. 26*: 406–414, 1968.

42. Keen, R.R.: Multiple Basal–Cell Nevoid Syndrome. Report of Two Cases. *J. Oral Surg. 27*: 404–408, 1969.

43. Holubar, K., Matras, H., and Smalik, A.V.: Multiple Basal Cell Epitheliomas in Basal Cell Nevus Syndrome. *Arch. Derm. 101*: 679–682, 1970.

44. McEvoy, B.F., H. Gatzek: Multiple Nevoid Basal Cell Carcinoma Syndrome. Radiologic Manifestations. *Brit. J. Radiol 42*: 24–28, 1969.

45. Etter, L.E.: Osseous Abnormalities of Thoracic Cage Seen in 40,000 Consecutive Chest Roentgenograms. *Amer. J. Roentgen. 51*: 359–363, 1944.

46. Ashbury, H.E., J.G. Wilding, and F.T. Rogers: Roentgenological Reports of Chest Examination Made of Registrants at U.S. Army Induction Station No. 6, Third Corps Area, Baltimore, Md. May 1, 1941 to March 31, 1942.

47. Eisenbud, L., H. Brooks, and S. Busch: Klippel–Feil Syndrome with Multiple Cysts of Jawbones. *Oral Surg. 5*: 659–666, 1952.

48. Mills, J. and J. Foulkes: Gorlin's Syndrome. A Radiological and Cytogenetic Study of 9 Cases. *Brit. J. Radiol. 40*: 366–371, 1967.

49. Erp, I.F.R., van, Naevus epitheliomatodes multiplex. *Dermatologica. 136*: 257–264, 1968.

50. Kedem, A. et al.: Basal Cell Nevus Syndrome Associated with Malignant Melanoma of the Iris. *Dermatologica. 140*: 99–106, 1970.

51. Pimenta, W.P., P.M.G. Pagnano, and H.J.S. Brandao: Sindrome do nevo–basocellular. *Anais Bras. Derm. 40*: 190–191, 1965.

52. Gunderson, C.H.: The Klippel–Feil Syndrome. Genetic and Clinical Re-evaluation of Cervical Fusion. *Medicine 46*: 491–512, 1967.

53. Becker, M.H., A.W. Kopf, and A. Lande: Basal Cell Nevus Syndrome. Its Roentgenologic Significance. Review of the literature and Report of Four Cases; *Amer. J. Roentgen. 99*: 816–825, 1967.

54. Bramley, P.A. and R.M. Browne: Recurring Odontogenic Cysts. *Brit. J. Oral Surg. 5*: 106–116, 1968.

55. Lile, H.A., J.F. Rogers and B. Gerald: The Basal Cell Nevus Syndrome. *Amer. J. Roentgen. 103*: 214–218, 1968.

56. Worth, H.M. and Wollin, D.G.: The Basal Cell Naevi and Jaw Cyst Syndrome. *Clin. Radiol. 19*: 416–420, 1968.

57. Swanson, A.E. and Q.D. Jacks: An Unusual Propensity for Odontogenic Cyst Formation. *J. Canad. Dent. Ass. 27*: 723–731, 1961.

58. Gerber, N.J.: Zur Pathologie und Genetik des Basalzell–Naevus Syndroms. *Humangenetik 1*: 354–373, 1965.

59. Gorlin, R.J., R.A. Vickers, E. Kelln, and J.J. Willaimson: The Multiple Basal-cell Nevi Syndrome. An Analysis of a Syndrome Consisting of Multiple Nevoid Basal-cell Carcinoma, Jaw Cysts, Skeletal Anomalies, Medulloblastoma and Hyporesponsiveness to Parathormone. *Cancer 18*: 89–104, 1967.

60. Dijk, E. van and J.F.H. Sanderink: Basal Cell Nevus Syndrome. *Dermatologica 134*: 101–106, 1967.

61. Taylor, W.B., D.E. Anderson, J.B.

Howell and C.S. Thurston: The Nevoid Basal Cell Carcinoma Syndrome. *Arch. Derm. 98*: 612–614, 1968.

62. Summerly, R. and Hale, A.J.: Basal Cell Naevus Syndrome. *Trans. St. John Derm. Soc. 51*: 77–79, 1965.

63. Smith, N.H.H.: Multiple Dentigerous Cysts Associated with Arachnodactyly and other Skeletal Defects. *Oral Surg. 25*: 99–107, 1968.

64. Stevanovic, D.V.: Nevoid Basal Cell Carcinoma Syndrome. *Arch. Derm. 96*: 696–698, 1967.

65. Berlin, N.I., E.J. Scott, W.E. Clendenning, H.O. Archard, J.B. Block, C.J. Witkop and H.A. Haynes: Basal Cell Nevus Syndrome. *Ann Intern. Med. 64*: 403–421, 1966.

66. Cernea, P., R. Kuffer, M. Baumont, C. Brocheriou, and F. Guilbert: Naevomatose baso–cellulaire. *Rev. Stomat. 70*: 181–226, 1969.

67. Bloom, R.A.: The Metacarpal Syndrome. *Brit. J. Radiol. 43*: 133–135, 1970.

68. Lausecker, H.: Beitrag zu den Naevo–Epitheliomen. *Arch. Derm. 194*: 639–666, 1952.

69. Davidson, F. and J.J. Key: Multiple Nevoid Basal Cell Carcinomata and Associated Congenital Abnormalities. *Proc. Roy. Soc. Med. 57*: 891, 1964.

70. Mordecai, L.R.: Basal Cell Nevus Syndrome. *J. Nat. Med. Ass. 58*: 32–34, 1966.

71. Meerkotter, V.A. and M. Shear: Multiple Primordial Cysts Associated with Bifid Rib and Ocular Defects. *Oral Surg. 18*: 498–503, 1964.

72. Jones, J.E., P.C. Desper, W.A. Welton, and E.B. Flink: The Nevoid Basal-Cell Carcinoma Syndrome. *Arch. Intern. Med. 115*: 723–729, 1965.

73. Cairns, R.J.: Commenting on Case of Caron, G.A.

74. Bataille, R., J.C. Vigneul and J. Marsen: Deux cas de naevomatose. *Rev. Stomat. 70*: 305–306, 1969.

75. Davidson, F.: Multiple Naevoid Basal Cell Carcinomata and Associated Congenital Abnormalities. *Brit. J. Derm. 74*: 439–444, 1962.

76. Ferrier, P.E. and W.L. Hinrichs: Basal Cell Carcinoma Syndrome. *Amer. J. Dis. Child. 113*: 538–545, 1967.

77. Abrahams, I.: Basal Cell Nevus Syndrome. *Arch. Derm. 92*: 747–748, 1965.

78. Shear, M. and Welton, E.: Cytogenetic Studies of the Basal Cell Carcinoma Syndrome. *J. Dent. Ass. S. Afr. 23*: 99–104, 1968.

79. Reed, J.C.: Nevoid Basal Cell Carcinoma Syndrome with Associated Fibrosarcoma of the Maxilla. *Arch. Derm. 97*: 304–306, 1968.

80. Binkley, G.W.: Basal Cell Nevi with Bone Anomalies and Dystopia Canthorum. *Arch. Derm. 90*: 104–106, 1964.

81. Kopp, W.K., J. Klatell, and M. Blake: Basal Cell Nevus Syndrome with Other Abnormalities. *Oral Surg. 27*: 9–14, 1969.

82. Clarkson, P. and H. Wilson: Two Cases of Basal–Cell Congenital Naevus. *Proc. Roy. Soc. Med. 53*: 295–296, 1960.

83. Veltman, G. and Adari, S.: Zur Klinik und Chromosomenanalyse der V. Phakomatose. XII Internat. Congress of Dermatology, Munich, 1967, Springer-Verlag. Berlin, Heidelberg, New York, pp. 575–576.

84. Nicotra, A.: La calcificazione e l'osteoma della falce del cervello, al controllo anatomo–radiologico e clinico. *Arch. Radiol.* (Napoli), *5*: 794, 1929.

85. Parnitzke, K.H.: *Endokranielle Verkalkungen im Rontgenbild. Ihre Deutung und Bedeutung im Dienste der klinischen*

Hirndiagnostik. G. Thieme, Leipzig, 1961.

86. Bruyn: Personal Communication, 1969.

87. Dyke, C.G.; Indirect Signs of Brain Tumor as Noted in Routine Roentgeno-examination. Displacement of the Pineal Shadow. A Survey of 3000 Consecutive Skull Examinations. *Amer. J. Roentgen. 23*: 598, 1930.

88. Stanton, J.B. and M. Wilkinson: Familial Calcification of the Petrosplenoidal Ligament. *Lancet 2*: 736, 1949.

89. Gross, P.P.: Epithelioma Adenoides Cysticum with Follicular Cysts of Maxilla and Mandible. Report of Case. *J. Oral Surg. 11*: 160–165, 1953.

90. Cawson, R.A. and G.A. Kerr: The Syndrome of Jaw Cysts, Basal Cell Tumors and Skeletal Anomalies. *Proc. Roy. Soc. Med. 57*: 799–801, 1964.

91. Formas, I.: Naevobasaliom. *Zschr. Haut-Geschl.-krkh. 42*: 131–140, 1967.

92. Rater, C.J., A.C. Selke, and E.F. Van Epps: Basal Cell Nevus Syndrome. *Amer. J. Roentgen. 103*: 589–594, 1968.

93. Tamoney, H.J., Jr.,: Basal Cell Nevoid Syndrome. *Amer. Surg. 35*: 279–283, 1969.

94. Cook, W.A.: Family Pedigree–Cancer, Cysts and Oligodontia. *Dent. Radiogr. Photogr. 37*: 27–35. 1964.

95. Moynahan, E.J.: Basal Cell Nevus Syndrome. *Trans. St. Johns Hosp. Derm. Soc. 50*: 187–188, 1964.

96. Graham, J.K., B.A. McJimsey, and J.C. Harden, Jr.: Nevoid Basal Cell Carcinoma Syndrome. *Arch. Otolaryng. 87*: 72–77, 1968.

97. Telle, B.: Multiple Basalioma bei einem jungen Mann. *Derm. Wschr. 151*: 1425–1431, 1965.

98. Oliver, R.M.: Basal–cell Nevus. *Arch. Derm. 81*: 284–285, 1960.

99. Anderson, D.E., W.B. Taylor, H.F. Falls, and R.T. Davidson: The Nevoid Basal Cell Carcinoma Syndrome. *Amer. J. Hum. Genet. 19*: 12–22, 1967.

100. Bazex, A., A. Dupre, M. Parant, and L. Bessiere: Epitheliomatose multiple, multiforme generalisee (type Ferrari). *Bull. Soc. Franc. Derm. Syph. 67*: 72–74, 1960.

101. Shear, M.: Primordial Cysts. *J. Dent. Ass. S. Afr. 15*: 211–217, 1960. 1960.

102. Philipsen, H.P.: Om keratocyster (kolesteatomer) i kaeberne. *Tandlaegebladet 60*: 963–980, 1956.

103. Thoma, K.H.: Polycystome. *Oral Surg. 12*: 484–488, 1959.

104. Thoma, K.H. and F.R. Blumenthal: Hereditary and Cyst Formation. *Amer. J. Orthodont. 32*: 273–281, 1946.

105. Laugier, P., A. Opperman, G. Pageaut: Syndrome naevique a predominance baso–cellulaire (5e phacomatose). *Ann. Derm. Syph.* (Paris) *93*: 361–372, 1966.

106. Bopp, C., L. Bakos, and H. Ebling: Sindrome Nevo baso celular. *Rev. Ass. Med. Rio Grande do Sul. 12*: 3–19, 1968.

107. Degos, R., J. Civatte, and M. Labrousse: Naevus baso–callulaire. *Bull. Soc. Franc. Derm. Syph. 73*: 360–361, 1966.

108. Batschwarov, B. and D. Minkov: Naevobasaliom, Mesenterialzysten und Maligom. *Derm. Wschr. 153*: 1294–1302, 1967.

109. Beahrs, O.H., E.S. Judd, and M.B. Dockerty: Chylous Cysts of the Abdomen. *Surg. Clin. N. Amer. 30*: 1081–1096, 1950.

110. Schweisguth, O., R. Gerard–Marchant and J. Lemerle: Naevomatose baso–cellulaire association a un rhabdomyosarcoma congenital. *Arch. Franc. Ped. 25*: 1083–1093, 1968.

111. McKelvey, L.E., C.R. Albright, and G. Prazak: Multiple Hereditary Familial Epithelial Cysts of Jaws with Associated Anomaly of Trichoepithelioma: Report of Case. *Oral Surg. 13*: 111–116, 1960.

Chapter 10

GARDNER'S SYNDROME

by Alvin Watne, M.D.

The association of visible and palpable soft tissue masses and bony tumors with the development of polyps of the colon was recognized by Devic and Bussy[1] in 1912 when they described a woman with osteomas of the mandible, sebaceous cysts of the scalp, subcutaneous lipomas and multiple polyposis coli.

Although a few similar cases had been reported prior to 1950[2, 3, 4] it was Elden J. Gardner who described the disease syndrome[5, 6]. Gardner's syndrome included multiple polyps of the lower digestive tract[7, 8] bone tumors (osteomas)[9, 10] connective tissue lesions (fibromas) and skin lesions (sebaceous cysts)[11]. MacDonald *et al*[12] reported that 118 cases had appeared in the literature by 1967 and there have been more reports of patients manifesting colonic polyposis with one or more of the other components of the syndrome.

Familial Incidence

The mode of inheritance of this syndrome appears to consistently follow an autosomal Mendelian dominant pattern. Gardner's original reports and follow-up data suggest that it results from a single defective gene, or from several separate but closely linked genes[8, 13]. In a review of 201 patients with familial polyposis, Smith[14] submitted that Gardner's syndrome represents the complete manifestation of a number of possible changes which might be present in any patient with multiple polyposis. McKusick[15] gave evidence to support the premise that this syndrome resulted from a single gene which was different from that responsible for simple familial polyposis.

We are presently following the members of four apparently unrelated families with the syndrome. The largest of these traces its ancestry back over five generations to some of the earliest settlers west of the Allegheny mountains. The genealogies of the four families (Fig. 1) represent a total of 143 persons who have been directly involved in the families; 114 of these people are under current investigation. Seventy-three of the members have thus exhibited one or more of the clinical features of the syndrome. Fifty-three patients have shown some type of soft tissue tumor, usually epidermal inclusion cysts or fibromas. Twenty-nine patients had osteomas or bony exostosis. However, the majority of the patients did not have the sophisticated x-ray survey required to identify small bony growths. Twenty-one patients had the entire triad of soft tissue tumors, bony tumors, and colonic polyposis.

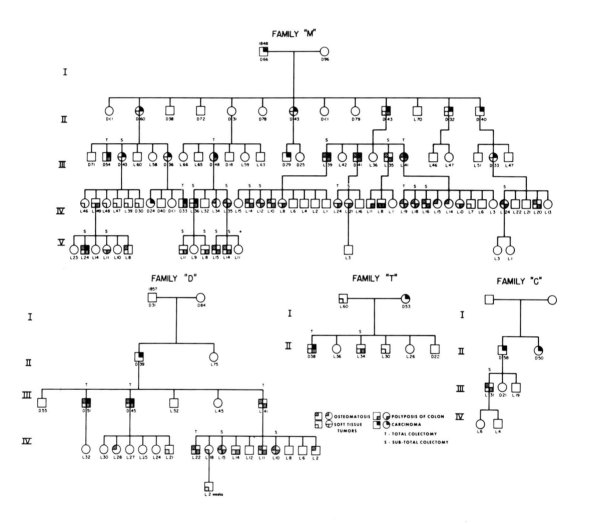

Figure 1. Genealogy of four unrelated families with Gardner's syndrome.

Twenty–six members have developed adenocarcinoma of the colon or rectum, and twenty–two of these are dead of their disease. The youngest patient with bowel cancer was 24 years old and the oldest patient to succumb to his cancer was the patriarch of family "M", a man born in 1848 who died of "bowel trouble" at the age of 66. Thirty–two patients have had a prophylactic colon resection for colonic polyposis. The sex distribution of the soft tissue tumors, osteomas, polyps, and carcinomas has been equal.

Clinical Features

The diagnostic features of the syndrome have shown a wide divergence in our patients. Great variations in the manifestations of the syndrome are also appearing in the literature.
Soft Tissue Tumors: The most common soft tissue tumors have been epidermal inclusion cysts. Paget[16], in 1853, was probably the first to mention the hereditary aspect of "sebaceous cysts." Cabot[2], Gardner, and Richards[11] and Oldfield[17] all emphasized the relation of sebaceous cysts and polyps of the colon. All of the members of family "M" who have undergone biopsy have shown such skin cysts. The presence of large cysts around the face, neck, and arms is characteristic of the syndrome (Fig. 2A, B, & C). These "lumps" were recognized by members of this family as a family trait. These cysts have at times been seen as large conglomerate subcutaneous masses covering an area as large as 12 centimeters in diameter. They have also been seen as rather small lesions representing sebaceous gland hyperplasia and may be overlooked (Fig. 3A, B). The cysts have been observed as young as a 14–day–old infant, but have generally appeared before puberty and continue to increase in size, even after colectomy for the polyposis.

The majority of patients in Family "D" have shown keloidal type of fibrous growths as their soft tissue tumors, (Fig. 4). These lesions tend to be localized to the trunk and extremities, and continue to appear and grow in size throughout life regardless of the status of the colon polyps. Unfortunately Family "D" members have shown retroperitoneal fibrosis, mesenteric fibrosis, hypertrophic scars, desmoid tumors, and fibrosarcomas. Three brothers in the third generation of Family "D" (Fig. 1, D.–III, 2, 3 & 6) have had repeated resections of abdominal wall and mesenteric fibrous tumors in addition to their colon cancers. Two of them eventually succumbed to their disease. One (D–III–2) died secondary to mesenteric fibrosis and bowel obstruction. Simpson, Harrison and Mayo[18] pointed out the serious nature of mesenteric fibrosis occurring in patients with Gardner's syndrome or familial polyposis and reported one patient who died from the intestinal obstruction and another who could not have a rectal carcinoma resected because of "unbelievable matting". The third brother (D–III–3) died from recurrent fibrosarcoma. The other brother underwent a total colectomy for the polyposis and in addition has a desmoid tumor which arose *de novo* in his right thigh (Fig. 5). His daughter (D–IV–10) underwent a subtotal colectomy and ileoproctostomy for colonic polyposis at the age of 15. Within one year she had developed a discrete mass in the abdominal wound scar and an ill–defined deep abdominal mass. At laparotomy she had severe retroperitoneal fibrosis (Fig. 6) and the abdominal wall mass was a low–grade

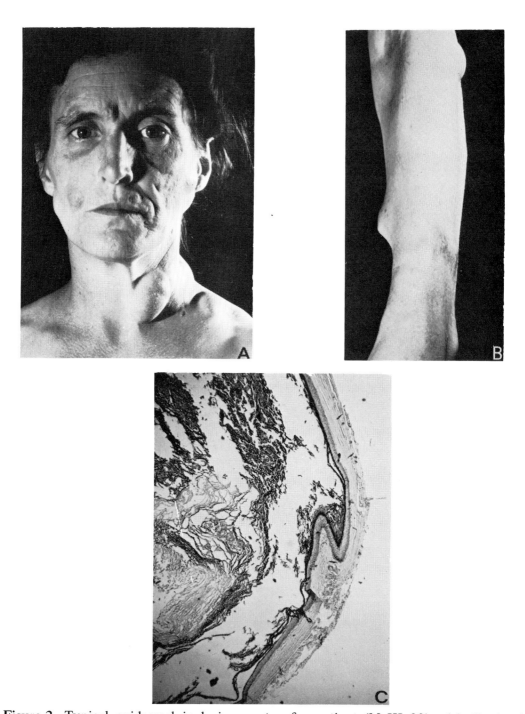

Figure 2. Typical epidermal inclusion cysts of a patient (M–III–20) with Gardner's syndrome

    A. Typical facial and neck cysts

    B. Cysts on the forearm

    C. Histology of epidermoid inclusion cyst. H & E stain, x 40.

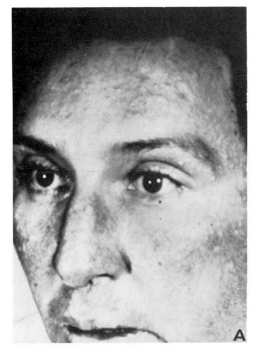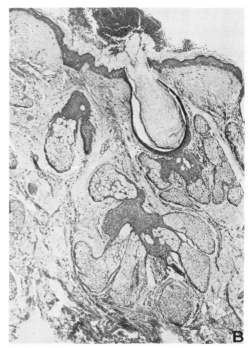

Figure 3. Sebaceous gland hyperplasia associated with Gardner's syndrome (T–II–1)
   A. Facial manifestation of sebaceous gland hyperplasia
   B. Histology of sebaceous gland hyperplasia H & E stain x 40.

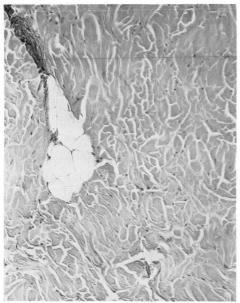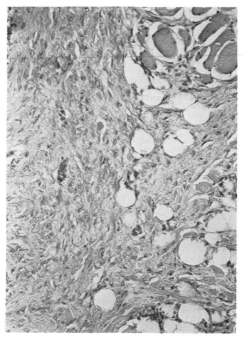

Figure 4. Keloidal overgrowth of fibrous tissue arising in abdominal surgical scar (D–IV–8) H & E stain, x 100

Figure 5. Desmoid tumor of thigh (D–III–6) H & E Stain, x 100

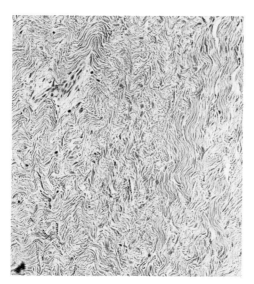

Figure 6. Retroperitoneal fibrosis arising one year after abdominal
colectomy (D–IV–10), H &
E stain, x 100

fibrosarcoma, desmoid type (Fig. 7).
In 1937 Miller and Sweet[19] reported a
patient with familial polyposis who developed a fibrosarcoma, desmoid type, of
the abdominal surgical scar. In 1943
Fitzgerald[3] reported a patient with recurrent desmoid tumors of the abdominal
wall and in 1945 Pugh and Nesselroad[20]
reported a patient with familial polyposis
and mesenteric fibrosis. O'Brien and
Wels[21] reported desmoid tumors in patients with familial polyposis. Smith[22]
reported a 26 year–old woman who died
as a result of a desmoid tumor that arose
de novo in her neck. He emphasized the
frequency of desmoid tumors in familial
polyposis, stating that it occurred in
3.5% of the patients with familial
polyposis compared to 0.03% for
the general population. Musgrove[23] reviewed the problem of extra–abdominal
desmoid tumors and believed their etiology could be from trauma or on an endocrine basis. Seventy per cent of his pa-

tients were female. He also believed
these patients exhibited some type of
"fibromatogenic principle". In a follow-
up of his original patients Gardner[13] noted the recurrence of fibromas and the development of a fibrosarcoma in the scar
on the back of a 2–year–old girl. A patient of Gumpel and Carballo[24] had a
9.5 lb. retroperitoneal fibrosarcoma
which apparently arose *de novo*. One of
Fader's patients had an abdominal fibro-
myxosarcoma[25]. Lipomas and leiomyo-
sarcomas have been reported[26], but we
have seen none in our patients. Retroperitoneal leiomyomas were reported in
familial polyposis by Clark and Parker[27]
Severe hemorrhage from a leiomyoma of
the jejunum was reported by Gumpel
and Carballo[24]. Collins[28] reported a
leiomyoma of the ileum. Guisto *et al*[29]
reported a leiomyosarcoma of the ascending colon of a patient with multiple
polyposis. Weston and Weiner[30] have
reported the association of colonic polyposis, bony exostoses, soft tissue tumors
and pigmented spots over the trunk. We

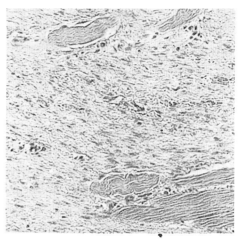

Figure 7. Low–grade fibrosarcoma, desmoid type arising in abdominal
wall scar one year after abdominal colectomy (D–IV–10) H
& E Stain, x 100.

have not seen this variation of the syndrome. Lipomas of the skin were reported by Collins[28] and Laberge *et al*[31]. Enterline[32] reported a liposarcoma in a patient with multiple polyposis.

Bony Tumors: The diagnosis of bone involvement requires a complete radiologic skeletal survey. The bone abnormalities observed most frequently with Gardner's syndrome are benign osteomatosis consisting of dense, bony proliferations of various sizes ranging from slight thickenings to large masses. They may involve almost all parts of the skeletal system.

Localized cortical thickening in the long tubular bones was the most common abnormality in a survey of our patients (Fig. 8)[33]. The short tubular bones were

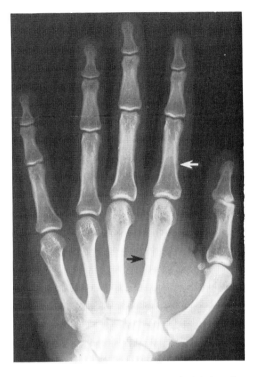

Figure 9. Localized cortical thickening of metacarpal and phalange of a patient with Gardner's syndrome after Chang et al.[33]

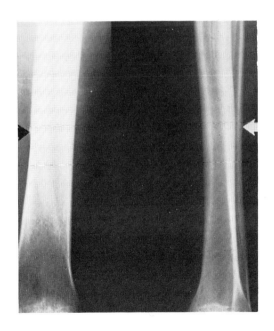

Figure 8. Localized cortical thickening of tibia & fibula of a patient with Gardner's syndrome. These bony growths were not clinically detectable. After Chang et al.[33]

also involved (Fig. 9). The frontal bone was the most frequent site of osteoma in the skull. Mandibular osteomas or central enostoses were frequently seen, as well as dental abnormalities. We have seen supernumerary teeth and unerupted teeth in 8 patients (Fig. 10). Fitzgerald's original patient[3] had multiple compound odontoma, torus palatinus, carious teeth and 37 rudimentary teeth and 2 permanent teeth embedded in the alveolar process. Fader *et al*[25] associated multiple impacted supernumerary and permanent teeth with the syndrome.

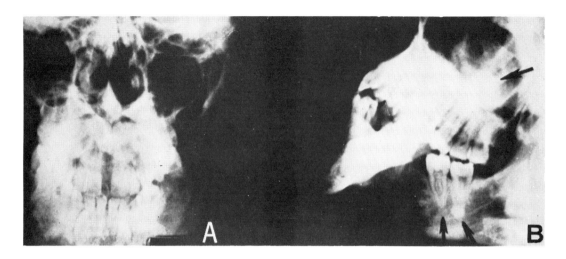

Figure 10. Dental abnormalities associated with Gardner's syndrome
        A. Frontal projection of mandible showing supernumerary and unerupted teeth.
        B. Oblique view showing enostoses involving central portion of mandible (arrows) and hypercernentosis after Chang et al.[33]

The cuboid bones were rarely involved and no obvious abnormalities were detected in the vertebrae. Our youngest patient with bone lesions was an 8–year old boy, who also had soft tissue tumors, but had not developed colon polyps. In our patients the soft tissue or bony tumors appear to precede the intestinal polyposis.

A member of family D (D–IV–3) underwent an above knee amputation at the age of 15 for osteogenic sarcoma. She has refused all follow–up care or examination, but is now 15 years post surgery and manifests no other stigmata of the syndrome. Two other patients with Gardner's syndrome and bone sarcoma have been reported[34]. Another family with multiple polyposis had members who developed pulmonary osteosarcoma, retroperitoneal liposarcoma and reticulum cell sarcoma.[35]

Colon Polyps: The finding of the soft tissue tumors and/or osteomas in patients with a family history suggestive of this syndrome should alert the physician to investigate the colon for the presence of polyps. We feel that this initial examination should include both a proctoscopic examination and a barium enema examination. We have never seen polyps diagnosed by barium enema that were not also visible at proctoscopy in our adult patients. However, we have seen the reverse situation in children. We have observed the development of polyps in young children following the identification of soft tissue and bony tumors, but we also have patients in their fourth and fifth decades with soft tissue tumors and no other manifestations of the disease (Fig. 1, M–IV–1, 3, 4, 5, 6). Colonic polyps have been demonstrated in 16 patients under the age of 15. LeFevre and Jacques[36] reported multiple colonic polyposis in an infant four months old. The polyps arise as very small excrescences and develop into typical mucosal polyps. (Fig. 11A, B, & C). In only one patient were these polyps grossly pedunculated (Fig. 12). Our patients showed no significant difference in the biologic behavior or location of the polyps when contrasted with patients with simple familial polyposis. The polyps were most prevalent in the rectum but were also scattered throughout the remainder of the colon with predominance at one or both colonic flexures. The disease starts with a few polyps present in the young child and these increase with age until a complete blanketing of the colonic mucosa has developed (Fig. 13). Of the patients that we have carefully examined only one boy (M–IV–27), 11 years of age has shown colon polyps without another stigmata of the syndrome. His brother (M–IV–28) had only one skin cyst present. The high rate of association of the components of the syndrome would tend to confirm the theories of McKusick[15] that a single gene, separate from that re-

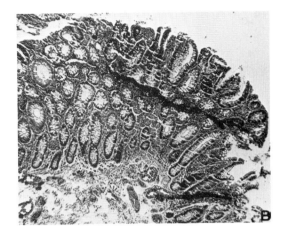

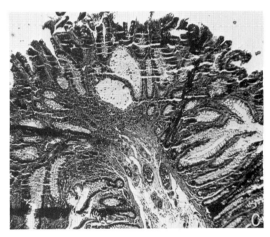

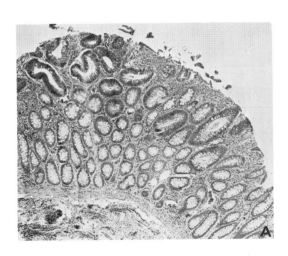

Figure 11. Stages of colonic polyp development associated with Gardner's syndrome. H & E Stain, x 100.

    A. Superficial mucosal excrescence, early stage of polyp formation.

    B. Adenomatous change involves all layers of mucosal cells, polyps are readily visible and palpable.

    C. Adenomatous polyp developing a pedunculated stalk, a relatively rare stage for Gardner's polyposis.

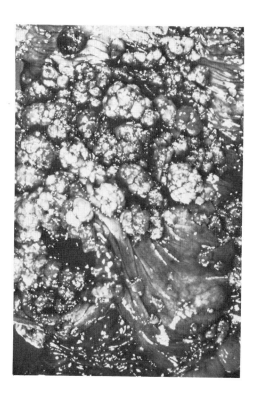

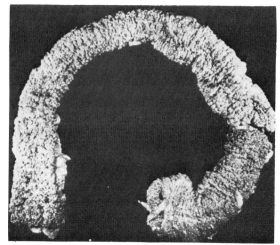

Figure 13. Gross specimen of abdominal colon of patient with Gardner's syndrome. The cobblestone appearance of the mucosal polyps is the usual type of colon polyposis seen with the syndrome.

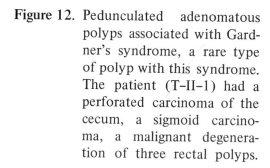

Figure 12. Pedunculated adenomatous polyps associated with Gardner's syndrome, a rare type of polyp with this syndrome. The patient (T–II–1) had a perforated carcinoma of the cecum, a sigmoid carcinoma, a malignant degeneration of three rectal polyps.

sponsible for familial polyposis, is involved. Pierce[37] showed a penetrance value of 49.43% for the siblings of patients with familial polyposis. It would appear that the penetrance value for the Gardner's syndrome is much higher. The potential for malignant degeneration of these polyps, if left untreated, is 100 percent. None of our patients with

polyps lived beyond the seventh decade without developing adenocarcinoma. When the cancers developed they were typical adenocarcinomas (Fig. 14) and invariably multiple. In family "M" there was a tendency for the bowel carcinomas to appear at an earlier age for each successive generation, the average ages for the generations being 66, 43, 40, 30 and 24 years respectively. The average at time of death of those members dying of adenocarcinoma was 41 years, virtually identical to that reported by Dukes as the average age of death from adenocarcinoma in patients with familial polyposis.[38]

Our patients have frequently demonstrated lymphoid hyperplasia, and, in two patients polypoid masses were present in the terminal ileum and were found on microscopic examination to be hyper-

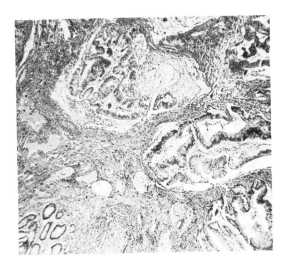

Figure 14. Adenocarcinoma of the rectum of a patient (M–III–20) with Gardner's syndrome. The woman also had 3 adenocarcinomas of the abdominal colon. H & E stain, x 100.

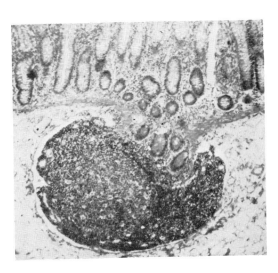

Figure 15. Hypertrophied lymphoid tissue of the distal ileum of a patient with Gardner's syndrome. H & E stain, x 100. Adapted from Watne et al CA 19: 267–275, 1969.

trophied lymphoid tissue. (Fig. 15). None of our patients have had true polyps or carcinomas of the small intestine, yet other authors have reported polyps and adenocarcinomas of the pancreas and ampulla of Vater in patients with Gardner's syndrome[2, 12], and Capps[39] a patient with familial polyposis of the colon who developed 5 synchronous colon carcinomas at age 14, four years later developed adenocarcinoma of the ampulla of Vater, and 13 years after his initial colon surgery developed a transitional cell carcinoma of the bladder.

Other Associated Findings with Gardner's Syndrome:

Throughout the literature there are occasional reports of other lesions associated in patients with Gardner's syndrome or familial polyposis. Additional skin lesions have included a squamous cell carcinoma of the chest in a 30–year–old male reported by Shiffman[40]. Fader[25] reported a woman who developed anaplastic carcinoma of the mandible. Gardner[13] reported a patient who manifested the syndrome including trichoepitheliomas along with sebaceous cysts. O'Brien and Wels[21] reported a patient who developed a fibrous tumor of the parotid gland at the age of nine years. Lieberman[41] remarked on the frequency with which patients with colon polyps give a history of having nasal polyps. While the majority of patients reported have been Caucasian, there are documented Negro patients[25, 35]. Weston and Weiner[30] reported the association of distinctive trunkal nevi with other manifestations of Gardner's syndrome. Yaffee[42] reported what he considered a variant of Gardner's syndrome involving skin nevi, fibromas, epidermal cysts and gastric polyps. The patient's maternal uncle had a frontal glioblastoma and polyposis coli, her father had an osteoma of the skull and Kaposi's sarcoma, and her paternal uncle had osteogenic sarcoma. The Cronkhite–Canada[43] syndrome includes polyps of the stomach, duodenum, ileum and colon along with abnormal pigmentation, alopecia and onchotrophia. Baughman *et al*[44] associated pigmented nevi, café au lait spots, colonic polyposis and brain tumors. He believed the inheritance as well as those patients previously reported by Turcot *et al*[45] to be on the basis of an autosomal recessive trait.

Camiel *et al*[46] reported pigmented nevi associated with one of their patients who developed thyroid carcinoma nine years before he was diagnosed as having Gardner's syndrome. The patient's father had colorectal polyposis and a brain tumor. Crail[47] presented a 24–year–old man who died of a medulloblastoma of the brain, with papillary carcinoma of the thyroid, present for 10 years, and had adenocarcinoma associated with colonic polyposis. Smith's[48] first patient developed follicular, papillary and solid adenocarcinoma of the thyroid gland ten years before he was recognized as having Gardner's syndrome. The author also reported two other patients with familial polyposis and papillary carcinoma of the thyroid gland[49]. Wermer[50] reported subcutaneous and bony lesions associated with endocrine adenomatosis. Cabot's[2] original patient had an adrenal adenoma, and Weiner[51] found a family where 19 of 20 patients with peptic ulceration showed some kind of endocrine adenomatosis. Many of the patients demonstrating Gardner's syndrome have had an associated problem of peptic ulcer,

3, 20, 27, 52, 53. Duodenal polyps were reported by McCaughan et al[53] and Kaplan[54]. The latter's patient also had a congenital anterior anus. Jones[55] reported a patient with a pectus excavatum and another with a urachal cyst. We have seen two patients in unrelated families with ectopic kidneys, and a young boy with a chordee of the penis. Weiner and Cooper[52] reported a patient with an absent right testicle. Capps *et al*[39] reported a patient with familial polyposis, who had a horseshoe kidney and developed a transitional cell carcinoma of the bladder. Hughes[56] reported a woman with Gardner's syndrome who developed hydronephrosis secondary to the severe retroperitoneal fibrosis that followed total proctocolectomy and ileostomy. The patient showed an elevated erythrocyte sedimentation rate, as is typically seen in idopathic retroperitoneal fibrosis. Comings and associates[57] have suggested that there may be a hereditary factor in retroperitoneal fibrosis, and the authors felt that the fibrodysplasias of Gardner's syndrome may be related to the syndromes of retroperitoneal fibrosis. One of Clark and Parker's patients[27] was an achondroplastic dwarf, and these patients show an increase in postoperative scarring.[58] Keloid scars contain an increased quantity of acid mucopolysaccharide, part of which is sensitive to hyaluronidase and part of which is resistant[59]. Gorlin and Chaudhry[26] reported the urinary acid mucopolysaccharides to be normal in patients with Gardner's syndrome. They also reported a normal Rebuck test for the inflammatory cycle and normal plasma electrophoresis patterns. Baughman *et al*[44] reported a normal serum immunoelectrophoresis pattern in one of their patients. Normal chromosome studies of the leukocytes have been reported[44, 55]. McCaughan *et al*[53] reported a normal 5-hydroxyindole acetic acid excretion in a Gardner's syndrome patient with bowel obstruction and an abdominal desmoid tumor after ileoproctostomy. The patient also had a normal Frog test and normal values of serum calcium and phosphorous. However, Trygstad *et al*[60] have demonstrated that two adults with Gardner's syndrome were resistant to parathyroid extract and a child with the syndrome showed a normal response. No genetic linkage has been established for patients with Gardner's syndrome but Veale[61] found a genetic linkage between the dominant gene of multiple intestinal polyposis and the locus for the MN blood genes.

Treatment:

Our recommended treatment of the colonic polyposis, where the degree of involvement and dependability of the patient permits, has been subtotal colectomy with ileoproctostomy immediately upon diagnosis. We have observed a progressive increase in the size and number of polyps present in the colon and rectum of patients with the disease. We have never seen a spontaneous regression of the colonic polyps without some type of surgical intervention. Extensive involvement of the rectum with polyps or cancer, progression of rectal polyps following ileoproctostomy, and personal irresponsibility of the patient are indications for total proctocolectomy with ileostomy. Twenty-one of our patients have undergone proctocolectomy with ileostomy. We have performed colectomy and ileoproctostomy in patients as young as 10 years of age without any growth or developmental problem. We prefer this operation to an anal ileostomy as described by Ravitch and Sabiston[62] or the cecoproctostomy as described by Lillehei and Wangensteen[63]. Five of the 12 patients with subtotal colectomy and ileoproctostomy have shown regression of the rectal polyps following surgery; and in one patient the polyps have disappeared. This is consistent with observations in patients with familial polyposis, where regression of the residual rectal polyps has occurred following subtotal colectomy with ileoproctostomy[64]. The exact etiological mechanism is not clear. Dunphy, Patterson, and Legg[65] proposed a growth-activating factor within the colon, and Cole, McKalen and Powell[66] favored an inhibiting role by the ileal contents.

Hubbard[67] documented the disappearance of rectal polyps after ileoproctostomy, and reviewing the literature found that cancer occurred in the remaining rectal stumps in 4% to 16% of the patients with familial polyposis. Turnbull[68] emphasized the importance of performing an ileoproctostomy and not an ileosigmoidostomy. The regrowth of polyps and development of rectal cancer may well occur in patients with Gardner's syndrome; thus, the performance of an ileoproctostomy does not remove the necessity for a yearly physical examination including proctoscopy. Progressive growth of the polyps, or the development of a carcinoma are indications for a proctectomy and ileostomy.

The problem of retroperitoneal fibrosis and the development of desmoid tumors or fibrosarcomas following colon surgery remains a serious complication and important aspect of Gardner's syndrome. Radiotherapy is of no value,[69] and carefully considered surgical excision remains our treatment of choice for these soft tissue tumors.

REFERENCES

1. Devic, A. & Bussy: Un cas de polypose adenomateuse generalisée à tout de l'intestin. *Arch Mal. App.* digest. 6: 278–289, 1912.

2. Cabot, R.C.: Case records of the Massachusetts General Hospital. Case No. 21061. *New Eng. J. Med.* 212: 263–267, 1935.

3. Fitzgerald, G.M.: Multiple composite odontomas coincidental with other tumorous conditions. Report of case. *J. Amer. Dent. Ass.* 30: 1408–1416, 1943.

4. Guptill, P.: Familial polyposis of the colon: Two families, five cases. *Surgery* 22: 286–304, Aug., 1947.

5. Gardner, E.J.: Mendelian pattern of dominant inheritance for a syndrome including intestinal polyposis, osteomas, fibromas and sebaceous cysts in a human family group. *Amer. J. Hum. Genet.* 2: Mendelione, L. Gedda, ed. pp. 321–329, 1955.

6. Gardner, E.J.: Inherited multiple neoplasia syndrome. Genetics Today. Proc. XI Intern. Cong. Genet. Vol. 1, p. 287, 1963.

7. Gardner, E.J. & Stephens, F.E.: Cancer of the lower digestive tract in one family group. *Am. J. Hum. Genet.* 2: 41–48, 1950.

8. Gardner, E.J.: A genetic and clinical study of familial polyposis, a predisposing factor for carcinoma of the colon and rectum. *Amer. J. Hum. Genet.* 3: 167–176, 1951.

9. Gardner, E.J. & Plenk, H.P.: Hereditary pattern for multiple osteomas in a family group. *Amer. J. Hum. Genet.* 4: 31–36, 1952.

10. Plenk, H.P. & Gardner, E.J.: Osteomastosis (Leontiasis Ossea) hereditary disease of membranous bone formation associated in one family with polyposis of the colon. *Radiology* 62: 830–840, 1954.

11. Gardner, E.J. & Richards, R.C.: Multiple cutaneous and subcutaneous lesions occurring simultaneously with hereditary intestinal polyposis and osteomas. *Amer. J. Hum. Genet.* 5: 139–147, 1953.

12. MacDonald, J.M., Davis, W.C., Crago, H.R., Beck, A.O.: Gardner's Syndrome and Periampullary Malignancy. *Amer. J. Surg.* 113: 425–430, March, 1967.

13. Gardner, E.J.: Follow-up study of a family group exhibiting dominant inheritance for a syndrome including intestinal polyps, osteomas, fibromas, and epidermal cysts. *Amer. J. Hum. Genet.* 14: 376–390, 1962.

14. Smith, W.G.: Multiple polyposis, Gardner's Syndrome and desmoid tumors. *Dis. Colon Rectum* 1: 323–332, 1958.

15. McKusick, V.A.: Genetic factors in intestinal polyposis. *J.A.M.A.* 182: 271–277, 1962.

16. Paget, J.: Lectures on Surgical pathology delivered at the Royal College of Surgeons of England. Edited by W. Turner. Presley Blakiston, 1012 Walnut Street, Philadelphia, p. 438, 1854.

17. Oldfield, M.C.: Association of familial polyposis of colon with multiple sebaceous cysts. *Brit. J. Surg.* 41: 534–541, 1954.

18. Simpson, R.D., Harrison, E.G. & Mayo, C.W.: Mesenteric fibromatosis in familial polyposis. A variant of Gardner's Syndrome. *Cancer 17*: 526–534, 1964.

19. Miller, R.H. & Sweet, R.H.: Multiple polyposis of the colon: A familial disease. *Ann. Surg.* 105: 511–515, 1937.

20. Pugh, H.L. & Nesselrod, J.P.: Multiple polypoid disease of colon and rectum. Ann. Surg. 121: 88–99, 1945.

21. O'Brien, J.P. & Wels, P.: The syn-

chronous occurrence of benign fibrous tissue neoplasia in hereditary adenosis of the colon and rectum. *New York J. Med.* 55: 1877–1880, 1955.

22. Smith, W.G.: Desmoid tumors in familial multiple polyposis. *Proc. Staff Meet. Mayo Clin.* 34: 31–38, 1959.

23. Musgrove, J.E.: Extra–Abdominal Desmoid Tumors. Thesis. Graduate School, U. of Minnesota, 1947.

24. Gumpel, R.C. & Carballo, J.O.: A new concept of familial adenomatosis. *Ann. Intern. Med.* 45: 1045–1058, 1956.

25. Fader, M., Kline, S.N., Spatz, S.S., Zubrow, H.J.: Gardner's Syndrome (intestinal polyposis, osteomas, sebaceous cysts) and a new dental discovery. *Oral Surg.* 15: 153–172, 1962.

26. Gorlin, R.J. & Chaundhry, A.P.: Multiple osteomatosis, fibromas, lipomas & fibrosarcomas of the skin and mesentery. Epidermoid inclusion cysts of the skin, leiomyomas and multiple intestinal polyposis. *New Eng. J. Med.* 263: 1151–1158, 1960.

27. Clark, F.B. & Parker, J.M.: Familial Polyposis of the Colon. *J. Maine Med. Ass.* 41: 331–336, 1950.

28. Collins, D.C.: The frequent association of other body tumors with familial polyposis. *Amer. J. Gastroent.* 31: 376–381, 1959.

29. Guisto, D.F., Thoshinsky, M.J. & Brizzolara, L.G.: Leiomyosarcoma of the ascending colon associated with multiple polyposis. *Amer. J. Surg.* 95: 1007–1010, 1958.

30. Weston, S.D. & Weiner, M.: Familial polyposis associated with a new type of soft tissue lesion (skin pigmentation) report of three cases and review of literature. *Dis. Colon Rectum* 10: 311–321, 1967.

31. Laberge, M.Y., Sauer, W.G. & Mayo, C.W.: Soft–tissue tumors associated with familial polyposis. *Proc. Staff Meet. Mayo Clinic* 32: 749–752, 1957.

32. Enterline, H.T., Culberson, J.D., Rocklin, D.B. & Brady, L.W.: Liposarcoma. *Cancer* 13: 932–950, 1960.

33. Chang, C.H., Piatt, E.D., Thomas, K.E. & Watne, A.L.: Bone abnormalities in Gardner's syndrome. *Amer. J. Roentgen.* 103: 645–652, 1968. 1968.

34. Hoffman, D.C. & Brooke, B.N.: Familial sarcoma of bone in a polyposis coli family. *Dis. Colon Rectum* 13: 119–120, 1970.

35. Fraumeni, J.F., Vogel, C.L. & Easton, J.M.: Sarcomas and multiple polyposis in a kindred. A genetic variety of hereditary polyposis? *Arch. Intern. Med.* 121: 57–61, 1968.

36. Le Fevre, H.W. Jr. & Jacques, T.F.: Multiple polyposis in an infant of four months. *Amer. J. Surg.* 81: 90–91, 1951.

37. Pierce E.R.: Some genetic aspects of familial multiple polyposis of the colon in a kindred of 1422 members. *Dis. Colon Rectum* 11: 321–329, 1968.

38. Dukes, C.E.: Familial intestinal polyposis. *Amer. Eugenics* 17: 1–29, 1952.

39. Capps, W.F. Jr., Lewis, M.I. & Gazzaniga, D.A.: Carcinoma of the colon, ampulla of Vater and urinary bladder associated with familial multiple polyposis. *Dis. Colon Rectum* 11: 298–305, 1968.

40. Shiffman, M.A.: Familial multiple polyposis associated with soft–tissue and hard–tissue tumors. *JAMA 179*: 514–522, 1962.

41. Lieberman, W. discussion of Collins, D.C.: The frequent association of other body tumors with familial polyposis. *Amer. J. Gastroent. 31*: 376–381, 1959.

42. Yaffee, H.S.: Gastric polyposis and soft tissue tumors: A variant of Gardner's

syndrome. *Arch. Derm. 89*: 806–808, 1964.

43. Cronkhite, L.W. & Canada, W.J.: Generalized gastrointestinal polyposis. An unusual syndrome of polyposis, pigmentation, alopecia and onchotrophia. *New Eng. J. Med. 252*: 1011–1015, 1955.

44. Baughman, F.A. Jr., List, C.F., Williams, J.R., Muldoon, J.P., Segarra, J.M. & Volkel, J.S.: The glioma–polyposis syndrome. *New Eng. J. Med.* 281: 1345–1346, 1969.

45. Turcot, J., Despres, J.P. & St. Pierre, F.: Malignant tumors of the central nervous system associated with familial polyposis of the colon: Report of two cases. *Dis. Colon Rectum 2*: 465–468, 1959.

46. Camiel, M.R., Mule, J.E., Alexander, L.L., & Benninghoff, D.L.: Association of thyroid carcinoma with Gardner's syndrome in siblings. *New Eng. J. Med. 278*: 1056–1058, 1968.

47. Crail, H.W.: Multiple primary malignancies arising in rectum, brain, and thyroid: report of case. *U.S. Navy Med. Bull. 49*: 123–128, 1949.

48. Smith, W.G.: Familial multiple polyposis: Research tool for investigating the etiology of carcinoma of the colon *Dis. Colon Rectum 11*: 17–31, 1968.

49. Balfour, D.C., Jr.: Personal communication reported by Smith, W.G., *Dis. Colon Rectum. 11*: 17–31, 1968.

50. Werner, P.: Genetic aspects of adenomatosis of endocrine glands. *Amer. J. Med. 16*: 363–371, 1954.

51. Werner, P.: Endocrine adenomatosis and peptic ulcer in a large kindred. *Amer. J. Med. 35*: 205–211, 1963.

52. Weiner, R.S. & Cooper, P.: Multiple polyposis of the colon, osteomatosis and tumors. *New Eng. J. Med. 253*: 795–799, 1955.

53. McCaughan, J.S., Soder, P.O, & Biddle, L.R.: Gardner's syndrome. *Dis. Colon Rectum 9*: 286–292, 1966.

54. Kaplan, B.J.: Gardner's syndrome: Heredofamilial adenomatosis associated with "soft" & "hard" fibrous tumors and epidermoid cysts. *Dis. Colon Rectum 4*: 252–262, 1961.

55. Jones, E.L. & Cornell, W.P.: Gardner's syndrome. Review of the literature and report on a family. *Arch. Surg. 92*: 287–300, 1966.

56. Hughes, L.E.: Abdominal fibrodysplasia and polyposis coli. *Dis. Colon Rectum 13*: 121–123, 1970.

57. Comings, D.E., Skubi, K.B., Van Eyes, J. & Motulsky, A.G.: Familial multifocal fibrosclerosis: Findings suggesting that retroperitoneal fibrosis, mediastinal fibrosis, sclerosing chalangetis, Riedel's thyroiditis, and pseudo–tumor of the orbit may be different manifestations of a single disease. *Ann. Intern. Med. 66*: 884–892, 1967.

58. Scott, D. & Stiris, G.: Osteogenesis imperfecta tarda. A study of three families with special reference to scar formation. *Acta Med. Scand. 145*: 237–257, 1953.

59. Hansen, G.A.: Survey of normal & pathological occurence of mucinous substances and mast cells in dermal connective tissue in man. *Acta Dermatovener 30*: 338–347, 1950.

60. Trygstad, C.W., Zisman, E. Witkop, C.J., and Barter, F.C.: Resistance to parathyroid extract in Gardner's syndrome. *J. Clin. Endocr. 28*: 1153–1159, 1968.

61. Veale, A.M.O.: Clinical and genetic problems in familial intestinal polyposis. *J. Brit. Soc. Gastroent. 1*: 285–290, 1960.

62. Ravitch, M.M., Sabiston, D.C., Jr.,: Anal Ileostomy and Preservation of Anal

Sphincter. *Surg. Gynec. Obstet.* 84: 1095–1099, 1947.

63. Lillehei, R.C. & Wangensteen, O.H.: Total and subtotal colectomies: A clinical evaluation. *Bull. Univ. Minn. Hosp. Staff Meet.* 25: 21–26, 1953.

64. Williams, R.O. & Fish, J.C.: Multiple polyposis, polyps regression and carcinoma of the colon. *Amer. J. Surg. 112*: 846–849, 1966.

65. Dunphy, J.E., Patterson, W.B. & Legg, M.A.: Etiologic factors in polyposis and carcinoma of the colon. *Ann. Surg. 150*: 488–498, 1959.

66. Cole, J.W., McKalen, A. & Powell, J.: The role of ileal contents in the spontaneous regression of rectal adenomas. *Dis. Colon Rectum 4*: 413–418, 1961.

67. Hubbard, T.B., Jr.: Familial polyposis of the colon: the fate of the retained rectum after colectomy in children. *Amer. Surg. 23*: 577–586, 1957.

68. Turnbull, R.B.: Discussion of McLachlin, A.D.: Familial intestinal polyposis. *Arch. Surg. 79*: 393–398, 1959.

69. Schweitzer, R.J. & Robbins, G.F.: A desmoid tumor of multicentric origin. *Arch. Surg. 80*: 489–494, 1960.

Chapter 11

THE GASTROINTESTINAL SYSTEM, SKIN, GENETICS, AND CANCER

by John Woodbury, M.D.

INTRODUCTION

Many skin diseases which the practitioner observes are limited to the skin and/or its appendages. However, cutaneous manifestations associated with underlying disease is certainly common and this is especially true in regard to the gastrointestinal tract.

The purpose of this chapter is to discuss briefly those several diseases with a known or suspected hereditary basis in which the skin and gastrointestinal tract are involved and where the skin disorder by nature of its characteristics suggests underlying gastrointestinal disease.

Tylosis

Tylosis palmaris et plantaris is characterized by a marked thickening of the epidermal horny layer of the palms (Figure 1) and soles and occasionally there are associated changes in the nails which may become thickened and malformed. This skin disorder has been very well described in several families[1-6] and represents an autosomal dominant mode of inheritance (additional discussion may be found in chapter 15).

There is an early onset form of tylosis which occurs during the first year of life and a late onset form which occurs after one year. The early onset form is more commonly observed but it is the late onset form in which a high incidence of esophageal carcinoma of the squamous cell type occurs.

Howell–Evans, et al[2&6] described two families in which 18 cases of esophageal carcinoma occurred in three generations. Tylosis was noted to be definitely present in 17 of the 18 cases and probably present in all 18. A life table was constructed for these two families in which it was predicted that 95 per cent of those members manifesting tylosis would develop carcinoma of the esophagus by age 65. Those members of the two families who did not manifest keratosis of the palms or soles did not develop esophageal carcinoma.

It is recognized that carcinoma of the esophagus, in the absence of tylosis, does not have a hereditary basis.[3]

Bean, et al[4] studied 230 patients with various internal malignancies and 699 control patients at the University of Minnesota to determine if there was an increased incidence of acquired palmar keratosis in patients with internal malignancy. In contrast to Dobson, et al[5] he did not find an increased incidence of keratosis of the palms in patients with internal malignant disease.

The distribution of carcinoma of the esophagus in the affected individuals is similar to carcinoma of the esophagus in the general population without tylosis. The distal esophagus is more commonly involved than the body and the proximal esophagus is least involved.

A premalignant lesion of the esophagus has not been described in patients with hereditary tylosis making the management of family members at risk difficult.

In a patient with hereditary tylosis of late onset, barium esophagram and esophagoscopy are certainly indicated in the presence of esophageal symptoms.

For the asymptomatic tylotic at risk, esophageal washings for cytology obtained through the use of nasogastric tube would be the most innocuous examination to employ in following these patients. Yearly barium esophagram could be associated with a considerable amount of irradiation and an early lesion might be missed.

In view of the new flexible esophagoscopes, esophagoscopy in experienced hands would seem to be the more desirable approach in an attempt to diagnose these patients early.

Esophagoscopy on a yearly basis would seem reasonable.

Ulcerative Colitis

Ulcerative colitis is an idiopathic diffuse non–specific inflammatory disease affecting primarily the mucous membrane of the rectum (idiopathic proctitis) in virtually all cases and in many involvement of the proximal colon to variable distances (idiopathic proctocolitis) as well. Mucosal ulcerations are frequently but not invariably present.

Although several hypotheses have been advanced, the etiology of the disease remains unknown.[7]

It is not rare for ulcerative colitis to occur in families. Kirschner and Spencer recorded an incidence of 6 per cent in a study of 1,084 cases from the University of Chicago. They also cited 14 instances in which more than two members of a family were involved with the disease.[8] Ulcerative colitis has been recorded in twins who were very likely monozygotic.[9] A genetic influence seems to be an important factor in a Southampton family studied by Morris. The distribution of the disease in this family is suggestive of an autosomal dominant pattern.[10] The role of heredity in this disease requires additional study; at present we can say that genetic factors seem to be important in some families but extra genetic factors seemingly are responsible for the majority of patients with this disease.

In the majority of cases ulcerative colitis is a chronic relapsing illness; however, the cardinal initial symptoms in most patients consists of diarrhea and bright red blood in the stool. Sixty percent of the patients in Tanden's series complained of abdominal pain. Less common symptoms are weight loss, fever, vomiting and, in a small percent, constipation.[11]

There are local complications arising directly out of the pathological changes in the bowel and systemic complications which are remote to the diseased bowel but specifically encountered in the disease.

Involvement of the integument is one such systemic complication. There are two skin conditions which are found with such frequency among patients with ulcerative colitis that they merit special consideration as systemic complications of the disease. They are erythema nodosum, and, in particular, pyoderma gangrenosum.[12]

A great variety of clinical forms of pyoderma have been described which may cause extensive vegetations or ulcerations of the skin. In its fully developed form the lesions of pyoderma gangrenosum are characteristic and when observed in patients with diarrhea and, in particular, those with associated rectal bleeding ulcerative colitis is the likely underlying disorder. The skin lesions frequently parallel the activity of the bowel disease and have been observed to regress or disappear following remission of the underlying bowel disease or following colectomy.

Although carcinoma of the colon in patients with ulcerative colitis does not represent the most common complication, nevertheless, it occurs with sufficient frequency to merit the critical attention of both patient and physician regarding this possibility.

The risk of cancer for an individual patient with idiopathic proctitis is very small and may be the same as that in the general population.[13] On the other hand a patient with total or near total involvement of the colon is at a high risk to develop a carcinoma of the colon. During the first 10 years of symptoms the risk is low, 0.4 per cent per annum. After this decade the annual risk rises sharply to 2 per cent per annum during the second decade and 5 per cent per annum for the remainder of the patient's life.[14] Thus, prophylactic colectomy is performed by many physicians for cancer control in patients with chronic disease of long duration.

Celiac Sprue

Celiac disease of infancy and adult celiac disease (non–tropical sprue, gluten induced enteropathy, idiopathic steatorrhea) are the same basic disease best termed celiac sprue.[15]

It is generally accepted that celiac sprue results from a specific response of the intestinal mucosa in the susceptible individual to gluten in the diet.

The median age of onset of symptoms is in the third decade; women outnumber men in a ratio of 2:1.[16]

There is evidence confirming the familial nature of celiac sprue but a definite mode of inheritance remains uncertain although it has been suggested that the disease may be inherited through a dominant gene with incomplete penetrance.[17]

Although patients frequently present with complaints of diarrhea, weakness, lassitude, weight loss and are found to have steatorrhea and anemia, many patients present with only one major manifestation of malabsorption. Such manifestations may be iron deficiency anemia,[18] bleeding secondary to Vitamin D malabsorption, osteomalacia, tetany,[19] and macrocytic anemia secondary to B^{12} and/or folate malabsorption.[20]

Eczema is a frequent cutaneous manifestation of celiac sprue and treatment with a gluten free diet improves both the malabsorption and the skin condition.[21]

The hypothesis that small bowel reticuloses may develop as a complication in patients with celiac sprue was suggested by Gough in 1962. This hypothesis is reinforced in the study of Harris[22] of 202 patients with adult celiac disease and idiopathic steatorrhea in which there was noted the development of lymphoma in 6.9 per cent of his patients which compares well with an incidence of 10 per cent reported by Austad[23] and 6.2 per cent by Benson.[19] The problem of malignancy in celiac sprue is not restricted to lymphomas. (In Harris's group there appeared to be an increased incidence of esophageal carcinoma.)

According to Harris, "the celiac patient in whom a lymphoma is most likely to develop is male, over 40 years of age, with a history of celiac disease for more than 10 years, and not on a gluten free diet."

Hereditary Polyposis

There is general agreement that there are three distinct varieties of intestinal polyposis that are genetically determined. These are:

1. Familial polyposis coli.[24–26]
2. Gardner's syndrome.
3. Peutz–Jeghers syndrome.

In addition to these well defined syndromes there are several other varieties of intestinal polyposis which have been described in which a definite mode of inheritance is highly probable or suspected.

4. Turcot' syndrome.[27]
5. Cronkhite–Canada syndrome.[28]
6. Familial polyposis of the entire gastrointestinal tract.[29]

Familial Polyposis Coli

Familial polyposis of the colon is recognized to be a dominant trait capable of being transmitted by both males and females, and therefore autosomal. The polypoid lesion is grossly and microscopically indistinguishable from the common discrete adenoma observed in the general population.

The frequency of familial polyposis noted by Reed and Neel was found to be one in 8,300 births.[30]

Unfortunately there are no characteristic symptoms. The propositus is usually found because of symptoms of rectal bleeding, pain, change in bowel habit or signs and symptoms secondary to the development of carcinoma of the colon. Therefore, the majority of patients with familial polyposis coli are diagnosed by examining the family members when a propositus has been detected.

The diagnosis of familial polyposis is established by sigmoidoscopy and barium enema examination. In the typical case presentation the polyps will appear grossly like the single nonhereditary adenomatous polyp. The polyps are usually fairly uniform in size averaging 0.5 cm. and will tend to carpet the entire colonic mucosa from the anus to the ileocecal valve.

Patients with this disease are particularly prone to the development of adenocarcinoma of the colon. The cancer is often multicentric in origin and exhibits an unusually rapid growth and spread.

Of the 218 patients observed by Lockhart–Mummery, 154 later developed carcinoma of the colon.[31] Because of the high risk of cancer of the colon in patients with familial polyposis few if any authorities disagree with colectomy as the form of treatment once the diagnosis is made.

However, disagreement exists as to the type of surgery which should be done.[32] There are those who prefer total colectomy with ileoproctostomy in an attempt to preserve continuity with the rectum and those who recommend ileoproctectomy with ileostomy.[33]

Jackman and Smith followed 86 patients with colectomy and ileoproctostomy for five years and noted that carcinoma of the rectum developed in 8.1 per cent.

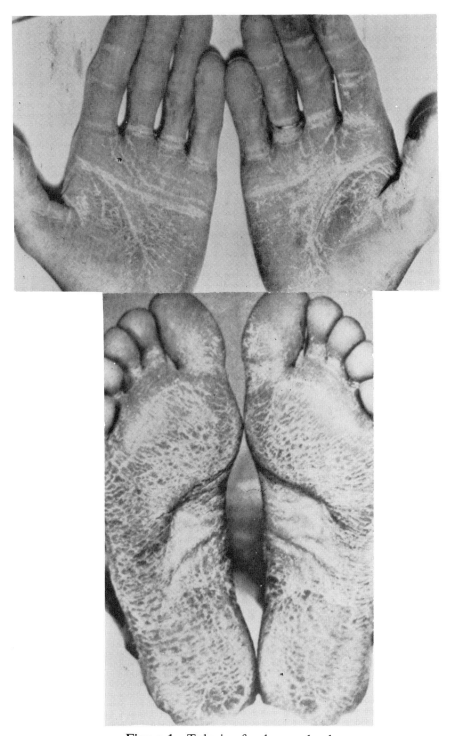

Figure 1. Tylosis of palms and soles.

(reprinted from Quarterly Journal of Medicine, Vol. 27, 1958, with permission of publishers.)

Factors which should be considered in favor of the latter procedure are the risks of carcinoma developing in the retained rectal stump, the necessity for repeated sigmoidoscopies and fulguration of recurring polyps with its attendant risks, the fear that in our mobile society the patient might be lost to followup, and the unmeasurable effect on the psyche because of the fear of developing a rectal carcinoma.

Gardner's Syndrome

Gardner and Richards reported seven members of the same family with exostoses, sebaceous cysts and polyposis.[34]

Examination of the published pedigrees leaves no doubt that this syndrome is transmitted as an autosomal dominant. The gene appears distinct from that determining familial polyposis coli in the absence of the skeletal and cutaneous manifestations of Gardner's syndrome.

The symptoms of this disorder, like familial polyposis coli, are not characteristic. The presence of epidermal cysts, osteomas, or lipomas of the skin should alert the observer that an underlying disease may be present. These findings in conjunction with polyps of the gastrointestinal tract provide strong evidence in favor of this syndrome. This syndrome is mentioned here only for the sake of completeness. An in depth discussion is found in Chapter 10.

Peutz–Jeghers Syndrome

Peutz–Jeghers syndrome is characterized by brown to black mucocutaneous macules usually involving the lips and oral cavity but can be seen over the face and tips of the fingers (Figure 2) and toes and associated with hamartomatous polyps of the small intestine.[35] Less frequently polyps are observed in the rectum, colon, stomach and appendix.[36]

Peutz–Jeghers syndrome is inherited as an autosomal dominant.[37] Both sexes are affected about equally and the disorder may present at both extremes of life.

The most common complication is intussusception, accounting for the frequently observed colicky abdominal pain. Gastrointestinal hemorrhage is commonly seen as a presenting complaint or in association with intussusception.

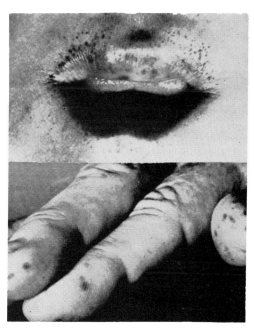

Figure 2. Patient with Peutz–Jegher's syndrome showing cutaneous pigmented macules of the lips, peri–oral area and of the distal portions of the fingers.

(reprinted from Butterworth and Strean: *Clinical Geno Dermatology* with permission of The Williams and Wilkins Company.)

Early in the description of this disease the polyps were thought to be precancerous because of epithelial elements being caught up in the bands of smooth muscle and were misinterpreted as invasive carcinoma. Most agree presently that these lesions are hamartomas and since earlier descriptions of the syndrome could not document the presence of lymphatic invasion or evidence of metastasis it was generally felt that this syndrome did not represent a premalignant condition.

According to Dozois,[38] of the 321 reported cases of Peutz–Jeghers syndrome 11 cases of malignancy are recognized; involving stomach (4 cases), duodenum (3 cases), colon and rectum (3 cases) and ileum (1 case).

Jejunal and colonic adenocarcinomas have been reported in association with the Peutz–Jeghers syndrome[40] and ovarian neoplasms, with a predeliction for granulosa cell tumors, may develop more frequently in women with the Peutz–Jeghers syndrome than in women in the general population.[39]

Gastrointestinal carcinoma is certainly an uncommon occurrence in Peutz–Jeghers syndrome and therefore this disorder should be treated conservatively.

Turcot's Syndrome

Turcot's syndrome (Glioma–Polyposis syndrome) represents an unusual association of tumors of the nervous system with polyposis of the colon. Turcot described two cases of diffuse polyposis of the colon in teenagers in whom there subsequently developed malignant tumors of the central nervous system. The first case was that of a 15–year–old Caucasian male who presented with diarrhea and bloody stools. He was found to have large polypoid lesions of the rectum, sigmoid and upper colon. At laparotomy a malignant tumor of the sigmoid was found. Three years later he died and the autopsy revealed a medulloblastoma of the spinal cord. The other case was a 13–year–old girl (sister of the aforementioned case) who presented with diarrhea and rectal bleeding. She was found to have colonic polyposis without evidence of carcinoma. She died suddenly at the age of 18 and at autopsy a glioblastoma of the left frontal lobe was found.

No associated abnormalities other than the central nervous system tumors were noted. This syndrome at present appears to be a distinct entity differing from Gardner's syndrome and familial polyposis coli.

Cronkhite–Canada Syndrome

Cronkhite–Canada syndrome was initially described in 1955. This syndrome consists of diffuse gastrointestinal polyposis, ectodermal changes and hypoproteinemia.

This syndrome has not been described in more than one member of the family. However, only a small number of cases have been described over the past fifteen years.

Patients with this disorder frequently present with weight loss, diarrhea, hyperpigmentation of the skin, changes in the nails (onychotropia), occasionally alopecia and infrequent abdominal pain.

Hypoproteinemia is a frequent finding and labeled albumin studies have confirmed a protein–losing enteropathy to be present.

The polyps are of the adenomatous type and are seen throughout the gastrointestinal tract. No evidence of malignant change has been noted in this disorder.

The mortality is high in this syndrome and usually secondary to the malabsorption syndrome with associated cachexia. Treatment at present is symptomatic.

Familial Polyposis of the Entire Gastrointestinal Tract

Familial polyposis of the entire gastrointestinal tract is an extremely rare condition. Although it is not definitely established, this disorder is thought to represent an autosomal dominant pattern of inheritance.

Polyps are present in the colon, small bowel and stomach. One patient reportedly was found to have a desmoid tumor of the abdominal wall.

Management should be directed toward correction of existent complications and priority given to prophylactic surgery of the colorectum since the colon in this disorder is predisposed to cancerous changes as in familial polyposis and Gardner's syndrome.

Idiopathic Hemochromatosis

Idiopathic hemochromatosis is an inborn error of iron metabolism. Males are much more frequently affected than females and the few affected females described in the literature are most often past the menopause. Patients are asymptomatic until the fourth and fifth decade when manifestations of tissue damage appear in the form of cardiac failure, cirrhosis and diabetes.

Familial cases of hemochromatosis have been described, and in studies on asymptomatic relatives of patients with hemochromatosis approximately half of the adult male siblings and of the male offspring over the age of 15 years had abnormally high serum iron levels and coefficients of iron saturation.[41]

In most instances this disease appears to be inherited as an autosomal dominant genetic defect with incomplete penetrance. On the other hand, Felts recently described two young sisters (parents normal) with hemochromatosis suggesting that there is also an autosomal recessive form of this disease.[42]

This disease develops over a period of years and is due to an abnormal accumulation of iron in the tissues of various organs. Although hemochromatosis affects many organ systems, 80 per cent of the cases present with pigmentation of the skin, diabetes mellitus and cirrhosis.[43]

The skin pigmentation is believed to be a result of increased melanin accounting for the slaty bluish–gray appearance of the involved areas. Only 10 to 15 percent show pigmentation of the mucous membranes.

The liver is involved in all cases and has been found to be palpably enlarged in 93 percent of cases. The spleen is palpable in about 50 percent of cases. Ascites and jaundice are much less frequently observed. About one–third of all patients later develop cardiac symptoms and approximately this number die of cardiac complications.

The diagnosis of hemochromatosis should be considered in all patients with increased pigmentation of the skin, enlarged liver and diabetes mellitus.

The most useful diagnostic tests are based on demonstration of abnormal iron metabolism.

Hepatoma is frequently observed in hemochromatosis. Edmondson noted that primary liver cancer complicated 18 percent of cases of hemochromatosis.[44]

Treatment of hemochromatosis consists of phlebotomies alone or in combination with chelating agents.[43]

BIBLIOGRAPHY

1. Shine, I., Allison, P.R. Carcinoma of the Oesophagus with Tylosis, (Keratosis palmaris et plantaris). *Lancet 1*: 951, 1966.

2. Howel–Evans, W., McConnell, R.B., Clark, C.A. and Sheppard, P.M. Carcinoma of the Esophagus with Keratosis palmaris et plantaris (Tylosis): A Study of Two Families. *Quart. J. Med. 27*: 413, 1958.

3. Mosbech, J. and Videbak, A. On the Etiology of Esophageal Carcinoma. *J. Nat. Cancer Inst. 15*: 1665, 1955.

4. Bean, S.F., Foxley, E.G. and Fusaro, R.M. Palmar Keratosis and Internal Malignancy. *Arch. Derm. 97*: 528, 1968.

5. Dobson, R.L., Young, M.R., Pinto, J.S. Palmar Keratosis and Cancer. *Arch. Derm. 92*: 553, 1965.

6. Harper, P.S., Harper, R.M.J. and Howel–Evans, A.W. Carcinoma of the Oesophagus with Tylosis. *Quart. J. Med. 155*: 317, 1970.

7. DeDombal, F.T., Burck, P.R.J., Watkinson, G. Actiology of Ulcerative Colitis. *Gut 10*: 270, 1969.

8. Kirschner, J.B., Spencer, J.A. Familial Occurrence of Ulcerative Colitis, Regional Enteritis and Ileocolitis. *Ann. Intern. Med. 59*: 133, 1963.

9. Lyons, C.H., Pastlethwait, R.W. Chronic Ulcerative Colitis in Twins. *Gastroenterology 10*: 545, 1948.

10. Morris, P.M. Familial Ulcerative Colitis. *Gut 6*: 176, 1965.

11. Tandon, B.M., Mather, A.K., Mohapotin, L.N., Tanden, H.D. and Wig, K.L. A Study of the Prevalence and Clinical Pattern of Specific Ulcerative Colitis in Northern India. *Gut 6*: 448, 1965.

12. Johnson, M.L., Wilson, H.T.H. Skin Lesions in Ulcerative Colitis. *Gut 10*: 255, 1969.

13. MacDougall, I.P.M. The Cancer Risk in Ulcerative Colitis. *Lancet, 2*: 655, 1964.

14. DeDombal, F.T., Watts, J. Mek., Watkinson, G. and Goligher, J.E. Local Complications of Ulcerative Colitis: Stricture, Pseudopolyposis, and Carcinoma of the Colon and Rectum. *Brit. Med. J. 1*: 1442, 1966.

15. Rubin, C.E., Dobbins, W.O., III. Peroral Biopsy of the Small Intestine: A Review of its Diagnostic Usefulness. *Gastroenterology 49*: 676, 1965.

16. Rubin, C.E., Brandborg, L.L., Phelps, P.C., and Taylor, H.C., Jr. Studies of Celiac Disease–I. The Apparent Identical and Specific Nature of the Duodenal and Proximal Lesion in Celiac Disease and Ideopathic Sprue. *Gastroenterology 38*: 28, 1960.

17. MacDonald, W.C. Dobbins, W.O., III, Rubin, C.E. Studies of the Familial Nature of Celiac Sprue Using Biopsy of the Small Intestine. *New Eng. J. Med. 272*: 448, 1965.

18. McGuigan, J.E., Volwiler, W. Celiac Sprue: Malabsorption of Iron in the Absence of Steatorrhea. *Gastroenterology 47*: 636, 1964.

19. Benson, G.D., Kowlessar, O.O. and Sleisinger, M.H. Adult Celiac Disease with Emphasis upon Response to the Gluten-free Diet. *Medicine 43*: 1, 1964.

20. Cooke, W.T., Fone, D.J., Cox, E.V., Meynell, M.J. and Gaddie, R. Adult Celiac Disease. *Gut 4*: 279, 1963.

21. Friedman, M., and Hare, P.J. Gluten–sensitive Enteropathy and Eczema. *Lancet 1*: 521, 1965.

22. Harris, O.D., Cooke, W.T., Thompson, H. and Waterhouse, J.A.H. Malignancy in Adult Coeliac Disease and Idiopathic Steatorrhea. *Amer. J. Med., 42*: 899, 1967.

23. Austad, W.I., Cornes, J.S., Gough, K.R., McCarthy, C.F. and Read, A.E. Steatorrhoea and Malignant Lymphoma: The Relationship of Malignant Tumors of Lymphoid Tissue and Celiac Disease. *Amer. J. Dig. Dis., 12*: 475, 1967.

24. Gardner, E.J.: A Genetic and Clinical Study of Intestinal Polyposis, a Predisposing Factor for Carcinoma of the Colon and Rectum. *Amer. J. Hum. Genet. 3*: 167, 1951.

25. Jeghers, H., McKusick, V.A. and Katz, K.H. Generalized Intestinal Polyposis and Melanin Spots of the Oral Mucosa, Lips and Digits. *New Eng. J. Med. 241*: 933, 1949.

26. Bachus, H.L., Tachdjian, V., Fergusson, L.K., Mouhran, K. and Chamberlain, C. Adenomatous Polyp of the Colon and Rectum, its Relation to Carcinoma. *Gastroenterology 41*: 225, 1961.

27. Turcot, J., Despres, J.P. and St. Pierre, F. Malignant Tumors of the Central Nervous System Associated with Familial Polyposis of the Colon: Report of Two Cases. *Dis. Colon Rectum 2*: 465, 1959.

28. Cronkhite, L.W., Canada, W.J. Generalized Gastrointestinal Polyposis. An Unusual Syndrome of Polyposis, Pigmentation, Alopecia and Onychatrophia. *New Eng. J. Med. 252*: 1011, 1955.

29. Yonemoto, R.H., Slayback, J.B., Byron Jr., R.L. and Rosen, R.B. Familial Polyposis of the Entire Gastrointestinal Tract. *Arch. Surg. 99*: 427, 1969.

30. Reed, T.E., Neel, J.F. Genetic Study of Multiple Polyposis of the Colon. *Amer. J. of Hum. Genet. 7*: 236, 1955.

31. Lockhart–Mummery, H.E., Dukes, D.E. and Bussey, H.J. The Surgical Treatment of Familial Polyposis of the Colon. *Brit. J. Surg. 43*: 476, 1956.

32. Flotte, E.T., O'Dell, F.C., Jr. and Coller, F.A. Polyposis of the Colon. *Amer. Surg. 144*: 165, 1956.

33. Smith, W.J., Jackman, R.J. Results of Treatment in Familial Multiple Polyposis. *Proc. Staff Meet. Mayo Clin. 31*: 304, 1956.

34. Gardner, E.J. and Richards, R.C.: Multiple Cutaneous and Subcutaneous Lesions Occurring Simultaneously with Hereditary Polyposis and Osteomatosis. *Amer. J. Hum. Genet. 5*: 139, 1953.

35. McKusick, V.A. Genetic Factors in Intestinal Polyposis. *JAMA 182*: 271, 1962.

36. Bartholomew, L.G., Dohlin, D.C. and Wough, J.M. Intestinal Polyposis Associated with Mucocutaneous Melanin Pigmentation (Peutz–Jeghers Syndrome). *Proc. Staff Mayo Clin. 32*: 675, 1957.

37. Jeghers, H., McKusick, V.A. and Katz, K.N. Geneological Intestinal Polyposis and Melanin Spots of Oral Mucosa, Lips and Digits. A Syndrome of Diagnostic Significance. *New Eng. J. Med. 241*: 993, 1949.

38. Dozois, R.R., Judd, E.S., Dahlin, D.C. and Bartholomew, L.G. The Peutz–Jeghers Syndrome: Is There a Predisposition to the Development of Internal Malignancy? *Arch. Surg. 98*: 509, 1969.

39. Dozois, R.R., Kempers, R.D., Dahlin, D.C., and Bartholomew, L.G. Ovarian Tumors Associated with the Peutz–Jeghers Syndrome. *Ann. Surg. 172*: 233, 1970.

40. Shibata, H.R. and Philips, M.J. Peutz–Jeghers Syndrome with Jejunal and Colonic Adenocarcinomas. *Canad. Med. Ass. J. 8*: 103, 1970.

41. Debre, R., Dreyfus, J.S., Frezal, J., Labie, D., Lamy, M., Maroterux, P. Schapira, F. Schapira, G. Genetics of Hemochromatosis. *Ann. Hum. Genet. 23*: 16, 1958.

42. Felts, J.H., Nelson, J.R., Herndon, C.N. and Spurr, C.L. Hemochromatosis in Two Young Sisters. *Ann. Intern. Med.* *67*: 117, 1967.

43. Finch, S.C. and Finch, C.A. Idiopathic Hemochromatosis, an Iron Storage Disease. A. Iron Metabolism in Hemochromatosis. *Medicine 34*: 381, 1955.

44. Edmondson, H.R. and Steiner, P.E. Primary Carcinoma of the Liver. A study of 100 cases among 48,900 Necropsies. *Cancer 7*: 462, 1954.

Chapter 12

IMMUNOLOGY, SKIN, GENETICS AND CANCER

by Guillermo Villacorte, M.D. and
Robert Townley

INTRODUCTION

The possible role of the immune mechanism in the pathogenesis of human cancer has long been considered,[1] but due to the obvious ethical and technical problems, it was not until recently that some significant advances came to the fore.

This chapter will be confined to a selective review of the more recent literature on cancer immunology and to some extent, touch on the dermatologic and genetic aspects of certain types of human cancer.

What follows is a brief description of the present concept of the normal immune response to put this discussion in its proper perspective.

THE NORMAL IMMUNE RESPONSE

Man has been endowed with intricate and highly developed protective mechanisms to ensure his anatomical and functional integrity. One of these is the immune defense system, schematically illustrated in Figure 1. Governing this system is another host's mechanism which is capable of discriminating *non-self* from *self.*[2] Depending upon the physico-chemical make-up and quantity of the *non-self,* the host may respond by means of the non–specific defense mechanism alone or may in addition call forth the specific immunologic reaction. The *non-self* that can evoke the latter host's response is termed an *antigen.*

Comprising the non–specific defense system are the anatomical barriers, e.g. the skin and mucous membrane together with their corresponding bactericidal glandular secretions, the inflammatory

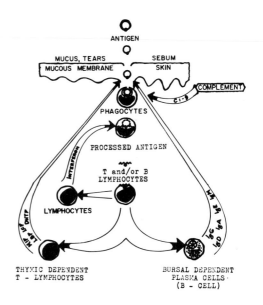

Figure 1. Schematic representation of the normal immune response.

reaction, and the interferon, a species specific, broad spectrum anti–viral substance that may very well be a part of the immune response.[3–5]

The transfer of the processed antigen from the receptor–bearing phagocytes to the T and/or B (*thymic* or *bursal*–derived) lymphocytes, which also possess surface immunoglobulin receptors, is believed to trigger the chain of events that characterizes the specific immunologic reaction. Again, depending on the nature of the antigen, the immune response may either be cellular or humoral or both.

Cellular immunity appears to be the host's principal protective shield against certain chemical and bacterial agents, viruses, and allogeneic or genetically dissimilar cells. It is thymic dependent, as evidenced by its impairment in infants with congenital absence of the thymus, and its restoration after thymic transplants.[6, 7] It is mediated by T–lymphocytes believed to have originated from the bone marrow stem cell and passed through or in some way influenced by the thymus. A characteristic histological feature of cellular immunity is the T–cell proliferation in the deep cortical area of the regional lymph node.[8] *In vitro* studies have demonstrated that interaction between previously sensitized lymphocytes and the sensitizing antigen results in the production of at least four soluble mediators of cellular immune response, e.g. transfer factor for delayed cutaneous hypersensitivity, lymphoblastogenic factor, macrophage inhibitory factor, and lymphocytotoxin.[9]

On the other hand, the B–cell mediated humoral antibody response appears to be relatively T–cell dependent.[6,7, 10, 11] Like interferon, immunoglobulins are synthesized both locally in the mucous

membrane[12–14] and systemically in the lymph nodes and spleen.[15, 16] There are now at least five known immunoglobulins, e.g. IgG, IgA, IgM, IgD and IgE. While the bulk of local or secretory antibody is made up of IgA,[13] the principal serum antibody is IgG.[17] The humoral antibody system functions by lysing, neutralizing and opsonizing the antigens with or without the participation of the complement components. Release of certain pharmacological mediators may result from one of these interactions.[18] Histamine liberation in allergic diseases is a good example.

In general, where the port of entry of the antigen is the mucous membrane, local antibody production precedes and probably influences the systemic humoral antibody response. When the latter becomes expedient, IgM is the earliest detectable antibody. This is followed by the appearance of IgG, and in cases where it was checked, also IgA. The positions of IgD and IgE in this sequence of events that characterizes the primary immune response, remain to be determined. In contrast to cellular immunity, humoral immune response is associated with lymphoid cell proliferation in the far cortical area and increased number of plasma cells in the medullary cords of the regional lymph nodes.[8]

A second encounter with the same antigen will evoke an accelerated and accentuated immune response, so–called anamnestic or secondary response. Because of the immediate availability of humoral antibody, phagocytosis is enhanced through opsonization. Similarly, rapid destruction or isolation of the antigen occurs in case of cellular immunity.

Relative inefficiency of the immunologic function has been observed during early infancy and senescence.[19, 20] The genetic aspect of the specific immune response has yet to be elucidated.[21]

TUMOR ANTIGEN

The mere implication that the immunologic mechanism has something to do with the host's defense against oncogenesis requires first of all the existence of tumor antigen. That this is indeed the case in most experimental neoplasms, is now well established. However, evidence for the presence of specific antigen in human cancer is just beginning to accumulate.

Transplantation studies in both syngeneic and allogeneic animals have revealed the phenomena of antigenic loss and antigenic gain. That is, a tumor may lose its organ specific antigen while gaining a new one, thereby becoming foreign to the host.[22, 23] This newly acquired tumor antigen is independent of the histocompatibility system. Its antigenicity varies, but has been observed to be generally of low degree. It may be the carcinogen itself as in the case of RNA virus induced tumors or a carcinogen–induced alteration of the normal cell constituent.

Physical, chemical or viral carcinogens can induce tumors with relative ease in animals. Tumors induced by a single strain of virus tend to have a common cross–reacting antigen, even in different animal species.[24] Contrariwise, neoplasms induced by a given physical or chemical carcinogen, even in the same animal, possess different non–cross–reacting tumor specific antigens.[25, 26]

The available data on human cancer seem to parallel the findings in virus induced experimental tumors insofar as the presence of a common antigen for a given type of malignancy is concerned. A cell membrane glyco–protein antigen which is identical to the normal fetal constituent during the first six months of life, has been demonstrated in all human adenocarcinomata arising from the entodermally–derived epithelium of the gastro–intestinal tract.[27] This so-called carcinoembryonic antigen seems to be relatively specific. It disappeared from the serum following surgical excision of the tumor,[28] and has not been detected in normal individuals. Normal pregnant women are the only other group of individuals who have detectable circulating anti–carcinoembryonic antibody. However, it is not inconceivable that such antibody could have been induced by fetal antigen which had somehow seeped through the placenta.

Other cases where similar antigenic reversion has been noted are primary hepatoma with its $alpha_1$ fetoprotein and lung cancers with their placental alkaline phosphatase isoenzyme.[29, 30] The $aplha_1$ fetoprotein appears to be less specific. It has been found in only about 50% of patients with primary hepatoma and has also been detected in other hepatic diseases.

Another cross–reacting tumor specific antigen has recently been demonstrated in malignant melanoma.[31] A cystic melanoma extract which has a beta globulin mobility on electrophoresis, was shown to induce *in vitro* blastogenesis in the donor's lymphocytes, as well as those from six other patients with metastatic malignant melanoma, but not those from normal subjects.

THE HOST'S RESPONSE TO THE TUMOR ANTIGEN

Given an antigen, the host's reaction may be envisaged as being no different from the normal pattern of immune response. However, it is apparent that the host's recognition apparatus is impaired in cancer patients,[32] and this could very well be responsible for the overall depression of the immunologic mechanism in such individuals. The macrophage itself appears to be even hyperactive when tested for its phagocytic activity in the presence of a normal recognition component.[33]

In vitro studies with interferon have demonstrated its capacity to inhibit both the intracellular replication of and the induction of cellular transformation by the oncogenic viruses.[34–37] There are some indications of a similar interferon activity *in vivo.*[38–41] Viruses are known interferon inducers, but whether the tumor itself has the same capability is not known.

Where demonstrable, both humoral and cellular immune response to the weak tumor antigens seem to be the case in man and animal alike.[27, 31, 42–45] Variation in the degree of responsiveness between these two types of immunity has also been observed, but it is becoming evident that the host's protection against cancer is dependent upon a competent cellular immune apparatus.[46, 47]

EFFECTS OF HOST'S RESPONSE ON TUMOR GROWTH

If, indeed, human neoplasms were due to oncongenic viruses, as evidence seems to suggest,[47a] then theoretically interferon would have a definite role in preventing tumor growth. Further developments in this area will hopefully be forthcoming.

Phagocytosis does not appear to have much influence on oncogenesis in the absence of a competent recognition mechanism.[32]

As pointed out previously, the immune response of cancer patients is generally depressed, but it is beginning to appear that intact delayed cutaneous hypersensitivity goes hand–in–hand with localized tumor.[46–48] In some patients with metastatic tumors, the cellular immune mechanism appears to be overwhelmed rather than suppressed. Partial excision tends to facilitate the eventual rejection of the rest of the tumor.[49, 50] The role of the humoral antibody system in the destruction of cancer cells has been controversial. Although *in vitro* experiments did demonstrate its opsonizing and complement–dependent cytoxic activities, *in vivo* studies have not been very encouraging.[51–54] Evidence seems to indicate that the humoral antibody may even actually enhance tumor growth.[55, 56] It is conceivable that the antibody in its attempt to protect, also jeopardizes the host by shielding the tumor specific antigen, thereby obviating the cellular immune response or preventing the interaction between the latter and the cancer cells.

EFFECTS OF CARCINOGENS ON THE IMMUNE RESPONSE

Data on the immunosuppressive properties of viral and chemical carcinogens are obviously restricted to those obtained from experimental animals. Oncogenic viruses can depress both the cellular and the humoral immunologic apparatus, although to a variable degree.[57–62] Their depressive actions appear to affect both the primary and secondary response of the humoral antibody system. It has also been shown that depression of the cellular immunity does not become evident until the appearance of the tumor.[63] Measles, rubella, and other common non–oncogenic human viruses are well known causes of anergy in man. The mechanism behind this phenomenon is poorly understood.

Most if not all chemical carcinogens are also immunosuppressants.[64–66] Like the oncogenic viruses, these chemicals are capable of depressing both humoral and cellular immune reactions. Among the physical carcinogens, x–irradiation is the known immuno–depressant.[67, 68]

EFFECTS OF CANCER ON THE IMMUNE RESPONSE

While the immunosuppressive effect of the carcinogens is well established, the same cannot be said for the tumor itself. The available clinical data purporting a depressed immunologic state in cancer patients were understandably gathered only after the diagnosis. A recent study yielded a suggestive evidence for a partly tumor–induced depression of the humoral antibody response in animals.[69] On the other hand, there are some indications that the immunologic apparatus of some cancer patients remains competent and the apparent impairment can be a result of its being overwhelmed by the fast-growing malignant cells.[49,69a] Partial removal of the tumor has been associated with improvement of the immune response.

IMMUNODEFICIENCY AND CANCER

The association between immunodeficiency states and cancer is now well established. Table 1 shows the frequently occurring malignancies in some of the primary immunodeficiency disorders.

Reticulum cell sarcoma, plasmacytoma and lymphosarcoma have been reported in transplantation patients receiving various kinds of immunosuppressives.[91] Senescence, immunodeficiency and cancer are also known to go hand–in–hand.[76]

Thymectomized BALB/c mice are susceptible to experimentally induced leukemia, and animals receiving anti–lymphocyte serum tend to develop reticulum cell sarcomata.[92]

The foregoing data tend to give support to the hypothesis that oncogenesis is dependent upon the state of the immuno-surveillance system.[93]

CANCER, AUTO–IMMUNE DISEASE AND IMMUNODEFICIENCY

Cancer and auto–immune disease share a common attribute, viz. the capacity to evoke an immunologic response directed against an erstwhile normal host's constituent. While the phenomen is not exactly identical in many respects, it is hard to ignore the seemingly parallel patterns between these two disorders. An increased incidence of spontaneous tumor has been noted in NZB/Bl mice which happen to be unusually susceptible to auto–immune diseases.[94, 95] Likewise, a diverse form of malignancy is known to occur in association with auto–immune diseases in man. Lymphomas have been found in patients with systemic lupus erythematosus, rheumatoid arthritis, Sjogren's syndrome and Hashimoto's disease.[96–99]

Both auto–immune disease and neoplasms are more common in individuals with immunodeficiency, and all these three entities have been found to occur with an unusual frequency in certain families.[70, 96, 97, 100–103]

Table I (References 70–90)

PRIMARY IMMUNODEFICIENCY DISEASES*	ESTIMATED INCIDENCE OF CANCER#	COMMONLY ASSOCIATED MALIGNANCIES
HUMORAL IMMUNODEFICIENCY		
X–linked recessive Agammaglobulinemia (Bruton's)	5%	Malignant lymphoma; acute lymphocytic leukemia; chronic myelogenous leukemia; Hodgkin's disease; sarcoma; carcinoma
Primary Hypogamma-globulinemia** (Acquired late–onset Agammaglobulinemia)	10%	Lymphoma; leukemia; Hodgkin's disease; Gl carcinoma; reticulum cell sarcoma; solid tissue fibrosarcoma; other epithelioma
COMBINED IMMUNODEFICIENCY		
Autosomal recessive Thymic Hypoplasia with Agammaglobulinemia (Swiss)	5%	Lymphoid malignancy (acute leukemia; lymphosarcoma; Hodgkin's disease)#
Autosomal recessive Ataxia–Telangiectasia–Immunodeficiency Syndrome (Louis–Bar's)	10%	Hodgkin's disease; reticulum cell sarcoma; small cell lymphosarcoma; dysgerminoma; frontal lobe glioma; acute lymphocytic leukemia; epithelioma
X–linked recessive Eczema–Thrombopenia–Immunodeficiency Syndrome (Wiskott–Aldrich)	10%	Malignant lymphoma; chronic myelogenous leukemia; malignant reticulo–endotheliosis; astrocytoma

*Partly based on WHO nomenclature (New Eng. J. Med. 283:656, 1970)
**May have combined immunodeficiency
#Gatti, R.A., Good, R.A.: Occurrence of Malignancy in Immunodeficiency Diseases. A Literature Review, Cancer, *28*: 89, 1971.

In Immunologic Deficiency Diseases in Man. Good R.A. & Bergsma, D. Eds. Birth Defects Original Article Series. Nat. Foundation Press. p. 443, 1968.

CANCER, GENETICS, SKIN & IMMUNITY

The importance of utilizing the readily available cutaneous manifestations of certain types of cancer for its diagnostic and genetic implications has been previously pointed out.[104, 105] Human cancer having specific dermatologic lesions and immunologic aberrations at the same time are listed in Table II.

The intimate association between the tumors of the lympho–reticular tissue and immunologic impairment is further borne out in the above data.

However, evidence indicates that the immunologic aberration follows rather than precedes the malignancy.[125]

The cutaneous lesions may be rare and may not manifest itself until later in the course of the tumor but are nevertheless specific in these particular cases. The dearth of genetic information is quite obvious.

THE STATUS AND FUTURE OF CANCER IMMUNOTHERAPY

There is no doubt that the present mode of cancer therapy has been far

TABLE II (Reference 104-124)

CANCER	GENETICS	SPECIFIC CUTANEOUS LESIONS*	IMMUNOLOGIC ABERRATIONS
Malignant melanoma	May be familial	Primarily a cutaneous malignancy arising from junctional nevi	Delayed hypersensitivity is intact when localized but impaired when metastatic. Auto–antigen–induced lymphoblastogenesis is intact.
Lympho–sarcoma	Unknown	Discrete or coalesced dull red, firm, deep papules, nodules or tumors	Impaired delayed hypersensitivity and both primary and secondary humoral response.
Acute leukemia	Unknown	Nodules and diffuse cutaneous infiltrate may be found	Impaired primary but normal secondary humoral antibody response
Chronic lympho-cytic leukemia	Unknown CH[1] chromosome	Same as above, with higher frequency	Impaired primary and secondary humoral antibody response
Hodgkin's disease	May be familial HL–A5 positive	Uncommon but may have papules, nodules or granulomatous or ulcerative plaques	Impaired delayed hypersensitivity and primary but normal secondary humoral immune response
Multiple myeloma	Unknown	Rare but may have dark red papules, nodules or tumors, which may ulcerate	Impaired primary and secondary humoral antibody response

*Specific or characteristic cancer cells are histologically demonstrable.

from adequate. Although surgical excision may be curative for localized tumors, it certainly is not the ideal treatment for widespread cancer. Both x–irradiation and chemotherapeutic measures are non–specific and tend to damage normal tissues, as well as compromise the already impaired immune mechanism and therefore even seem illogical forms of therapy. Nevertheless, the judicious utilization of these measures, either singly or in combination may yet lead to cancer cure in those patients whose immunologic apparatus are merely overwhelmed rather than depressed.

Based on the foregoing discussion, humoral antibody, be it passively administered or actively induced, appears to have a limited value in cancer immunotherapy. Results of preliminary studies have been discouraging and its potential tumor enhancing effect is always to be reckoned with.[54, 55, 126]

Reconstitution of the defective cellular immune response in cancer patients, with histocompatible bone marrow graft has been attempted. So far, the allogeneic bone marrow transplants have not been very successful because of severe graft–versus–host reactions.[127] The non–specific stimulation of cellular immunity with BCG vaccine has also shown some encouraging results.[128] Another possibility is the utilization of specific anti–tumor lymphocytes, which have been demonstrated to be effective at least in experimental animals.[129–131] Thus, it appears that the immunotherapeutic measures aimed at restoring cellular immunocompetency alone or in combination with the other standard regimen, would be the logical approach to cancer management in the future.

SUMMARY AND CONCLUSION

The present concept of tumor immunology has been summarized. There is now some evidence for the existence of tumor specific antigen common to a given type of human cancer. Such antigens have been shown to evoke both humoral and cellular immune response, and therefore have diagnostic significance in immuno-competent cancer patients. Tumor immunity seems to depend on an intact cellular immune mechanism. Individuals with metastatic tumors tend to have either an overwhelmed or a depressed immunologic system. While the immunosuppressive properties of the experimental carcinogens are well established, those of the tumor itself remain to be elucidated. Impairment of both recognition and immune mechanisms might occur before, during or after carcinogenesis. The apparent intimate inter–relationship between cancer, autoimmune diseases and immunologic deficiency states tend to support the concept of immunosurveillance.

Immunotherapy alone or in combination with the standard regimen seems to be the logical approach to cancer management. However, cure and prevention can only be realized when the epidemiology, genetics and etiopathogenesis of human cancer have been decisively delineated through an all–out concerted effort.

REFERENCES

1. Erlich, P.: In Collected Papers. 2: 557, 1957. Pergamon Press.

2. Boyden, S.: Cellular Recognition of Foreign Matter. *Int. Rev. Exp. Path.* 2: 311, 1963.

3. Lockhart, R.Z., Jr.: Biological Properties of Interferons; Criteria for Acceptance of a Viral Inhibitor as an Interferon. In Interferon, p. 1. Finter, N.B., Ed., W.B. Saunders Co., Philadelphia, 1966.

4. Green, J.A., Copperband, S.R., Kleinman, L.F., and Kibrick, S.: Immune Stimulation of Interferon in Human Leukocyte Cultures by Non–viral Antigens. *Ann. N.Y. Acad. Sci. 173:* 736, 1969.

5. Stinebring, W.R. and Absher, P.M.: Production of Interferon Following an Immune Response. *Ibid. 173*: 714, 1969.

6. August, C.S., Rosen, F.S., Filler, R.M., Janeway, C.A., Markowski, B., and Kay, H.E.M.: Implantation of a Foetal Thymus, Restoring Immunological Competence in a Patient with Thymic Aplasia (DiGeorge's Syndrome). *Lancet ii*: 1210, 1968.

7. Cleveland, W.W., Fogel, B.J., Brown, W.T., and Kay, H.E.M.: Foetal Thymic Transplant in a Case of DiGeorge's Syndrome. *Ibid. ii*: 1211, 1968.

8. Gatti, R.A. and Good, R.A.: Immunological Deficiency Diseases. *Med. Clin. N. Amer. 54:* 281, 1970.

9. Lawrence, H.S.: Transfer Factor and Cellular Immune Deficiency Disease. *New Eng. J. Med. 283:* 411, 1970.

10. Kretschmer, R., Say, B., Brown, D. and Rosen, F.S.: Congenital Aplasia of the Thymus Gland (DiGeorge's Syndrome). *Ibid. 279:* 1295, 1968.

11. Porter, H.M.: Immunologic Studies in Congenital Agammaglobulinemia with Emphasis on Delayed Hypersensitivity. *Pediatrics 20:* 958, 1957.

12. Ogra, P.O., Karzon, D.T., Righthand, F., and MacGillvray, M.: Immunoglobulin Response in Serum and Secretions After Immunization with Live and Inactivated Poliovaccine and Natural Infections. *New Eng. J. Med. 279:* 893, 1968.

13. Tomasia, T.B., Jr.: Human Immunoglobulin A. *Ibid. 279*: 893, 1968.

14. Butler, W.T., Rossen, R.D., and Waldmann, T.A.: The Mechanism of Appearance of Immunoglobulin A in Nasal Secretions in Man. *J. Clin. Invest. 46*: 1883, 1967.

15. Rowley, D.A.: The Formation of Circulating Antibody in the Splenectomized Human Being Following Intravenous Injection of Heterologous Erythrocytes. *J. Immunol. 65*: 515, 1950.

16. McMaster, P.D., and Hudack, S.S.: The Formation of Agglutinins Within Lymph Nodes. *J. Exp. Med. 61*: 783, 1935.

17. Fahey, J.L.: Heterogeneity of Gamma–globulins. *Adv. Immunol 2:* 42, 1962.

18. Schild, H.O., Hawkins, D.F., Mongar, J.L., and Herxheimer, H.: Reactions of Isolated Human Asthmatic Lung and Bronchial Tissue to a Specific Antigen. *Lancet ii:* 376, 1951.

19. Zak, S.J., and Good, R.A.: Immunochemical Studies of Human Serum Gamma-globulins. *J. Clin. Invest. 38*: 579, 1959.

20. Gross, L.: Immunological Defect in Aged Population and its relationship to cancer. *Cancer 18*: 201, 1965.

21. Clarke, C.A., Price Evans, D.A., Harris, R.B., McConnell, R.B., and Woodrow, J.C.: Genetics in Medicine: A Review. *Quarterly J. Med. 37:* 220, 1968.

22. Haughton, G., and Amos, D.B.: Immunology of Carcinogenesis. *Cancer Res. 28:* 1839, 1968.

23. Foley, E.J.: Antigenic properties of Methylcholanthrene Induced Tumors in Mice of the Strain of Origin. *Ibid.*

13: 835, 1953.

24. Old, L.J., and Boyse, E.A.: Antigens of Tumors and Leukemias Induced by Viruses. *Fed. Proc. 24*: 1009, 1965.

25. Klein, G., and Klein, E.: Antigenic Properties of Other Experimental Tumors. *Cold Spring Harbor Symp. Quant. Biol. 27*: 463, 1962.

26. Globerson, A., and Feldman, M.: Antigenic Specificity of Benzpyrene Induced Sarcoma. *J. Nat. Cancer Inst.* 32: 1229, 1964.

27. Gold, P., Gold, M., and Freedman, S.O.: Cellular location of Carcinoembryonic Antigens of the Human Digestive System. *Cancer Res.* 28: 1331, 1968.

28. Thompson, D.M.P., Krupey, J., Freedman, S.O., and Gold, P.: The Radioimmunoassay of Circulating Carcinoembryonic Antigen of the Human Digestive System. *Proc. Nat. Acad. Sci. 64:* 161, 1969.

29. Alpert, M.E., Uriel, J., and De Nechaud, B.: Alpha$_1$ Fetoglobulin in the Diagnosis of Human Hepatoma. *New Eng. J. Med. 278*: 984, 1968.

30. Stolbach, L.L., Krant, M.J., and Fishman, W.H.: Ectopic Production of and Alkaline Phosphatase Isoenzyme in Patients with Cancer. *Ibid. 281:* 757, 1969.

31. Jehn, U.W., Nathanson, L., Schwartz, R.S., and Skinner, M.: In Vitro Lymphocyte Stimulation by a Soluable Antigen from Malignant Melanoma. *Ibid. 283:* 329, 1970.

32. Pisano, J.C., Di Luzio, N.R., and Salky, N.K.: Absence of Macrophage Humoral Recognition Factor (s) in Patients with Carcinoma. *J. Lab. Clin. Med. 76:* 141, 1970.

33. Salky, N.K., Di Luzio, N.R., Levin, A.G., and Goldsmith, H.S.: Phagocytic Activity of the Reticuloendothelial System in Neoplastic Disease. *J. Lab. Clin.*

Med. 70: 393, 1967.

34. Gauntt, C.J. and Lockhart, R.Z., Jr.: Inhibition of Mengo Virus by Interferon. *J. Bacteriol. 91:* 176, 1966.

35. Gauntt, C.J. and Lockhart, R.Z., Jr.: Destruction of L Cells by Mengo Virus: Use of Interferon to Study the Mechanism. *J. Virol. 2:* 567, 1968.

36. Allison, A.C.,: Interference with, and Interferon Production by Polyoma Virus. *Virology 15:* 47, 1961.

37. Finter, N.B., Ed., Interferon, W.B. Saunders Co., Philadelphia, 1966.

38. Gresser, I., Coppey, J., Falcoff, E., and Fontaine, D.: Interferon and Murine Leukemia I. Inhibitory Effect of Interferon Preparations on Development of Friend Leukemia in Mice. *Proc. Soc. Exp. Biol. Med. 124:* 84, 1967.

39. Gresser, I., Fontaine, D., Coppey, J., Falcoff, R., and Falcoff, E.: Interferon and Murine Leukemia. II. Factors Related to the Inhibitory Effect of Interferon Preparations on Development of Friend Leukemia in Mice. *Proc. Soc. Exp. Biol. Med. 124:* 91, 1967.

40. Zeleznick, L.D. and Bhuyan, B.K.: Treatment of Leukemic (L–1210) Mice with Double–stranded Polyribonuceotides. *Proc. Soc. Exp. Biol. Med. 130:* 126, 1969.

41. De Clercq, E., and Merigan, T.C.: Current Concepts of Interferon and Interferon Induction. *Ann. Rev. Med. 21:* 17, 1970.

42. Klein, G.: Tumor–specific Transplantation Antigens. *Cancer Res. 28:* 625, 1968.

43. Batchelor, J.R.: The use of Enhancement in Studying Tumor Antigens. *Ibid; 28:* 1410, 1968.

44. Hellstrom, I., Hellstrom, K.E., Pierce, G.E., and Yang, J.P.S.: Cellular and Humoral Immunity to Different Types of Human Neoplasms. *Nature*

220: 1352, 1968.

45. Southam, C.M.: The Immunologic Status of Patients with Non–lymphomatous Cancer. *Cancer Res. 28:* 1433, 1968.

46. Alexander, P., and Fairley, G.H.: Cellular Resistance to Tumours. *Brit. Med. Bull. 23:* 86, 1967.

47. Klein, G.: Experimental Studies in Tumor Immunology. *Fed. Proc. 28:* 1739, 1969.

47a. Gallo, R.C.; Yang, S.S., and Ting, R.C.: RNA Dependent DNA Polymerase of Human Acute Leukemic Cells. *Nature 228:* 927, 1970.

48. Fass, L., Herberman, R.B., and Ziegler, J.: Delayed Cutaneous Hypersensitivity Reactions to Autologous Extracts of Burkittlymphoma Cells. *New Eng. J. Med. 282:* 776, 1970.

49. Wilson, R.E., Hager, E.B., Hampers, C.L., Corson, J.M., Merrill, J.P. and Murray, J.E.: Immunologic Rejection of Human Cancer Transplanted with a Renal Allograft. *New Eng. J. Med. 278:* 479, 1968.

50. Eilber, F.R. and Morton, D.L:. Impaired Immunologic Reactivity and Recurrence Following Cancer Surgery. *Cancer 25:* 362, 1970.

51. Hellstrom, K.E. and Moller, G.: Immunological and Immunogenetic Aspects of Tumor Transplantation. *Progr. Allergy 9:* 158, 1965.

52. Gold, P.: Circulating Antibodies Against Carcinoembryonic Antigens of the Human Digestive System. *Cancer 20:* 1663, 1967.

53. Gorer, P.A.: The Antigenic Structures of Tumors. *Immunology 1:* 345, 1961.

54. Milner, J.E., Evans, C.A., and Werser, R.S.: Immunity and the Treatment of Cancer. *Lancet ii:* 816, 1964.

55. Kaliss, N.: Immunological enhancement. *Int. Rev. Exp. Path. 8:* 241, 1969.

56. Hellstrom, K.E. and Hellstrom, I: Cellular Immunity Against Tumor Antigens. *Advances Cancer Res. 12*: 167, 1969.

57. Peterson, R.D.A., Hendrickson, R., and Good, R.A.: Reduced Antibody Forming Capacity During the Incubation Period of Passage A Leukemia in C3H Mice. *Proc. Soc. Exp. Biol. Med. 114:* 517, 1963.

58. Dent, P.B., Peterson, R.D.A., and Good, R.A.: A Defect in Cellular Immunity During the Incubation of Passage A Leukemia in C3H Mice. *Ibid. 119:* 869, 1965.

59. Salomon, M.H., and Wedderburn, N.: The Immunodepressive Effect of Friend Virus. *Immunology 10*: 445, 1966.

60. Cremer, N.E.: Selective Immunoglobulin Deficiencies in Rats Infected with Moloney Virus. *J. Immunol. 99:* 71, 1967.

61. Cremer, N.E., Taylor D.O.N., and Hagens, S.J.: Antibody Formation, Latency and Leukemia: Infection with Maloney Virus. *Ibid. 96:* 495, 1966.

62. Siegel, B.V. and Morton, J.I.: Depressed Antibody Response in the Mouse Infected with Rauscher Leukemia Virus. *Immunology 10:* 559, 1966.

63. Stjernsward, J.: Immunodepressive Effect of 3–Methylcholanthrene. Antibody Formation at the Cellular Level and Reaction Against Weak Antigenic Homografts. *J. Nat. Cancer Inst. 35:* 885, 1965.

64. Rubin, B.A.: Carcinogen–induced Tolerance to Homotransplanatation. *Progr. Exp. Tumor Res. 5:* 217, 1964.

65. Malmgren, R.A., Bennison, B.E., and McKinley, T.W.: Reduced Antibody Titers in Mice Treated with Carcinogenic and Cancer Chemotherapeutic Agents.

Proc. Soc. Exp. Biol. Med. 79: 484, 1952.

66. Berenbaum, M.C.: Effects of Carcinogens on Immune Processes. *Brit. Med. Bull. 20:* 159, 1964.

67. Kaplan, H.S. and Brown, M.B.: A Quantitative Dose–response Study of Lymphoid–tumor Development in Irradiated C57 Black Mice. *J. Nat. Cancer Inst. 13:* 185, 1952.

68. Taliaferro, W.H.: Modification of the Immune Response by Radiation and Cortisone. *Ann. N.Y. Acad. Sci. 69:* 745, 1957.

69. Kearney, R. and Hughes, L.E.: The Effect of Tumour Growth on Immune Competence. A Study of DMBA Mammary Carcinogenesis in the Rat. *Brit. J. Cancer 24:* 319, 1970.

69a. Old, L.J., Boyse, E.A., Clarke, D.A., and Carswell, E.A.: Antigenic Properties of Chemically Induced Tumors. *Ann. N.Y. Acad. Sci. 101:* 80, 1962.

70. Page, A.R., Hansen, A.E., and Good, R.A.: Occurrence of Leukemia and Lymphoma in Patients with Agammaglobulinemia. *Blood 21:* 197, 1963.

71. Gelleman, E.F. and Vietti, T.J.: Congenital Hypogammaglobulinemia Preceding Hodgkin's Disease: A Case Report and Review of the Literature. *J. Pediat. 76:* 131, 1970.

72. Reisman, L.E., Mitani, M., and Zuelzer, W.W.: Chromosome Studies in Leukemia. I. Evidence of the Origin of Leukemic Stemlines from Aneuploid Mutants. *New Eng. J. Med. 270:* 591, 1964.

73. Fudenberg, H.H., and Solomon, A.: "Acquired Agammaglobulinemia" with Autoimmune Hemolytic Disease: Graft–versus–host Reaction? *Vox Sang. 6:* 68, 1961.

74. Douglas, S.D., Goldberg, L.S., and Fudenberg, H.H.: Clinical, Serologic and Leukocyte Function Studies on Patients with Idiopathic "Acquired" Agammaglobulinemia and Their Families. *Amer. J. Med. 48:* 48, 1970.

75. Green, I., Litwin, S., Adlersberg, R., and Rubin, I.: Hypogammaglobulinemia with Late Development of Lymphosarcoma. *Arch. Intern. Med. 118:* 592, 1966.

76. Hermans, P.E., Huizenga, K.A., Hoffman, H.N., Brown, A.L., and Markowitz, H.: Dysgammaglobulinemia Associated with Nodular Lymphoid Hyperplasia of the Small Intestine. *Amer. J. Med. 40:* 78, 1966.

77. Gatti, R.A. and Good, R.A.: Aging, Immunity, and Malignancy. *Geriatrics 25:* 158, 1970.

78. Huber, J.: Experience with Various Immunologic Deficiencies in Holland. In Immunologic Deficiency Diseases in Man. Good, R.A. and Bergsma, D., Eds. Birth Defects Original Articles Series, National Foundation Press, p. 53, 1968.

79. Boder, E. and Sedgwick, R.P.: Ataxia–telangiectasia: A Review of 101 Cases. In Cerebellum, Posteur and Cerebral Palsy. Walsh, G., Ed. London: Heinemann, p. 110, 1963.

80. Dunn, H.G., Meuwissen, H., Livingstone, C.S., and Pump, K.K.: Ataxia–telangiectasis. *Canad. Med. Ass. J. 91:* 1106, 1964.

81. Peterson, R.D.A., Kelly, W.D., and Good, R.A.: Ataxia–telangiectasia. Its Association with a Defective Thymus, Immunological Deficiency Disease and Malignancy. *Lancet 1:* 1189, 1964.

82. Shuster, J., Hart, Z., Stimson, C.W., Brough, A.J., and Poulik, M.D.: Ataxia-telangiectasia with Cerebellar Tumor. *Pediatrics 37:* 776, 1966.

83. Hecht, F., Koler, R.D., Rigas, D.A., Dahnke, G.S., Case, M.D., Tisdale, V., and Miller, R.W.: Luekemia and Lympho-

cytes in Ataxia– telangiectasia. *Lancet 2:* 193, 1966.

84. Smeby, B.: Ataxia–telangiectasia. *Acta Paediat. (Uppsala) 55:* 239, 1966.

85. Haerer, A.F., Jackson, J.F., and Evers, C.G.: Ataxia–telangiectasia with Gastric Adenocarcinoma. *JAMA 210:* 1884, 1969.

86. Coleman, A., Leikin, S., and Guin, G.H.: Aldrich's Syndrome. *Clin. Proc. Child. Hosp. (Wash.) 17:* 22, 1961.

87. Kildeberg, P.: A Case of Aldrich's Syndrome. *Acta Paediat. (Uppsala) 140:* 120, 1961.

88. ten Bensel, R.W., Stadlan, E.M., and Krivit, W.: The Development of Malignancy in the Course of the Aldrich Syndrome. *J. Pediat. 68:* 761, 1966.

89. Jeunet, F., and Good, R.A.: Thyoma, immunologic Deficiencies and Hematological Abnormalities. In Immunologic Deficiency Diseases in Man. Good, R.A. and Bergsma, D., Eds. Birth Defects Original Articles Series, National Foundation Press, p. 192, 1968.

90. Gafni, J., Michaeli, D., and Heller, Il.: Idiopathic Acquired Agammaglobulinemia Associated with Thymoma. Report of Two Cases and Review of the Literature. *New Eng. J. Med. 263:* 536, 1960.

91. Penn, I., Hammond, W., Brettschneider, L., and Starzl, T.E.: Malignant Lymphomas in Transplantation Patients. *Transpl Proc. I:* 106, 1969.

92. Allison, A.C., and Law, L.W.: Effects of Antilymphocyte Serum on Virus Oncogenesis. *Proc. Soc. Exp. Biol. Med. 127:* 207, 1968.

93. Burnet, F.M.: The Concept of Immunosurveillance. *Exp. Tumor Res. 13:* 1, 1970.

94. Bielschowsky, M., and Bielschowsky, F.: Reaction of the Reticular Tissue of Mice with Autoimmune Haemolytic Anemia to 2–amino–fluorene. *Nature 194:* 692, 1962.

95. Mellors, R.C.: Autoimmune Disease in NZB/Bl Mice. II. Autoimmunity and Malignant Lymphoma. *Blood 27:* 435, 1966.

96. Cammarata, R.J., Rodman, G.P., and Jensen, W.N.: Systemic Rheumatic Disease and Malignant Lymphoma. *Arch. Intern Med. 111:* 330, 1963.

97. Talal, N. and Bunim, J.J.: The Development of Malignant Lymphoma in the Course of Sjögren's Syndrome. *Amer. J. Med. 36:* 529, 1964.

98. Ranstrom, S.: Malignant Lymphoma of the Thyroid and its Relation to Hashimoto's and Brill–Symmers Disease. *Acta. Chir. Scand. 113:* 185, 1957.

99. Cureton, R.J.R., Harland, D.H.C., Hosford, J., and Pike, B.: Reticulosarcoma in Hashimoto's Disease. *Brit. J. Surg. 44:* 561, 1957.

100. Fudenberg, H.H.: Immunologic Deficiency, Autoimmune Disease, and Lymphoma; Observation, Implications, and Speculations. *Arthritis Rheum. 9:* 464, 1966.

101. Ginsberg, A. and Mullinax, F.: Pernicious Anemia and Monoclonal Gammopathy in a Patient with IgA Deficiency. *Amer. J. Med. 48:* 787, 1970.

102. Schwartz, R.S. and Costea, N.: Autoimmune Hemolytic Anemia; Clinical Correlations and Biological Implications. *Seminars Hemat. 3:* 2, 1966.

103. Freeman, A.I., Sinks, L.F., and Cohen, M.M.: Lymphosarcoma in Siblings, Associated with Cytogenetic Abnormalities, Immune Deficiency, and Abnormal Erythropoiesis. *J. Pediat. 77:* 996, 1970.

104. Lynch, H.T.: Skin, Heredity, and Cancer. *Cancer 24:* 277, 1969.

105. Lynch, H.T. and Szentivanyi, J.: Genetics as Guide to Early Diagnosis and Cancer Control – Cutaneous Syndrome. *Cutis 6:* 179, 1970.

106. Lewis, G.M. and Wheeler, C.E., Jr. Practical Dermatology. 3rd Ed. W.B. Saunders Co., Philadelphia, 1967, p. 549.

107. Fass, L., Ziegler, J.L., Herberman, R.B., and Kiryabwire, J.W.M.: Cutaneous Hypersensitivity Reactions to Autologous Extracts of Malignant Melanoma Cells. *Lancet 1:* 116, 1970.

108. Geller, W.: A Study of Antibody formation in Patients with Malignant Lymphomas. *J. Lab. Clin. Med. 42:* 232, 1953.

109. Heath, R.B., Fairley, G.H., and Malpas, J.S.: Production of Antibodies Against Viruses in Leukemia and Related Disorders. *Brit. J. Haemat. 10:* 365, 1964.

110. Fairley, G.H. and Scott, R.B.: Hypogammaglobulinemia in Chronic Lymphatic Leukemia. *Brit. Med. J. 2:* 920, 1961.

111. Hudson, R.P. and Wilson, S.J.: Hypogammaglobulinaemia and Chronic Lymphatic Leukaemia. *Cancer 13:* 200, 1960.

112. Silver, R.T., Utz, J.P., Fahey, H., and Frei, E.: Antibody Responses in Patients with Acute Leukemia. *J. Lab. Clin. Med. 56:* 634, 1960.

113. Shaw, R.K., Szwed, C., Fahey, J.L., Frei, E. Morrisoin, E., and Utz, J.P.: Infection and Immunity in Chronic Lymphocytic Leukemia. *Arch. Intern. Med. 106:* 467, 1960.

114. Barr, M. and Fairley, G.H.: Circulating Antibodies in Reticuloses. *Lancet 1:* 1305, 1961.

115. Lytton, B., Hughes, L.E., and Fulthorpe, A.J.: Circulating Antibody Response in Malignant Disease. *Ibid 1:* 69, 1964.

116. Lamb, D., Pilney, F., Kelly, W.D., and Good, R.A.: A Comparative Study of the Incidence of Anergy in Patients with Carcinoma, Leukemia, Hodgkin's Disease and Other Lymphomas. *J. Immunol. 89:* 555, 1962;

117. Schier, W.W., Roth, A., Ostroff, G., and Schrift, M.H.: Hodgkin's Disease and Immunity. *Amer. J. Med. 20:* 94, 1956.

118. Hughes, L.E. and Mackay, W.D.: Suppression of the Tuberculin Response in Malignant Disease. *Brit. Med. J. 2:* 1346, 1965.

119. Solowey, A.C. and Rapaport, F.T.: Immunologic Responses in Cancer Patients. *Surg. Gynec. Obstet. 121:* 756, 1965.

120. Aisenberg, A.C.: Immunologic Status of Hodgkin's Disease. *Cancer 19:* 385, 1966.

121. Levin, A.G., McDonough, E.F., Jr., Miller, D.G. and Southam, C.M.: Delayed Hypersensitivity Response to DNFB in sick and healthy persons. *Ann. N.Y. Acad. Sci. 120:* 400, 1964.

122. Miller, D.G.: Patterns of Immunological Deficiency in Lymphomas and Leukemias. *Ann. Intern. Med. 57:* 703, 1962.

123. Zinnerman, H.H. and Wendell, H.H.: Recurrent Pneumonia in Multiple Myeloma and some Observations on Immunologic Response. *Ann. Intern. Med. 41:* 1152. 1954.

124. Lawson, H.A., Stuart, C.A., Paull, A.M., Phillips, A.M., and Phillips, R.W.: Observations on the Antibody Content of the Blood in Patients with Multiple Myeloma. *New Eng. J. Med. 252:* 13, 1955.

125. Southam, C.M.: Evidence for Cancer–specific Antigens in man. *Progr. Exp. Tumor Res. 9:* 1, 1967.

126. Alexander, P.: Immunotherapy of

Cancer: Experiments with Primary Tumours and Syngeneic Tumour Grafts. *Progr. Exp. Tumor Res. 10:* 22, 1968.

127. Mathe, G., Amiel, J.L., Schwarszenberg, L., Schneider, M., Cattan, A., Schlumberger, J.R., Nowza, K., and Hrask, Y.: Bone Marrow Transplantation in Man. *Transpl. Proc. 1:* 16, 1969.

128. Mathe, G., Amiel, J.L., Schwarzenberg, L., Schneider, M., Cattan, A., Schlumberger, J.R., Hayat, M., and Vassal, F.: Active Immunotherapy for Acute Lymphoblastic Leukemia. *Lancet 1:* 697, 1969.

129. Alexander, P., Connell, D.I., and Mikulska, Z.B.: Treatment of a Murine Leukemia with Spleen Cells or Sera from Allogeneic Mice Immunized Against the Tumor. *Cancer Res. 26:* 1508, 1966.

130. Alexander, P., Delorme, E.J., and Hall, J.G.: The effect of Lymphoid Cells from the Lymph of Specifically Immunized Sheep on the Growth of Primary Sarcomata in Rats. *Lancet. 1:* 1186, 1966.

131. Alexander, P., Delorme, E.J., Hamilton, L.D.G., and Hall, J.G.: Effect of Nucleic Acids from Lymphoid Cells of Specifically Immunized Donors on the Growth of Primary Sarcomata in Rats. *Nature 213:* 569, 1967.

Chapter 13

MULTIPLE MUCOSAL NEUROMATA SYNDROME*

by Neil Schimke, M.D.

INTRODUCTION

Most clinicians are rather casual in their examination of the mucosal surfaces of the body. Obvious congenital anomalies or inflammatory lesions can hardly be overlooked, but more subtle alterations, such as those involving abnormal pigmentation, faulty dentition or minor structural change are frequently missed. The thorough physician who carefully examines the mucous membranes may be rewarded with the discovery of important physical findings, perhaps indicative of more significant internal disease. For example, oral pigmentation is an integral feature of Peutz–Jeghers syndrome and idiopathic Addison's disease. Gingival fibromas may occur with tuberous sclerosis or with Gardner's syndrome, and actually may suggest the diagnosis in a mildly affected patient. The presence of conjunctival or buccal telangiectasia in a comatose patient may facilitate an accurate assessment of the cerebrovascular status of an individual with hereditary hemorrhagic telangiectasia. A whole host of congenital abnormalities of the oral cavity, often hereditary in nature, have been described as part of more complex syndromes, other facets of which may have malignant potential (1).

Neurofibromatosis or von Recklinghausen's disease is known to affect both the skin and the mucosal surfaces, although the latter are rarely involved in the absence of extensive cutaneous lesions[2]. Recently, a syndrome has been described in which the mucocutaneous hallmarks of the disorder are mucosal neuromas which occur in association with peripheral neurofibromas, a rather uncommon type of thyroid carcinoma, and bilateral pheochromocytomas (2 – 4). Despite some common features, the mucosal neuroma syndrome appears to be distinct both from von Recklinghausen's disease and from certain other endocrine neoplasia syndromes.

Clinical Features

The facial features of affected patients are distinctive and quite unlike their normal relatives (Figures 1 & 2). The characteristic mucosal neuromas primarily involve the lips and anterior part of the tongue (Figure 3) but they may be seen on the buccal, gingival, nasal, or conjunctival mucosa (Figure 4) (3). The lesions may be flat or pedunculated. The tarsal plates may be thickened, and the lashes displaced, giving the eyes a hooded,

*Supported in part by Clinical Research Center Grant FR–67 and Program Project Grant GM15956-03.

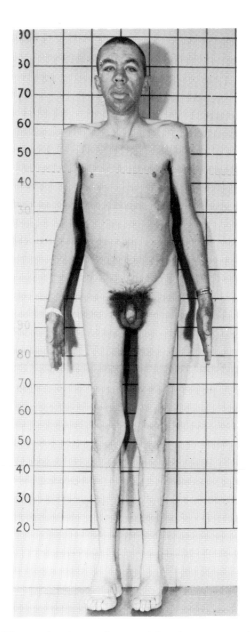

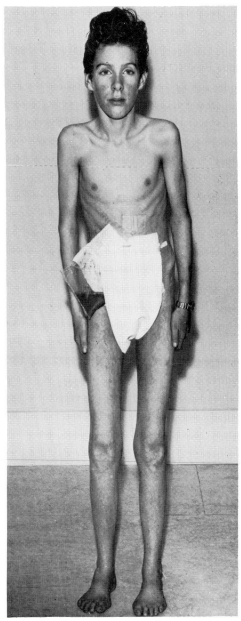

Figure 1. A patient with the mucosal neuroma syndrome. Note the heavy facial features and the Marfan–like habitus.

Figure 2. A younger patient with the same syndrome. Despite the age difference, the patient strongly resembles Figure 1 (From Normann, T. and Otnes, B.: Intestinal ganglioneuromatosis, diarrhoea and medullary thyroid carcinoma. *Scand. J. Gastroent.* 4: 553, 1969).

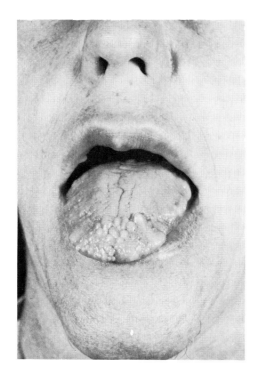

Figure 3. The tongue of this patient is studded with mucosal neuromas (Reproduced through the courtesy of the New Eng. J. Med.).

sleepy appearance (Figure 5). The corneal nerves may be strikingly enlarged (Figure 6). The labial involvement is often so extensive that the lips appear swollen and out of proportion to the remainder of the face. There is some variability in the age of onset of the neuromas, but in at least some cases the tumors have been present from birth (4). Microscopically, the mucosal nodules are essentially composed of nerve fibers with an appearance similar to plexiform neuromas. (Figure 7 & 8).

The mandible may appear prognathic, and on palpation has a somewhat rubbery consistency, the result of soft tissue rather than bony overgrowth. The prominence of the lower jaw occasionally is so marked as to suggest acromegaly, but growth hormone values have not been elevated. Some patients have shown freckling or frank café–au–lait pigmentation elsewhere on the body, and in a few cases, documented cutaneous neurofibromas have been seen (5). Intractable diarrhea may be a presenting symptom (6). Intestinal gangliomatosis has been reported on a number of occasions, and large bowel involvement may be extensive enough to suggest the radiographic diag-

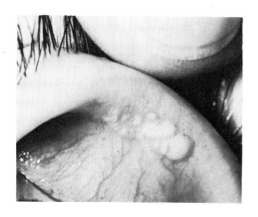

Figure 4. Typical conjunctival neuromata in an affected patient.

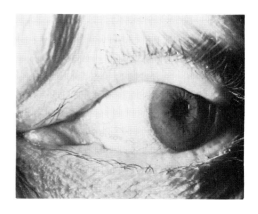

Figure 5. Note the thickened lid margins and displaced lashes.

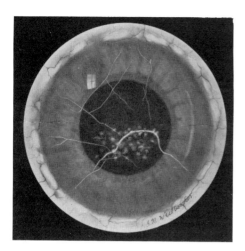

Figure 6. Thickened corneal nerves, stromal infiltrates and nodular perilimbal conjunctiva are typical ocular findings in the mucosal neuroma syndrome (Figures 4, 5 & 6 from Knox, D.L., Payne, J.W. and Hartmann, W.H.: Thickened corneal nerves and eyelids as signs of neurofibromatosis and medullary thyroid carcinoma. *Prog. Neuro–ophthalmology,* Vol. 2 of Proc. Second Int. Cong. Neuro–genetics & Neuro–ophthalmology, Montreal, Sept. 1967, p. 262).

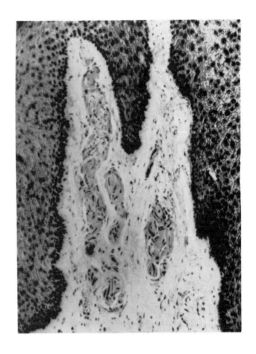

Figure 7. Histologic section of tongue nodule showing numerous nerve bundles.

nosis of ulcerative colitis (Figure 9) (4, 6, 7). Alternatively, the barium enema may be more compatible with megacolon, although ganglion cells are invariably found on biopsy, (3, 8) and histologic sections show proliferation of the nerve elements (Figure 10). Diverticulosis has been described (3, 7, 9). The patients are frequently tall and slender with long legs, a body habitus that

may simulate the Marfan syndrome (Figure 1) (10). Pes cavus, pectus excavatum and kyphosis have been reported, and muscular hypotonicity and lax joints are not uncommon. However, no ocular or cardiovascular abnormalities compatible with the Marfan syndrome have ever been found.

While the physical features are quite striking, the patient often first consults a physician because of a lump or mass in the thyroid region. A radioiodine scan may show one or more fuctionless nodules, although the patients are usually euthyroid. Exploratory surgery invariably reveals a thyroid carcinoma, frequently multifocal, and local lymph nodes may

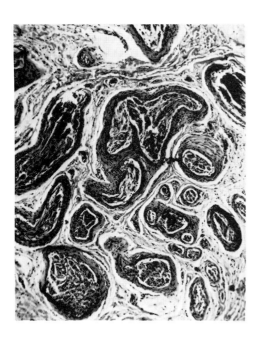

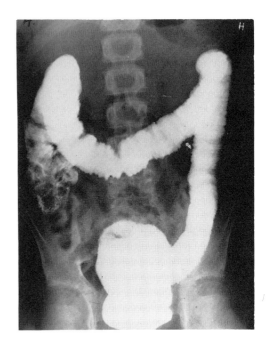

Figure 8. Higher power photomicrograph of Figure 7 showing mass of axons surrounded by thickened perineurium and epineurium (Figures 7 & 8 from Gorlin, Sedano, H.O., Vickers, R.A. and Cervenka, J.: Multiple mucosal neuromas, pheochromocytoma and medullary carcinoma of the thyroid – a syndrome. *Cancer* 22: 293, 1968).

Figure 9. Barium enema showing the radiographic appearance of intestinal gangliomatosis. The haustral markings are lost and the picture resembles ulcerative colitis.

be extensively involved. The thyroid tumor is of the solid or medullary type, and characteristically contains an amyloid stroma (Figure 11). The tumor cells frequently are found in nests or rosettes, but spindle cells are common, and pleomorphism even within the same tumor is not exceptional. The tumor may appear quite anaplastic, but long-term survival has been reported (11). The neoplasm metastasizes to every organ of the body, and lung, liver and bone are common distant sites. It has now been rather conclusively demonstrated that the tumor source is the parafollicular or C–cell of the thyroid (12, 13). The parafollicular cell in turn is thought to be of ultimobranchial origin, the cellular remnants of which in man have fused with the thyroid gland. However, controversy still surrounds the derivation of the parafollicular cell, since histochemical

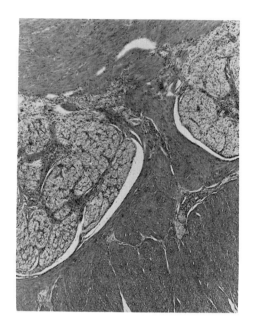

Figure 10. Photomicrograph of histologic section from the colon. The nerve elements are proliferated. (Figures 9 & 10 from Normann, T. and Otnes, B.: Intestinal gangliomatosis, diarrhoea and medullary thyroid carcinoma. *Scand. J. Gastro.* 4: 553, 1969).

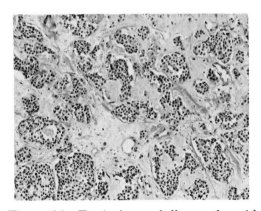

Figure 11. Typical medullary thyroid carcinoma. Note the nests of cells surrounded by a dense amyloid stroma (H & E × 165).

studies suggest the embryologic anlage may be neural crest tissue (14). It is possible that neural crest cells migrate into and become admixed with the ultimobranchial body, an epithelial pharyngeal pouch derivative.

Whatever the embryologic origin, the parafollicular cell has been firmly established as the source of the calcium–lowering hormone, calcitonin (15, 16). Extremely high levels of this hormone have been found in the medullary thyroid tumor, and the more recent development of radioimmunoassay techniques has revealed an elevated concentration of calcitonin in the peripheral blood of some medullary carcinoma patients (16, 17). The physiologic significance of calcitonin in man is not well understood; it seems evident that continued hypersecretion of this substance may lower serum calcium concentration significantly enough to elicit compensatory parathyroid hyperplasia and even adenoma formation (3). On occasion, symptoms of hyperparathyroidism may even be the presenting complaint of a patient with medullary thyroid carcinoma. Other hormonally active substances including ACTH, serotonin and prostaglandins have been isolated from the medullary thyroid carcinoma, and ectopic hormone production has been extensive enough to result in both Cushing's and the carcinoid syndrome (3, 18). Excess serotonin and prostaglandin secretion also has been implicated in the diarrhea afflicting some individuals, since removal of the tumor has resulted in decreased intestinal motility in some, but not all patients (19). Since many patients have intestinal gangliomatosis as well, the diarrhea could have either neural or hormonal pathogenetic components, and in some cases both mechanisms may be operative.

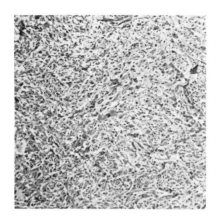

Figure 12. Histologic section of a pheo-chromocytoma showing the somewhat pleomorphic pattern (H & E × 135).

The remaining component of this syndrome is the pheochromocytoma, and the adrenal medullary lesion is commonly bilateral and multifocal. The signs and symptoms of catecholamine excess are familiar to most physicians and consist of attacks of weakness, nausea, headache, flushing sensations, palpitations, sweating and diarrhea. Elevated urinary levels of catecholamines or metabolic products of epinephrine or norepinephrine such as vanilmandelic acid (VMA) are characteristically found. Occasionally, the adrenal tumors may be asymptomatic and discovered accidentally at laporatomy or even at autopsy. Provocative tests with histamine, tyramine or glucagon may be successful in evoking release of pressor amines from the tumors, but negative responses have been seen. It is possible that the vasodilating activity of prostaglandins elaborated by a simultaneously occurring medullary thyroid cancer on occasion may inhibit the vascular re-

sponse to catecholamines (19). Microscopically, the adrenal tumors are typical pheochromocytomas (Figure 12). Less than 10% are reported to metastasize but in view of the ubiquitous nature of chromaffin tissue, the diagnosis of metastatic disease is often tenuous.

Genetics

The entire symptom complex has been described in relatively few patients, and most cases have been sporadic. Both sexes are affected, although available reports show a preponderance of females. An affected father and daughter have been reported (2), and a large family has been described in which some members suffered from the complete syndrome whereas others were less severely affected (5). The pedigree pattern was compatible with autosomal dominant inheritance. Variability in clinical expression is characteristic of autosomal dominant disorders, and some intrafamilial differences are to be expected. There is such a strong physical resemblance between the sporadic and the familial cases that most of the isolated cases probably represent new dominant mutations (20).

The occasional presence of cutaneous neurofibromas suggests a relationship with von Recklinghausen's disease. However, a large survey of patients with the latter diagnosis has revealed no increased incidence of thyroid carcinoma (21), and neurofibromas and café–au–lait pigmentation have been noted with such disorders as tuberous sclerosis and the von Hippel–Lindau syndrome. Pheochromocytomas have been reported in conjunction with the latter syndrome as well as with von Recklinghausen's disease (20). The phacomatoses are known to be genetically distinct autosomal dominant disorders, and the phenotypic overlap between them is probably related to different gene action on the common neuroectodermal tissue during a relatively short period of embryologic development. Most of the currently available evidence suggests that the mucosal neuroma syndrome is also a genetic derangement of neural crest derivatives, or in other words, a familial chromaffinomatosis (3, 5). Consequently, phenotypic overlap with the phacomatoses might be expected to occur.

Familial pheochromocytoma has been described without neurofibromatosis or medullary thyroid carcinoma, and the thyroid tumor has also been noted independently in familial aggregates (22). Whether these familial endocrine disorders, both inherited as autosomal dominants are truly genetically distinct from one another and from the mucosal neuroma syndrome is uncertain. The variable age of onset of the endocrine tumors, even within a given family, renders decisions regarding genetic independence difficult. In view of the increasing amount of genetic heterogeneity being uncovered almost daily within a given category of disease (e.g., the mucopolysaccharidoses, the mucolipidoses, the glycogen–storage diseases), a number of discrete heritable defects in neural crest development could easily exist. The mucosal neuroma syndrome might constitute one of a spectrum of entities with an identical pattern of inheritance and similar phenotypic abnormalities (23). It should be evident, however, that a patient presenting with any evidence of neural crest dysfunction should be completely evaluated from the point of view of the entire chromaffin system.

Since parathyroid adenomas have been described with the mucosal neuroma syndrome, some workers have felt that this disorder is merely one facet of Werner's syndrome of multiple endocrine adenomatosis. As previously mentioned, the parathyroid tumor would appear to be compensatory in the mucosal neuroma syndrome, whereas it is the most common type of primary endocrine lesion in Werner's syndrome (24). Moreover, pheochromocytomas have not been reported. Thyroid tumors are uncommon in Werner's syndrome, and none of the thyroid tumors have been of medullary type. Tumors of the pituitary, pancreas and adrenal cortex (except those due to ectopic ACTH production by the medullary thyroid tumor) have not been found in the mucosal neuroma syndrome. It appears that the autosomal dominant Werner's syndrome, or multiple endocrine neoplasia, type 1, is distinct from the mucosal neuroma symptom complex. The independence of these two syndromes has been stressed by some workers who prefer to designate the mucosal neuroma syndrome as multiple endocrine neoplasia, type 2 (25). In view of the possibility that a number of discrete heritable disorders presently may be misclassified as part of the mucosal neuroma syndrome, the use of numerical designations would seem to add little nosologic clarification.

Therapy

Most of the therapy must be directed toward the endocrine tumors. The thyroid carcinoma is multifocal and total thyroidectomy is the treatment of choice. Prophylactic thyroidectomy, with successful results, has been accomplished in a child with some of the mucocutaneous features of the mucosal neuroma syndrome and a positive family history (26).

A potentially useful diagnostic test involving measurement of serum calcitonin levels after infusions of calcium or glucagon recently has been developed (27). Preliminary studies suggest that calcitonin levels are higher after provocative testing in patients with medullary carcinoma, and thus may prove useful in the early diagnosis of this tumor in high-risk family members. Because of the tendency of the tumor to spread locally early and to metastasize widely relatively late, at least limited node dissection would seem to be of value. Radioiodine may be useful if surgery is contraindicated, but the effect is probably that of a non-specific irradiation, since the parafollicular cell is not known to have any particular avidity for iodine. Triiodothyronine-induced regression of both primary and metastatic lesions has been reported on one occasion (28). Why this should occur is not immediately clear. A recent report notes stromal amyloid in a mixed tumor with features of both papillary and follicular carcinoma, suggesting that the presence of amyloid may not be as specific as originally thought (29). The hormone-induced regression of the thyroid tumor may have been due to the fact that the neoplasm was not of the parafollicular type but was derived from thyroid epithelium and thus was predictably responsive to exogenous thyroid suppression.

Treatment of the pheochromocytomas is also surgical. Mention has already been made of the potential difficulties that may be encountered with provocative tests. Perirenal air insufflation has been used with some success, and occasionally an intravenous pyelogram may reveal a filling defect or some external distortion of the renal architecture. After the diagnosis is established, an abdominal surgical approach should be used since both adrenals must be explored, and if biochemical tests suggest a pheochromocytoma is present and no adrenal lesion is found, the sympathetic ganglia and the organ of Zuckerkandl should be examined. If the tumor is so extensive that removal is impossible or frozen sections show malignancy, drug therapy with a combination of alpha and beta blocking agents may be used to control symptoms. A substituted tyrosine derivative has been identified that interferes with the rate-limiting conversion of tyrosine to DOPA and thus to epinephrine and norepinephrine (30). This substance also may have some therapeutic utility in advanced cases.

Parathyroid hyperplasia, if present, may diminish after thyroidectomy. Unfortunately, parafollicular cells may also be found within the parathyroids and thymus (31), and calcitonin-producing tissue recently has been detected within the adrenal medulla (32), suggesting that this approach to hyperparathyroidism may not always be efficacious. Partial or complete parathyroidectomy may be required if symptoms are severe enough, although previous neck surgery renders such a procedure exceedingly difficult.

The mucosal neuromas require no therapy, other than cosmetic surgery. No malignant degeneration as yet has been described. Peripheral neurofibromas, if present, should be observed for sarcomatous transformation, but this is probably rare. Little can be done about the intestinal gangliomatosis, since it is likely not to be localized enough for surgical correction. Recognition of the mucosal neuroma syndrome with its potential for autonomic dysfunction may save the patient from needless gastrointestinal surgery.

Diarrhea has been reported in roughly one-third of the patients with medullary thyroid carcinoma. The diarrhea is of the rapid-transit type, and water and electrolytes constitute the major fecal loss. The small bowel mucosa is usually normal. Thyroidectomy diminished the diarrhea in some patients, and the recurrence of this symptom is often coupled with the appearance of metastases. Other patients do not respond to thyroidectomy so readily, and a combination of codeine and codethyline has been used effectively (19).

Obviously, effective therapy requires long term follow-up of the patient, especially if the entire syndrome is not present upon initial examination. Careful neck palpation and radioiodine scan coupled with periodic monitoring of the blood pressure and catecholamine excretion are mandatory preventive measures. Prophylactic thyroid surgery, especially in children with the syndrome, or in cases where the patient is unreliable, might be considered in some circumstances.

Finally, most evidence favors the familial aggregation of the mucosal neuroma syndrome. Once the proband is identified, all first degree relatives must be evaluated, and the appropriate therapeutic measures undertaken. The pedigree pattern may warrant investigation of collateral relatives as well, and examination of pertinent death certificates and autopsy material may be rewarding. Just as with the index case, longitudinal follow-up of the family must be instituted and close cooperation with other physicians in other locales is essential. Since it is not certain how many distinct entities actually comprise the mucosal neuroma syndrome, any patient with one facet of the syndrome should be considered at risk for any or all of the other lesions, and any potentially affected relative also should be approached in this same comprehensive fashion. In this manner, the dimensions of the mucosal neuroma syndrome can be identified and the presence or absence of clinical and genetic heterogeneity can be accurately delineated.

REFERENCES

1. Gorlin, R.J. and Pindborg, J.J.: *Syndromes of the Head and Neck.* McGraw-Hill, New York, 1964.

2. Williams, E.D. and Pollack, D.J.: Multiple mucosal neuromata with endocrine tumors: a syndrome allied to von Recklinghausen's disease. *J. Path. Bact.* 91: 71, 1966.

3. Schimke, R.N., Hartmann, W.H., Prout, T.E. and Rimoin, D.L.: Syndrome of bilateral pheochromocytoma, medullary thyroid carcinoma and multiple neuromas. *New Eng. J. Med. 279:* 1, 1968.

4. Gorlin, R.J., Sedano, H.O., Vickers, R.A. and Cervenka, J.: Multiple mucosal neuromas, pheochromocytoma and medullary carcinoma of the thyroid — a syndrome. *Cancer 22:* 293, 1968.

5. Ljungberg, O., Cederquist, E. and von Studnitz, W.: Medullary thyroid carcinoma and phaeochromocytoma: a familial chromaffinomatosis. *Brit. Med. J.* 1: 279, 1967.

6. Normann, T. and Otnes, B.: Intestinal ganglioneuromatosis, diarrhoea and medullary thyroid carcinoma. *Scand J. Gastroent.* 4: 553, 1969.

7. Russell, D.S. and Rubenstein, L.J.: *Pathology of Tumors of the Nervous System.* Edward Arnold, Ltd., London, 1963, p. 271.

8. Weiler, J., Lacour, J., Gérard-Marchant, R., Tubiana, M., Parmentier, C., Milhaud, G. and Bock, J.: Les épithélio-

mas médullaries a strom amylöide du corps thyroide. *Path–Biol.* 17: 995, 1969.

9. Mielke, J.E., Becker, K.L. and Gross, J.B.: Diverticulitis of the colon in a young man with Marfan's syndrome. *Gastroenterology* 48: 379, 1965.

10. Cunliffe, W.J., Hudgson, P., Fulthorpe, J.J., Black, M.M., Hall, R., Johnston, I.D.A. and Shuster, S.: A calcitonin–secreting medullary thyroid associated with mucosal neuromas, Marfanoid features, myopathy and pigmentation. *Amer. J. Med.* 48: 120, 1970.

11. Fletcher, J.R.: Medullary (solid) carcinoma of the thyroid gland. *Arch. Surg.* 100: 257, 1970.

12. Williams, E.D.: Histogenesis of medullary carcinoma of the thyroid. *J. Clin. Path.* 19: 114, 1966.

13. Gonzalez–Licea, A., Hartmann, W.H. and Yardley, J.H.: Medullary carcinoma of the thyroid. *Amer. J. Clin. Path.* 49: 512, 1968.

14. Ljungberg, O.: Two cell types in familial medullary thyroid carcinoma. *Virchows Arch. Path. Anat.* 349: 312, 1970.

15. Melvin, K.E.W. and Tashjian, A.H.: The syndrome of excessive thyrocalcitonin produced by medullary carcinoma of the thyroid. *Proc. Nat. Acad. Sci. 59*: 1216, 1968.

16. Cunliffe, W.J., Black, M.M., Hale, R., Johnston, I.D.A., Hudgson, P., Shuster, S., Gudmundsson, T.V., Joplin, G.F., Williams, E.D., Woodhouse, N.J.Y., Galante, L. and MacIntyre, I.: A calcitonin–secreting thyroid carcinoma. *Lancet 2*: 63, 1968.

17. Clark, M.B., Boyd, G.W., Byfield, P.G.H. and Foster, G.V.: A radioimmunoassay for human calcitonin *M. Lancet 2*: 74, 1969.

18. Williams, E.D., Karin, S.M.M. and Sandler, M.: Prostaglandin secretion by medullary carcinoma of the thyroid. *Lancet* 1:22, 1968.

19. Bernier, J.J., Rambaud, J.C., Cattan, D. and Prost, A.: Diarrhoea associated with medullary carcinoma of the thyroid. *Gut* 10: 980, 1969.

20. Rimoin, D.L. and Schimke, R.N.: *Genetics of the Endocrine System,* Mosby, St. Louis, 1971 (in press).

21. Crowe, F.W., Schull, W.J. and Neel, J.V.: *Multiple Neurofibromatosis,* C.C. Thomas, Springfield, Ill., 1956.

22. Schimke, R.N. and Hartmann, W.H.: Familial amyloid–producing medullary thyroid carcinoma and pheochromocytoma: a distinct genetic entity. *Ann. Int. Med.* 63: 1027, 1965.

23. Schimke, R.N.: Familial tumor endocrinopathies. *Birth Defects (Original Article Series),* 1971 (in press).

24. Ballard, H.S., Frame, B. and Hartsock, R.J.: Familial multiple endocrine adenoma–peptic ulcer complex. *Medicine* 43: 481, 1964.

25. Steiner, A.L., Goodman, A.D. and Powers, S.R.: Study of a kindred with pheochromocytoma, medullary thyroid carcinoma, hyperparathyroidism and Cushing's disease: Multiple endocrine neoplasia, type 2. *Medicine* 47: 371, 1968.

26. Mandelstam, P., Rush, B.F., Jr., Mabry, C.C. and Bartlett, R.C.: Prophylactic thyroidectomy in a 4½–year–old boy with a family history of oral and mucous membrane neuromas, medullary carcinoma of the thyroid, pheochromocytoma, hyperparathyroidism and diarrhea. *Proc. Central Soc. Clin. Res.* 43: 36, 1979 (abst).

27. Tashjian, A.H., Howland, B.B., Melvin, K.E.W. and Hill, C.S., Jr.: Immunoassay of human calcitonin. *New Eng. J. Med.* 283: 890, 1970.

28. Wahner, H.W., Cuello, C. and Aljure, F.: Hormone–induced regression of medullary (solid) thyroid carcinoma. *Amer. J. Med.* 45: 789, 1968.

29. Polliack, A. and Freund, U.: Mixed papillary and follicular carcinoma of the thyroid gland with stromal amyloid. *Amer. J. Clin. Path.* 53: 592, 1970.

30. Jones, N.F., Walker, G., Ruthven, C.R.J. and Sandler, M.: α–methyl–p–tyrosine in the management of phaeochromocytoma. *Lancet* 2: 1105, 1968.

31. Galante, L., Gudmundsson, T.V., Mathews, E.W., Tse, A., Williams, E.D., Woodhouse, N.J.Y. and MacIntyre, I.: Thymic and parathyroid origin of calcitonin in man. *Lancet* 2: 537, 1968.

32. Kaplan, E.L., Armaud, C.D., Hill, B.J. and Peskin, G.W.: Adrenal medullary calcitonin–like factor: a key to multiple endocrine neoplasia, type 2. *Surgery* 68: 146, 1970.

Chapter 14

MISCELLANEOUS DISORDERS, GENETICS, SKIN, AND CANCER

by Henry T. Lynch, M.D.

A number of disorders of known or presumed hereditary etiology show a variable degree of predisposition to cancer. Interest in this aspect of the cancer problem is of recent origin, but it has become more intensified during the past decade as virologic and immunologic studies of cancer have added to our knowledge of hereditary factors in this disease. Undoubtedly, in due time the precise etiology of these conditions will become more clear, and hopefully as a result, we should learn more about their specific predisposition to cancer. Certainly a systematic investigation of any disease which is strongly associated with cancer could provide important clues to carcinogenesis.[1]

It is the purpose of this chapter to present a variety of conditions wherein evidence for either hereditary etiology or for cancer association is less clear-cut than that for other diseases discussed in this book. Some will be seen only on rare occasions, i.e. Werner's syndrome, Sjogren's syndrome, scleroderma and dermatomyositis, while others such as systemic lupus erythematosus will be seen more frequently. Though the etiology and the total neoplastic propensity of these disorders is unclear, it would certainly be remiss if we failed to call attention to them.

Werner's Syndrome

In his original description of the syndrome which now bears his name, Werner,[2] reported the following findings in four siblings: short stature and cataracts; skin changes which included atrophy, hyperkeratosis, tautness, and ulceration, involving primarily the feet but also the hands; other findings have included involvement of muscles, joint changes, early menopause, early graying of hair, and a premature and progressive senility.[2]

For many years Werner's syndrome was considered essentially the same disorder as that described by Rothmund[3] (Rothmund's syndrome). However, as a result of a comprehensive study by Thannhauser[4] a clear delineation was made between Werner's and Rothmund's syndromes. Epstein and associates[5] reviewed the subject thoroughly, and described a sibship which included three patients with Werner's syndrome. In addition, they analyzed 122 other cases from the world literature. Based on these extensive studies of Werner's syndrome, they characterized the primary features of the syndrome as including "... symmetrical retardation of growth with absence of the adolescent growth spurt, graying of the hair, atrophy and hyperkeratosis of the skin, generalized loss of hair, alteration of the voice, cataracts (subcapsular and cortical, usually posterior), ulcerations of the feet, and mild diabetes in about half the cases . . . (other features included) . . . atrophy of the muscle, fat and bone of the extremities, vascular calcification, soft tissue (usually periarticular) calcification, and generalized osteoporosis . . . 'Hypogonadism' . . . (in both sexes) was frequently present". Significantly, approximately 10 per cent of these patients showed malignant neoplasms, the majority of which were sarcomas as opposed to carcinomas. Meningiomas were also found frequently.

The diagnosis of Werner's syndrome cannot usually be made until after the age of 30 since the cardinal features of this syndrome, namely, cataracts and skin ulcerations are not often present until after this age. However, knowing that the syndrome is present in other members of the family could provide an increased index of suspicion so that an earlier diagnosis might be possible.

In spite of 65 years of accumulated clinical experience with Werner's syndrome, its basic metabolic defect remains an enigma. Theoretical considerations for its etiology have ranged from defects in ectoderm, which were first described by Werner, to primary endocrinopathies, implicating the parathyroid or pituitary glands,[6] to most recent considerations of enzymatic defects.[5, 7, 8] Though endocrinologic disturbances have been observed frequently in Werner's syndrome, particularly those involving the gonads, and diabetes mellitus, clear evidence for an underlying endocrinopathy has never been firmly established. Indeed, recent work by Riley and associates has tended to discount an endocrinopathic hypothesis.[9]

The mode of inheritance in Werner's syndrome is consistent with an autosomal recessive factor.[5] An intriguing aspect of Werner's syndrome is that its full effects are not expressed until the third or fourth decade of life. Epstein[10] has compared this phenomenon with that which occurs in ochronosis which is an unrelated, but also an autosomal recessively inherited disorder having alkaptonuria as a complication; this involves the staining of cartilage by metabolic products derived from homogentisic acid. As in Werner's syndrome, the deleterious effects of ochronosis do not occur until relatively late in life, at which time degenerative changes in cartilage may occur.

Some of the principal clinical features in Werner's syndrome, especially premature senescence, are well illustrated in a patient described by Riley and associates.[9] They reported a 34 year-old mentally retarded Negro male, (Fig. 1) who was hospitalized because of cataracts and ulceration of the skin of the ankle. This patient showed premature graying and thinning of his hair, (during his mid-twenties). Physical findings revealed short stature and a general physical appearance much older than his chronological age of 34. Pubic and axillary hair were sparse. The skin of the face was taut, dry, and atrophic; the nose was beak–shaped, (an observation also found in other patients with Werner's syndrome). The skin of the extremities was taut, limiting extension at the knees and the elbows. Hyperkeratosis was present on the soles of his feet along with the mentioned ulceration of the right ankle. His voice was high–pitched. It is of interest that this patient was the product of an incestuous union (father–daughter union), and his mother was mentally retarded.

The association of malignant neoplasms in patients with Werner's syndrome has

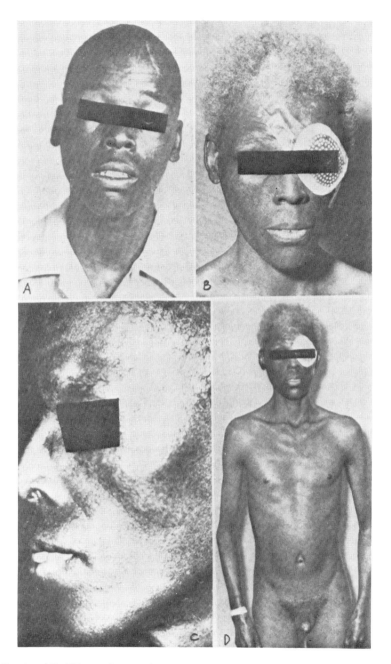

Figure 1. Patient with Werner's syndrome. A. The patient at age 24; B. The same patient at age 34 showing the marked aging; C. Demonstrates the characteristic beaking of the nose; D. Shows the slender tapering of the extremities, tight skin, and normal external genitalia. Reproduced by permission of Thomas R. Riley, M.D. and the Editor, *Annals of Internal Medicine 63*: 285, 1965.

been documented by several investigators.[7, 10–17] Due to the small number of descriptions of patients with Werner's syndrome the reported occurrences of malignant neoplasms represent an unusually high incidence, particularly of sarcoma. It has been suggested that possibly the somatic aging which characterises Werner's syndrome may be a critical factor in the pathogenesis leading to increased incidences of malignant neoplasms.[9]

Collagen Disease and Cancer

An intriguing association of cancer with collagen diseases such as lupus erythematosus, dermatomyositis, and scleroderma has come to the forefront particularly because of increased knowledge concerning autoimmune phenomena.[18-21] To evaluate this association researchers are indeed fortunate to have an experimental model available, specifically, certain New Zealand Black (NZB) in–bred strains of mice, wherein spontaneous lymphoma and autoimmune hemolytic anemia arise.[22] Studies of both mice and man are predicated upon the fact that normal immune mechanisms are dependent upon the normal functioning of lymphocytes and plasmacytes. In certain situations, however, abnormal lymphocytes may proliferate and in turn may produce abnormal globulins which may react with normal tissues of the host and lead to the production of an "autoimmune state" as is thought to be the case in some of the collagen diseases of man. A similar set of circumstances may occur in certain cancers such as multiple myeloma and chronic lymphocytic leukemia in which abnormal globulins or lymphocytes react abnormally to certain antigenic stimulation. Carry-

ing this analogy one step further, we then see a relationship between certain autoimmune states associated with cancer and an immunoproliferative disorder. Thus this entire system could be related to a breakdown in the host defense against cancer, namely, the production of abnormal lymphocytes and plasmacytes followed by the elaboration of defective globulin antibodies resulting in decreased resistance to cancer. Thus we see in a schematic manner in Figure 2, a "bridge" between collagen disease and cancer.

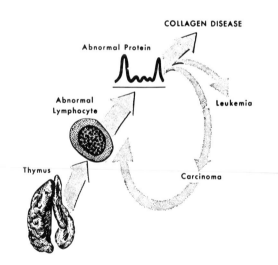

Figure 2. Drawing showing possible relationship between "collagen" disease, leukemia, and carcinoma which might be mediated through abnormal lymphocytes producing abnormal globulins. Reproduced by permission of Robert P. Barden, M.D. and Editor of *Radiology 92*: 972, 1969.

Systemic Lupus Erythematosus (SLE)

Systemic lupus erythematosus is a multi-system disease characterized by intermittent fever, arthritis, arthralgia, arteritis, phlebitis in the central nervous system, renal disease (lupus nephritis), and multiple cutaneous manifestations which include the characteristic malar erythema of the so-called "butterfly area" of the face. Tuffanelli and Dubois[23] reported in 1964, on cutaneous manifestations in L.E. based on findings from western countries; more recently Tay[24] presented similar findings on Chinese patients from Singapore. Table 1 is modified from the work of Tay and summarizes his findings as well as those of Tuffanelli and Dubois, and clearly illustrates the wide spectrum of skin manifestations in this disease.

Evidence has been rapidly accumulating relevant to the immunopathogenesis of SLE which has posed strong theoretical implications concerning the known association between connective tissue disease, immunological deficiency, and lymphoma. The concepts have been recently crystallized in a paper by Smith and associates[25] wherein they describe a patient with SLE, dysgammaglobulinemia and lymphoma, and in addition, present a review of the literature pertinent to eight patients with SLE and lymphoma. The authors suggest that a spectrum of immune abnormalities may be present in patients with SLE. They propose the presence of a selective immunoglobulin deficiency of connective tissue disease in general, and in association an inter-relationship with neoplasm or lymphoma in conditions such as dermatomyositis and Sjogren's syndrome.

Features of interest in their own patient with SLE included a high titer of IgM, antinuclear antibodies, profuse development of extracellular hematoxylin material, and an apparent restricted ability to form LE cells. The patient also manifested cryoglobulinemia which was shown to be related predominantly to the presence of IgM. Histopathologically, connective tissue disease, dysgammaglobulinemia, and lymphoma coexisted in this patient, findings which cast serious implications for the potential importance of an immunopathogenic relationship among these disorders.

Recently, provocative evidence for a viral etiology in SLE has come to the fore. Some of this work is being performed at the University of Texas Southwestern Medical School under the direction of Dr. Eric R. Hurd. Specifically, he has demonstrated viral antibody levels in SLE patients, and has shown the presence of cytoplasmic myxovirus-like tubular structures in the tissues of SLE patients. An interesting aspect of this work is that it could possibly demonstrate one further link between viruses and cancer and in this case in a known pre-cancerous autoimmune disease which appears to have a familial occurrence in certain kindreds. The mode of inheritance for SLE is not clear, though autosomal dominance has been suggested in several pedigrees.[26-28] In addition to the mentioned excess of lymphomas in SLE, increased occurrences of thymic tumors have been recorded.[29, 30]

Dermatomyositis

Dermatomyositis is a rare disorder which is considered by many clinical investigators to be a nonsuppurative form of polymyositis. This disease may present as an acute, subacute, or chronic disease process. It is frequently characterized by pain, tenderness, and weakness of muscles. There are variable systemic manifestations, and the pathology of this disease is characterized by inflammatory and degenerative changes primarily of skin and muscle which may lead to an associated atrophy, weakness, and tenderness. The principal involvement includes the musculature of the shoulder girdle, arms, and the gluteal and femoral areas. Such postures may result as drooping of the head and difficulty in sitting up or assuming an erect position. Intermittent fever may be a striking finding in some patients. Skin changes in the form of erythema and puffy edematous swellings of the eyelids ("heliotrope bloating") may occur; other cutaneous findings include minute telangiectasia, erythematous patches on the face and extremities (particularly upper) with brown pigmentation which may mimic the appearance and anatomic distribution of those found in lupus erythematosus. Similar vasomotor disturbances as found in Raynaud's disease may occur following exacerbations of dermatomyositis. Superficial epidermal exfoliation, mild pruritis, and occasionally poikiloderma may occur.[31] The skin changes in dermatomyositis, however, are not diagnostic, and may often resemble those of a non–specific or a toxic dermatitis.

Dermatomyositis and generalized scleroderma may be differentiated clinically during certain phases of their course. Such differentiation poses a particularly difficult problem in the acute edematous phases of each disease when multiple histologic sections may be required in order to locate a characteristic region diagnostic for dermatomyositis.[32] Calcinosis, with deposition of calcium in the proximal muscles of the shoulders, and pelvic girdle, is a common finding in children with dermatomyositis. This process may develop into a universal calcinosis as opposed to the calcinosis found in scleroderma which is usually limited to the hands and the feet.

Findings concerning the association between cancer and dermatomyositis vary considerably. For example, in a review of the literature to 1959, Williams[33] reported on approximately 92 cases of dermatomyositis of which 15 percent were associated with some form of malignant neoplastic disease. However, we believe a more accurate appraisal of cancer association will be obtained when a distinction is made between the *adult* and the *juvenile* forms of the disease (onset before age 20).[34, 35] Specifically, cancer appears in as many as 50 percent of patients with the adult variety of dermatomyositis. The most commonly occurring types of malignant neoplasms include cancer of the gastrointestinal tract, sarcomas of soft tissues, lymphoma, multiple myeloma, and malignant melanoma.[36–38]

The mechanisms involved in carcinogenesis in dermatomyositis are not known. Theoretical possibilities include the following: 1) tumor catabolic products may serve as allergenic agents for initiation of dermatomyositis. There is some evidence that extracts of tumor injected intradermally produce sensitivity in patients to their own tumors; 2) antinuclear antibodies have been found in patients with dermatomyositis suggesting the possible involvement of autoimmunity and hence involving in some way the development of sensitivity to nucleoprotein as a possible mechanism. The latter situation might possibly explain the documented cases of improvement in the clinical course of dermatomyositis following tumor extirpation, radiation therapy, or chemotherapy.

The genetics of dermatomyositis are

complex, and as yet a specific mode of inheritance cannot be determined.[39, 40] In one large kindred, two female first cousins manifested this disease. An interesting finding was an increased occurrence of rheumatoid arthritis and certain serum protein abnormalities, thus suggesting a relationship between dermatomyositis and other connective tissue disorders.[40]

Scleroderma

Scleroderma is a generalized multisystem disease, though skin is the primary target organ. Indeed the name scleroderma referred to by its German name "Hautsclerem" means hide–bound skin. The term "acro" as in acroscleroderma has been used to differentiate systemic forms of scleroderma associated with acrosclerosis from the more diffuse generalized form of systemic scleroderma.

Scleroderma may not always be present as a clearcut entity and indeed there may well be inter–relationships or transitions between scleroderma, lupus erythematosus, and dermatomyositis.[41] In addition, some clinicians think that scleroderma and Raynaud's phenomenon may be integral parts of systemic scleroderma.[42] Specifically, scleroderma may be subdivided into a generalized form with systemic manifestations and a localized variety which frequently lacks systemic manifestations, the latter having a more favorable prognosis. In the generalized form, changes in internal organs are believed to result primarily from vascular changes, most prominent of which are thickening of the walls of vessels with subsequent ischemia. The esophagus is probably most frequently implicated in the generalized systemic form of the disease. Shortening of this organ occurs, due in part to atrophy of its musculature. The average age of onset of scleroderma is in the third and fifth decades with females more often affected than males.

An increased incidence of malignant neoplasms is apparently associated with scleroderma. A premorbid cancerous state may be promulgated by the sclerodermatic process. For example, in bronchiolar carcinoma associated with scleroderma, the malignancy appears to be secondary to dense pulmonary fibrosis caused by scleroderma.[43] On the other hand, malignant neoplasms per se may give rise to systemic manifestations with a syndrome mimicking dermatomyositis, polyarthritis, and scleroderma.[44]

The specific mode of inheritance of scleroderma remains unclear at this time. A few instances of familial manifestations of this disease have been reported. For example, in one report the disorder was confirmed in two brothers while their sister and mother were "probably" affected, although the diagnosis was not certain.[45] Burge and associates[46] recently reviewed the genetic literature on scleroderma. They found four documented instances of familial scleroderma, and eight cases in which the documentation was less complete. These authors included their own family study wherein two sisters manifested scleroderma, one of whom died at age 16 from her disease.

Additional studies will be necessary before the role of genetics in the etiology of scleroderma can be more clearly comprehended. Meanwhile, one must consider the possible relationship of this disease with other forms of collagen vascular disease, particularly lupus erythematosus, in which genetic factors have been observed. This suggests that heredity may play an important role in this entire group of diseases.

Sjögren's Syndrome

Sjögren, a Swedish ophthalmologist described in 1933 a series of patients who manifested keratoconjunctivitis sicca with additional disorders of the lacrimal and salivary glands, xerostomia and rheumatoid arthritis. These findings have subsequently been considered a syndrome now known by Sjögren's name. This condition is associated with other collagen disorders including systemic lupus erythematosus, polyarteritis, polymyositis, progressive systemic sclerosis, and Raynaud's phenomenon. Sjögren's syndrome is characterized clinically by dryness and keratosis of mucous membranes most prominently in the mouth, conjunctiva, nose, throat and occasionally the urinary bladder and vagina. The symptoms may be rather disturbing to the patient, and be manifested as a conjunctivitis sicca with burning and photophobia and a stringy mucoid discharge. Occasionally corneal ulceration and loss of visual acuity may occur. The salivary and lacrimal glands may become inflamed and exquisitely tender; in addition they may be palpably enlarged yet yield a paucity of secretory material. Anemia and achlorhydria may also occur. There have been cases of granuloma annulare. The teeth are often in poor repair with frequent caries and a tendency to break. The fingernails are often brittle; there is dryness of the scalp and alopecia is common. Osteoporosis occurs with increased frequency in these patients. Biochemically, one finds an extremly high frequency of hypergammaglobulinemia, and many show the presence of rheumatoid factor, antinuclear factors, precipitating antibodies, and anti–IGm. Because of these occurrences, Sjögren's syndrome is considered as an autoimmune disease.[47]

Malignant lymphoma is often associated with Sjögren's syndrome. In one series of 58 patients with Sjögren's syndrome, 3 incidences of reticulum cell sarcoma occurred.[48] Another patient with Sjögren's syndrome was found to have malignant lymphoma of the salivary glands.[49] In another report, a patient with the syndrome was found to have adenocarcinoma of the parotid gland.[50] The genetics of Sjögren's syndrome remain unclear; however, support for a hereditary predisposition rests on its frequent association with known hereditary collagen diseases.

Bloom's Syndrome (congenital telangiectatic erythema and stunted growth)

Bloom's syndrome is an exceedingly rare autosomal recessively inherited disorder which occurs predominantly among individuals of Jewish extraction.[51] Chromosomal abnormalities include a high incidence of chromosome breakage and rearrangements.[52, 53]

The principal cutaneous lesions include congenital telangiectatic erythema of the face, particularly in the "butterfly distribution" with significant sensitivity to sunlight. Indeed, the facial appearance closely resembles that of lupus erythematosus. Erythema may occasionally occur over the dorsum of the hands and forearms. Associated skin anomalies have included *café au lait* spots, ichthyosis, acanthosis nigricans, hypertrichosis, and keratosis pilaris. In addition, these patients are almost invariably short in stature, slender, with a fine–featured face and a doliocephalic head.[51]

There is a high predilection for leukemia. For example, 3 of 23 patients with Bloom's syndrome died from leukemia at ages 12, 23, and 25. A fourth patient had lingual carcinoma.[54]

Chediak–Higashi Syndrome

The Chediak–Higashi syndrome is inherited as an autosomal recessive.[55] The cardinal feature of the syndrome involves an anomalous granulation in the polymorphonuclear leukocytes in the peripheral blood, inclusion bodies in myeloid series in the bone marrow, and irregular masses resembling Dohle bodies in the granulocytes.[31] Variable cutaneous manifestations have been described including fair complexion, dilution of hair color, hyperpigmentary response to sunlight, and excessive sweating.

Electron microscopic studies have recently shown a relationship between the pigmentary abnormality in this disorder and gigantism of the melanosomes which is similar to the gigantism of the leukocytic granules.[56] This generalized involvement of lysosomal granules has also been described by Lutzner and associates[57] in Aleutian mink which manifest a disorder quite similar to the Chediak–Higashi syndrome in man.

Findings in other organ systems include retinal albinism associated with photophobia and nystagmus, recurrent infections associated with fevers which may not be related to infection, and, less frequently, hepatosplenomegaly, lymphadenopathy, and neurologic manifestations including mental retardation, convulsions and neuropathy.

Autopsy studies have shown infiltration in viscera and lymph nodes "interpreted as compatible with a malignant lymphoma."[55] Lymphoma in association with this disease has been described by others.[58–60] Dent and associates[61] suggest that the lymphoma asso-

ciated with this disorder may result from an inordinate susceptibility to an infectious agent. Specifically, they found abundant virus–like particles in peripheral leukocytes from 2 of their patients. The particles resembled the Bernhard type C virus which has been associated with animal leukemia and lymphoma. They speculate that an increased fragility of lysosomal membranes in certain viral infections might result in an "abnormal release of lysosomal enzymes, which in turn would lead to the development of neoplastic changes within the cell . . ."[61]

The occurrence of the Chediak–Higashi syndrome, not only in Aleutian mink[62] but also in a herd of albino cattle,[63] has been of interest to geneticists and pathologists, though, to date, lymphoma has not been found in animals with this syndrome.[64]

Albinism

Albinism is characterized by a partial or total absence of pigmentation, most noteworthy in the skin, hair and, eyes ("pink eye"). The melanocytes of the skin are amelanotic. There appear to be several phenotypic varieties of albinism presumably due to different genetic mutations. Thus, some forms of albinism may be of the so–called "pure" type while others may be associated with impairment of vision, hearing, or mental retardation. Inheritance in the majority of cases of albinism is autosomal recessive.[65]

The skin of patients with albinism tends to show premature aging as noted by increased occurrence of actinic chelitis, telangiectasia, keratoses, and cancer, particularly squamous cell carcinoma. In some respects, the skin parallels that found in xeroderma pigmentosum.[66]

Fanconi's Aplastic Anemia (Congenital Pancytopenia)

Fanconi's anemia is inherited as an autosomal recessive; in addition, chromosome studies of fibroblasts, lymphocytes, and bone marrow have shown a high incidence of chromosomal structural aberrations including chromatid and isochromatid breaks, exchanges, and endoreduplications.[67, 68]

The cardinal findings in Fanconi's anemia include pancytopenia, bone marrow hypoplasia, and congenital anomalies. The latter may include hypoplasia of the thumbs, absence of the radius, strabismus, microcephaly, microphthalmia, dwarfism, and hypogenitalism. In addition, patients often show a spotty or patchy brown pigmentation of the skin. Indeed, the skin manifestations in some patients may appear similar to those found in patients with dyskeratosis congenita.[69] Some authors consider the conditions identical.[70] Family studies have revealed that relatives in at least one of these families have manifested features of both diseases, suggesting that they are genetically related.[71] The clinical picture is thought to be determined by the extent of mesodermal abnormalities (Fanconi's syndrome) versus ectodermal manifestations (dyskeratosis congenita). Cytogenetic studies of patients with dyskeratosis congenita should add clarification to the classification of these disorders.

Cancer shows an increased occurrence in Fanconi's anemia though existing data is insufficient for calculating meaningful incidence figures. The most frequently occurring malignant neoplasm in this disease is acute leukemia.[67,68] Interestingly, two of the patients described by Bloom and associates[67] died from acute monocytic leukemia six months and six years

respectively after the original diagnosis of pancytopenia. Swift and Hirschhorn,[72] on the other hand, reported a 30–year–old woman with squamous cell carcinoma of the skin of the anus and carcinoma in situ (Bowen's disease) of the vulva.

Aldrich Syndrome (Wiskott–Aldrich Syndrome)

The Aldrich syndrome is inherited as a sex–linked recessive.[73] The onset of this disease is in infancy, often earlier than four months. The disorder is characterized by generalized chronic eczema, erythroderma, thrombocytopenia, petechiae, purpura, recurrent infections including pyoderma, furuncles, and purulent otitis media with the majority of deaths resulting from overwhelming viral and bacterial infections. A lack of resistance to infection in this disease is thought to be due to a severe immunologic deficiency.[74, 75]

Cancer, particularly of the reticuloendothelial system, has been shown to be increased in the Aldrich syndrome, though true incidence estimates are not yet available.[73–75] An unusual family has been described by Basel and associates[73] in which 4 brothers, in a sibship of 7, manifested this disease. Two of these brothers died from neoplastic disease; one at age 3 showed findings consistent with myelogenous leukemia (necropsy), while his brother died at age 6 with findings resembling anaplastic reticulum cell sarcoma (necropsy). In their literature review, they found a boy of 20 months and another 2½ years old with malignant reticuloendotheliosis, a boy aged 7 years and 10 months with astrocytoma of the brain, and two 8–year–old boys with malignant lymphoma.

Bruton's Sex–Linked Agammaglobulinemia

Bruton's agammaglobulinemia is inherited as a sex–linked recessive. Affected males begin to show evidence of immunologic deficiency at about 6 months of age as evidenced by multiple recurrent infections such as pneumonia, suppurative otitis media, and meningitis. Skin manifestations include severe pyodermas, cellulitis, furunculosis, and conjunctivitis. Death often results from fulminant infections.

The pathogenesis of the immunologic deficiency in this disease has been ascribed to a defect in the formation of the immunoglobulin–producing system.[75]

Malignant lymphoma occurs in this disorder with a frequency significantly greater than expected in the general population.[76, 77] Page *et al*[76] described 2 children with sex–linked agammaglobulinemia and malignant lymphoma from a population comprising 24 children with congenital agammaglobulinemia. They compared the risk for malignant lymphoma in a comparable pediatric age group from their region and calculated that the risk for this disease in association with sex–linked agammaglobulinemia is highly significant.

Vitiligo and Gastric Carcinoma

Gastric carcinoma inexplicably has shown a marked decline in incidence in the United States during the past 30 years. In contrast, increased incidences of stomach cancer have occurred in the Japanese and in the inhabitants of Iceland.[78] However, while these data are undoubtedly of epidemiologic interest, they nevertheless fail to shed light on the possible role of hereditary factors. However, existing data show an approximately

three–fold increase in gastric carcinoma in the relatives of gastric cancer probands over that in controls.[79, 80] In addition, several pedigrees show concordance for gastric carcinoma in identical twins.[81] Another interesting association with possible genetic implications includes the correlation between blood group A and gastric carcinoma.[82,83] Finally, pernicious anemia shows a statistical correlation with gastric carcinoma, and individual pedigrees have shown an association among achlorhydria, gastric carcinoma, and pernicious anemia in relatives of gastric cancer probands.[84]

It is therefore of interest that vitiligo has been reported to shown an increased incidence in patients with pernicious anemia as well as with gastric carcinoma.[85, 86]

Tylosis and Esophageal Cancer (Keratosis Palmaris et Plantaris)

Tylosis denotes a hyperkeratosis of a body surface. In the case of patients with so–called keratosis palmaris et plantaris, hyperkeratosis involves the palms and soles. This is a diffuse symmetrical cornification of the horny layer of the epidermis on the surfaces. This condition has been known for many years to behave as an autosomal dominant trait, and in the overwhelming majority of cases it is completely benign. However, a study by Howel–Evans and associates in 1958[87] found tylosis of the palms and soles to be associated with carcinoma of the esophagus in an exceedingly large number of members of two families. The investigators constructed a life table of these families wherein it was predicted that 95 per cent of relatives with tylosis would develop carcinoma of the esophagus by age 65. Interestingly, in 1970,

Harper, Harper and Howel–Evans[88] updated their findings on these families for the twelve year interval of 1958 to 1970 and found that the predicted 95 percent occurrence of carcinoma of the esophagus in patients with tylosis was unfortunately occurring in accordance with their earlier predictions. Specifically, six new cases of esophageal carcinoma occurred in this twelve year interval and all in members who had tylosis. In short, no occurrences of esophageal cancer were found in patients without tylosis.

The tylosis in these families is characterized by a later age of onset than that seen in the usual hereditary occurrence of tylosis in the absence of esophageal cancer. Indeed several individuals developed tylosis as late as middle age. In addition, in some members of these esophageal cancer families, tylosis may be confined to the feet; indeed, two women who have died since 1958 of esophageal cancer, had tylosis restricted to their feet. Of further interest is the fact that when carcinoma of the esophagus occurs in families with tylosis, it occurs about ten years earlier than the usual age at onset of esophageal cancer in the general population.

Many problems have evolved concerning the management of members of these kindreds who are at risk for carcinoma of the esophagus. For example, in 1958 it was not felt justified to undertake regular preventive measures in individuals at risk, since the possibility for successful surgical cure was considered too small when compared to the risk of creating fear of cancer. However, as cancer continued to develop in family members followed by death in every case despite awareness of the condition by family doctors a reappraisal was made.

In addition, it was learned that the majority of family members were already aware of and worried about the risk of developing cancer and therefore were more reassured than alarmed by the prospect of having periodic medical evaluation of their problem. As might be expected, many members who did not have tylosis were also worried about the possibility of developing esophageal cancer; genetic counseling was able to provide them with some degree of reassurance. The approaches to preventive care have included barium swallows, esophagoscopy, and more recently, esophageal exfoliative cytology studies. In the case of the x–ray evaluation, investigators were concerned about the possibility of excessive x–ray exposure to an esophagus that was already harboring a predisposition to development of carcinoma; in the case of the performance of esophagoscopy, there was also the consideration of the attendant risks of this procedure, although it is now being performed on individuals who have tylosis and are receiving an anesthetic for any reason. It seems that a practical measure however, would be periodic screening with exfoliative cytology. In addition, members of the family have been advised to abstain from smoking and to minimize their alcohol consumption, since these factors have been clearly shown to be associated with carcinoma of the esophagus. However, practically speaking, the results show that these practices were not being followed by many members of the family. In addition, one of the youngest individuals to develop esophageal cancer, namely a 30–year–old patient, neither smoked nor drank. This raised serious question as to the efficacy of stressing the restrictions on smoking and consuming alcohol to these family members. Currently, the view is that there should be a constant awareness of the problem by both doctors and patients so that at the slightest indication of gastrointestinal symptoms an investigation of the esophagus is undertaken. In addition to these findings, the authors also reported two new cases of carcinoma of the esophagus associated with tylosis in different unrelated families.

In a family described by Shine and Allison[89] tylosis was found in association with congenital abnormality of the esophagus and esophageal cancer in the proband. This association of tylosis with congenital abnormality of the esophagus was present in two and possibly three generations; an autosomal dominant mode of inheritance was given for this particular family.

Cytogenetic studies in patients with tylosis and esophageal cancer have not been rewarding since they have been essentially normal.

Esophageal cancer in the absence of tylosis has failed to show any significant familial tendency.[90]

Tylosis and Cancer Other Than Esophageal Cancer

Huriez and associates[91] reported on tylosis of an unusual type known as "sclerotylosis" which occurred in three families in France. In this particular type of tylosis, hyperkeratosis of the hands and feet is present accompanied by atrophic changes of the skin and nails and, interestingly, a frequent occurrence of malignancy in the affected skin. Indeed, 7 out of 44 affected individuals developed malignant tumors in the skin, while seven other members expired from internal cancers of various anatomic sites including the tongue, tonsil, breast, and

uterus. Finally, no cases of esophageal cancer have been found in the families with this unusual form of tylosis, i.e. sclerotylosis. This type of tylosis is probably inherited as an autosomal dominant and appears to be located on a separate chromosomal locus from that of the usual type of tylosis and more particularly that associated with esophageal cancer.

Palmar and Plantar Seed Keratoses

There has been a suggested association between the presence of palmar and plantar seed keratoses and internal malignancy. For example, Dobson and associates[92] suggested that palmar keratoses occurred four times as frequently in patients with cancer than in those patients that did not manifest cancer. However, a later study by Bean and associates[93] showed that keratoses occured just as commonly in those with as those without malignancy. Finally, in a most recently reported study, Rhodes[94] surveyed 500 patients over the age of 40 years attending a dermatology clinic. He found that 62 per cent of these patients had "seed" keratoses on their palms or their soles. However, there was no statistically significant association found between the presence of keratoses and internal malignancy. However, there was a slight, but non–significant excess with keratoses and basal cell carcinoma.

Keratoacanthoma

Keratoacanthoma has also been referred to as so–called "molluscum sebaceum," and "self–healing carcinoma"; these may be solitary or multiple. The lesions usually just appear as red macules which progress rapidly to papules and nodules. The mature lesion is typically circular, firm, and pearly in appearance with a rolled and notched rim surrounding an umbilicated crater–like center, which, on gross examination, may mimic squamous cell carcinoma.[95, 96] The lesions have a predilection for the face, particularly the nose, lips, and cheeks though other areas of the body including the hands, wrists, and forearms and less frequently the scalp, thighs, genitalia, and buttocks may be involved. An interesting characteristic of the lesion is its propensity for exceedingly rapid growth followed by spontaneous involution.

This condition is almost always benign though there have been documented cases of squamous cell carcinoma[97–99] and basal cell epithelioma.[100,101] Finally, in a recent report by Burge and Winkelmann[102] a patient with keratoacanthoma was described in which there was an associated basal and squamous cell carcinoma.

The etiology of keratoacanthoma is not clear for all occurrences, though examples of its appearance in two or more members of families have been described.[103, 104] The mode of inheritance for this lesion appears to be consistent with an autosomal dominant pattern.[1]

Epidermolysis Bullosa Dystrophica

Epidermolysis bullosa dystrophica is a relatively rare hereditary disorder which may be inherited in some families as an autosomal dominant while in others it may be inherited as an autosomal recessive factor.[105] One of the striking features of this disease is the occurrence of lesions in the skin after mild trauma with a predilection for moist hyperhidrotic areas such as occur on the feet.

Other areas exposed to trauma including the extensor surfaces of joints are also frequent sites of lesions. The skin manifestations are characterized by the development of vesicles and bullae which occasionally may involve mucous membranes. The blisters show a tendency to become hemorrhagic followed by bluish atrophic scars. Dystrophy and loss of the nails are frequent. Patients with this condition also have a tendency to show teeth involvement wherein they may become rudimentary, mottled, or diminished in number. Esophageal strictures are occasionally encountered in patients with epidermolysis bullosa dystrophica. This may involve any part of the esophagus.[106]

Leukoplakia and carcinoma may occur on mucous membranes; multiple, basal, and squamous cell carcinomas of the skin have also been described in patients with this disorder.[107, 108]

Kaposi's Sarcoma (Multiple Idiopathic Hemorrhagic Sarcoma of Kaposi)

Kaposi's sarcoma is an obscure disease with distinctive cutaneous manifestations though other systems including the gastrointestinal tract may be involved. Any area of the skin may be involved with this disease though the most frequent sites of predilection are the extremities and particularly the legs and the feet. Early in the course of this disease, the lesions appear as reddish, purplish, or bluish–brown nodules with rubbery or firm consistency; their distribution may be unilateral, but later are often symmetrical. Lesions may appear simultaneously on the hands and feet. The process tends to course along the veins or lymphatics. Purpura, secondary infections, and edema occur frequently.[32]

These lesions show a strong predilection for the development of sarcoma.[1] Recent interest has been focused upon a broadening spectrum of malignant neoplasms associated with Kaposi's sarcoma. For example, O'Brien[109] reviewed 63 patients with Kaposi's sarcoma and found that among this group, 18 patients died of a second primary malignant neoplasm. Second primary cancers included five cases of Hodgkin's disease, three of lymphosarcoma, three of carcinoma of the colon, and one each of multiple myeloma, malignant melanoma, carcinoma of the prostate, carcinoma of the tongue, carcinoma of the tonsil, carcinoma of the pancreas, and carcinoma of the breast. It was of interest that the mortality from the second primary cancer was higher than the mortality of the disease itself. Other investigators have also called attention to the frequent coexistence of malignant lymphoma, Hodgkin's disease, and leukemia with Kaposi's sarcoma.[110, 111]

While the epidemiology of Kaposi's sarcoma remains an enigma, there are several interesting features about this disease that merit attention. These facts are enumerated as follows: 1) There is a significant sex ratio of male to female involvement (about 10:1); 2); there are certain geographic, racial, and ethnic predilections with increased occurrences among northern Italians, Ashkenazi Jews from Russia and Poland, and the Bantus of South Africa. With respect to the latter, this lesion is about 10 times as frequent among the Bantus as among the whites living in this region and is the most common cancer of the extremities in this group;[6] 3) multiple familial occurrences of this lesion have been observed with findings consistent with that of an autosomal dominant gene showing incomplete penetrance;[110, 112] 4) and finally, common environmental factors interacting with a susceptible genome must be given careful consideration in any etiologic hypothesis for this disease.[110]

Dermatoglyphics

One of the objectives of genetic studies is to find biochemical or physical markers which might prove to be helpful in identifying individuals at risk for a specific trait or disease. Dermatoglyphics is an important discipline which is not often known to the physician, but is utilized frequently by geneticists in the study of a variety of disorders. Cancer has been no exception in the quest for identifying markers which might be present in the dermal ridges of the hands. For example, the simian crease and other dermatoglyphic abnormalities in the hands of children with Down's syndrome has been known for a relatively long period of time. In turn, a significant association between Down's syndrome and leukemia has been confirmed during the past decade.[113]

Studies of dermatoglyphics in leukemia in the absence of Down's syndrome have been controversial though more investigation in this area is obviously necessary.[114, 115] For example, Verbov[116] has recently reviewed the subject and has presented findings from 110 patients with leukemia. In this group he was able to discern dermatoglyphic patterns in males with leukemia which differed from those of a normal control group. Important findings included an increased frequency of finger whorls and a decreased frequency of ulnar loops in patients with acute leukemia. There was also an increased frequency of radial loops and a

TABLE 1

Cutaneous Manifestations of S. L. E.

		Present Series (62 cases)		Tuffanelli's Series (520)
		No. of Cases	Percentage	Percentage
1	Butterfly rash	40	64.6	57.6
2	Diffuse alopecia	26	41.8	21.3
3	Photosensitivity	20	32.3	32.7
4	Maculopapular rash	14	22.6	19.0
5	Raynaud's phenomena	10	16.1	18.4
6	Purpura/ecchymosis	8	12.9	19.8
7	Hyperpigmentation/depigmentation	8	12.9	8.4
8	Livedo reticularis	6	9.6	———
9	Petechial haemorrhages	6	9.6	2.1
10	Leg ulcers/skin ulcers	6	9.6	5.1
11	Telangiectasia	5	8.0	— — —
12	Periungual haemorrhage	5	8.0	1.1
13	Herpes zoster	4	6.4	3.2
14	Palatal haemorrhage	4	6.4	1.3
15	Erythema nodosa	4	6.4	6.5
16	Mucous membrane involvement	3	4.8	9.1
17	Thrombophlebitis	3	4.8	4.6
18	Psoriasiform rash	3	4.8	0.6
19	Non–specific dermatitis	2	3.2	2.1
20	Conjunctivitis	2	3.2	6.5
21	Paronychia	2	3.2	———
22	Hyperkeratotic follicular papules	2	3.2	———
23	Hyperkeratosis palmaris et plantaris	2	3.2	———
24	Urticaria	1	1.6	6.9
25	Cicatricial alopecia	1	1.6	5.6
26	Gangrene	1	1.6	1.3
27	Subcutaneous nodules	1	1.6	5.0
28	Subcutaneous calcinosis	1	1.6	———
29	Periorbital oedema	1	1.6	4.8
30	Bullous formation	1	1.6	———

Table 1 is published with permission of C.H. Tay, M.D. and the Publisher of *Aust. J. Derm. 11*: 30, 1970.

decreased frequency of arches in chronic leukemia, more particularly in patients with chronic lymphocytic leukemia. These findings are included because of recent interest in the genetics of leukemia.[117–119] and the fact that a variety of dermatolgoic lesions have been secondarily associated with these diseases.

Ethnic Factors

The association of skin cancer with prolonged exposure to sunlight has been confirmed repeatedly by numerous investigators in different parts of the world.[120] It is generally accepted that wavelengths between 2800 and 3200 Å are primarily responsible for skin cancer formation and for phototoxic sunburn responses.[121] The factors affecting this fraction include the sun angle which is closely related to the time of day, the season of the year, and the latitude of exposure. The point is that in spite of physical quantitative factors relevant to solar radiation exposure to individuals at a given time residing in a specific area, one might sort out individuals differentially in any particular population who will be more likely to be at risk for the development of skin cancer.

It has been established that skin cancer occurs most frequently on areas which are most likely to receive sun exposure, namely the head, neck, arms, and hands. Pigmentation appears to provide a major protective role from the effects of solar radiation in that members of races with heavy pigmentation do not react to the sun with sunburn as do people with lightly pigmented skin. Skin cancer occurs more frequently in individuals of Nordic extraction with fair complexion, blue eyes, and blond or red hair. In addition, with a high degree of statistical significance, studies have shown that individuals of Celtic antecedents (Scotch, Irish, and Welsh) develop skin cancer more frequently than individuals of other ethnic origins. Silverstone's studies,[122, 123] performed in 1964 in three different areas of Queensland, Australia, revealed a significantly greater number of tumors in Celtic people than that which was expected based on distribution of the local population. In addition, the onset of cancer appeared to be about ten years earlier than in the other ethnic populations in that area. It was believed that the susceptibility to skin cancer in the Celtics was related to an inherited inability of the skin to protect them in the usual fashion against the carcinogenic effect of ultraviolet light radiation. Racial and ethnic groups used for comparison in this study included Australians born of Mediterranean or South American ancestry, Asiatics, and Aboriginals of mixed ancestral background. The likelihood of susceptibility of skin cancer increased with the degree of Celtic ancestry.

Finally, skin cancer appears to occur with greater frequency in all lightly pigmented individuals who engage in outdoor occupations, such as farming, outdoor construction work, fishing, etc.

1. Lynch, H.T.: Hereditary Factors in Carcinoma. In Recent Results in Cancer Research, vol. *12*, P. Rentchnick, ed., New York, Springer–Verlag, 1967; P. 186.

2. Werner, O: Ueber Katarakt in Verbindung mit Sklerodermie, (Doctoral Dissertation, Kiel University): Schmidt & Klaunig, Kiel, 1904.

3. Rothmund, A.: Ueber Cataracte in Verbindung mit einer Eigenthümlichien Hautdegeneration, *Arch. Ophthal.,* (Berl, 14, 1, St.,): 159–182, 1868.

4. Thannhauser, S.J.: Werner's Syndrome (Progeria of the Adult) and Rothmund's Syndrome: Two types of Closely Related Heredo–Familial Atrophic Dermatosis with Juvenile Cataracts and Endocrine Features, A Critical Study with Five New Cases, *Ann. Intern. Med.,* 23: 559–626, 1945.

5. Epstein, C.J., Martin, G.M., Schultz, A.L., and Motulsky, A.G.: Werner's Syndrome; A Review of Its Symptomatology, Natural History, Pathologic Features, Genetics, and Relationship to the Natural Aging Process, *Medicine* (Balt.), *45*: 177–221, 1966.

6. Oppenheimer, B.S., and Kugel, V.H.: Werner's Syndrome; Heredofamilial Disorder with Scleroma, Bilateral Juvenile Cataract, Precocious Graying of Hair and Endocrine Stigmatization, *Trans. Ass. Amer. Physicians, 49*: 358–370, 1934.

7. Boyd, M.W.J., and Grant, A.P.: Werner's Syndrome (Progeria of the Adult), Further Pathological and Biochemical Observations, *Brit. Med. J.,* 2: 920–925, 1959.

8. Petrohelos, M.A.: Werner's Syndrome; A Survey of Three Cases, with Review of the Literature, *Amer. J. Ophthal.,* 56: 941, Dec., 1963.

9. Riley, T.R., Wieland, R.G., Markis, J., et al: Werner's Syndrome, *Ann. Intern. Med.,* 63: 285–294, Aug., 1965.

10. Epstein, C.J.: Werner's Syndrome, *Ann. Intern. Med.,* 63: 343–345, 1965.

11. Ellison, D.J., and Pugh, D.W.: Werner's Syndrome, *Brit. Med. J.,* 2: 237, June 1955.

12. Muller, L., and Anderson, B.: Werner's Syndrome; Survey Based on Two Cases, *Acta Med. Scand. (Suppl.) 283, 146:* 1– 17, 1953.

13. Agatston, S.A., and Gartner, S.: Precocious Cataract and Scleroderma (Rothmund's Syndrome; Werner's Syndrome); Report Case, *Arch. Ophthal.* (Chicago), *21*: 492–496, March, 1939.

14. Oppenheimer, B.S., and Kugel, V.H.: Werner's Syndrome: Report of the First Necropsy and of Findings in a New Case, *Amer. J. Med. Sci., 202*: 629–642, Nov., 1941.

15. Jacobson, H.G., Rifkin, H., and Zucker–Franklin, D.: Werner's Syndrome: A Clinical Roentgen Entity, *Radiology, 74*: 373–385, March, 1960.

16. Boatwright, H., Wheeler, C.E., and Cawley, E.P.: Werner's Syndrome, *Arch. Intern. Med.* (Chicago), *90*: 243–249, Aug., 1952.

17. McKusick, V.A.: Medical Genetics 1962, *J. Chron. Dis. 16*: 457–634, June, 1963.

18. Causey, J.Q.: IgG Paraproteinemia Associated with Bronchogenic Carcinoma, *Arch. Intern. Med.* (Chicago), *119*: 407–410, April, 1967.

19. Dameshek, W.: Chronic Lympocytic Leukemia – An Accumulative Disease of Immunologically Incompetent Lymphocytes, *Blood, 29*: 556–584, April, 1967.

20. Deaton, J.G., and Levin, W.C.: Systemic Lupus Erythematosus and Acute Myeloblastic Leukemia; Report of Their Coexistence and a Survey of Possible Associating Features, *Arch. Intern. Med.* (Chicago), *120*: 345–348, Sept. 1967.

21. Thompson, J.S.: Immunity and Systemic Lupus Erythematosus, *Postgrad. Med. 37*: 619–627, June, 1965.

22. Mellors, R.C.: Autoimmune Disease in NZB–B1 Mice; II. Autoimmunity and Malignant Lymphoma, *Blood, 27*:

435–448, April, 1966.

23. Tuffanelli, V.L., Debois, E.L.: Cutaneous Manifestations of Systemic Lupus Erythematosus, *Arch. Derm.* (Chicago), *90*: 337–386, Oct., 1964.

24. Tay, C.H.: Cutaneous Manifestations of Systemic Lupus Erythematosus: A Clinical Study from Singapore, *Aust. J. Derm., 11*: 30–41, April, 1970.

25. Smith, C.K., Cassidy, J.T., and Bole, G.G.: Type I Dysgammaglobulinemia, Systemic Lupus Erythematosus and Lymphoma, *Amer. J. Med., 48*: 113–119, Jan., 1970.

26. Brunjes, S., Zike, K., and Julian R.: Familial Systemic Lupus Erythematosus; A Review of the Literature with a Report of Ten Additional Cases in Four Families, *Amer. J. Med., 30*: 529–536, 1961.

27. Leonhard, T.: Family Studies in Systemic Lupus Erythematosus, *Acta Med. Scand. (Suppl.), 416*: 1–156, 1964.

28. Pollack, V.E.: Antinculear Antibodies in Families of Patients with Systemic Lupus Erythematosus, *New Eng. J. Med., 271*: 165–171, 1964.

29. Barnes, R.D.: Thymic Neoplasms Associated with Refractory Anaemia, *Guy. Hosp. Rep. 114*: 73–82, 1965.

30. Beickert, A.: Lupus–erythematosus – Syndrome Bei Lymphogranulomatose, *Schweiz. Med. Wschr., 88*: 668–669, 1958.

31. Andrews, G.C., and Domonkos, A.N.: *Diseases of the Skin,* 5th ed., Philidelphia, W.B. Saunders Company, 1964; P. 749.

32. Montgomery, H.: *Dermatopathology,* New York, Hoeber Medical Division, Harper and Rowe, 1967, pp. 1247.

33. Williams, R.C.: Dermatomyositis and Malignancy; A Review of the Literature, *Ann. Intern. Med. 50*: 1174, 1959.

34. Arundell, F.D., Wilkinson, R.D., and Haserick, J.R.: Dermatomyositis and Malignant Neoplasms in Adults; A Survey of 20 Years' Experience, *Arch. Derm., 82*: 772–775, 1960.

35. Curtis, A.C., Heckaman, J.H., and Wheeler, A.H.: Study of the Autoimmune Reaction in Dermatomyositis, *JAMA, 178*: 571–573, 1961.

36. Christianson, H.B., Brunsting, L.A., and Perry, H.O.: Dermatomyositis: Unusual Features, Complications, and Treatment, *Arch. Derm., 74*: 581–589, 1956.

37. Grace, J.T., and Dao, T.L.: Dermatomyositis in Cancer: A Possible Etiological Mechanism, *Cancer, 12*: 648–650, 1959.

38. Katz, A., and Digby, J.W.: Malignant Melanoma and Dermatomyositis, *Canad. Med. Ass. J., 93*: 1367–1369, 25, Dec., 1965.

39. Lambie, J.A., and Duff, I.F.: Report of Familial Occurrence of Dermatomyositis and a Family Survey, *J. Lab. Clin. Med., 58*: 935–936, 1961.

40. Lambie, J.A., and Duff, I.F.: Familial Occurrence of Dermatomyositis: Case Reports and a Family Survey, *Ann. Intern. Med., 59*: 839–847, 1963.

41. Kierland, R.R.: The Collagenoses: Transitional Forms of Lupus Erythematosus, Dermatomyositis, and Scleroderma, *Mayo. Clinic Proc., 39*: 53, Jan., 1964.

42. Farmer, R.G., Gifford, R.W., Jr., and Hines, E.A., Jr.: Prognostic Significance of Raynaud's Phenomenon and Other Clinical Characteristics of Systemic Scleroderma: A Study of 271 Cases, *Circulation, 21*: 1088–1095, June, 1960.

43. Montgomery, R.D., Stirling, G.A., Hamer, N.A.: Bronchiolar Carcinoma in Progressive Systemic Sclerosis, *Lancet, 1*: 586–587, March, 1964.

44. Basten, A., and Bonnin, M.: Scleroderma in Carcinoma, *Med. J. Aust.,* *1*: 452, 1966.

45. McAndrew, G.M., and Barnes, E.G.: Familial Scleroderma, *Ann. Phys. Med.,* *8*: 128–131, Nov., 1965.

46. Burge, K.M., Perry, H.O., and Stickler, G.B.: "Familial" Scleroderma, *Arch. Derm.* (Chicago), 99: 681–687, 1969.

47. Denko, C.W., and Bergenstal, D.M.: The Sicca Syndrome (Sjögren's Syndrome); A Study of Sixteen Cases, *Arch. Intern. Med.* *105*: 849–858, 1960.

48. Talal, N., and Bunim, J.J.: The Development of Malignant Lymphoma in the Course of Sjögren's Syndrome, *Amer. J. Med. 36*: 529–540, 1964.

49. Rothman, S., Block, M., and Hauser F.V.: Sjögren's Syndrome Associated with Lymphoblastoma and Hypersplenism, *Arch. Derm. Syph. 63*: 642–643, 1951.

50. Delaney, W.E., and Balogh, K., Jr.: Carcinoma of the Parotid Gland Associated with Benign Lymphoepithelial Lesion (Mikulicz's Disease) in Sjögren's Syndrome, *Cancer 19*: 853–860, 1966.

51. Bloom, D.: The syndrome of congenital telangiectatic erythema and stunted growth, *J. Pediat. 68*: 103–113, 1966.

52. German, J., Archibald, R., and Bloom, D.: Chromosomal breakage in a rare and probably genetically–determined syndrome of man, *Science 148*: 506–507, 1965.

53. Rauh, J.L., and Soukup, S.W.: Bloom's Syndrome, *Amer. J. Dis. Child. 116*: 409–413, 1968.

54. German, J.: Bloom's syndrome, Presented to 3rd International Congress of Human Genetics, Chicago, Ill., September 5–10, 1966.

55. Kritzler, R.A., Terner, J.Y., Lindenbaum, J., Magidson, J., Williams, R., Preisig, R., and Phillips, G.B.: Chediak–Higashi syndrome: Cytologic and serum lipid observations in a case and family, *Amer. J. Med. 36*: 583–594, 1964.

56. Windhorst, D.B., Zelickson, A.S., and Good, R.A.: Chediak–Higashi syndrome: hereditary gigantism of cytoplasmic organelles, *Science 151*: 81–83, 1966.

57. Lutzner, M.A., Tierney, J.H., and Benditt, E.P.: Giant granules and widespread cytoplasmic inclusions in a genetic syndrome of Aleutian mink, *Lab. Invest. 14*: 2063, 1965.

58. Efrati, P., and Jonas, W.: Chediak's anomaly of leukocytes in malignant lymphoma associated with leukemic manifestations: case report with necropsy, *Blood 13*: 1063–1073, 1958.

59. Mauri, C., and Silingardi, V.: L'anomalia di Beugez Cesar-Steinbrinck–Chediak–Higashi, *Recent Progr. Med.* (Roma) *37*: 577–612, 1964.

60. Page, A.R., Berendes, H., Warner, J., and Good, R.A.: The Chediak–Higashi syndrome, *Blood 20*: 330–343, 1962.

61. Dent, P.B., Fish, L.A., White, J.G., and Good, R.A.: Chediak–Higashi syndrome: Observations on the nature of the associated malignancy, *Lab. Invest 15*: 1634–1643, 1966.

62. Leader, R.W., Padgett, G.A., and Gorham, J.R.: Studies of abnormal leukocyte bodies in the mink, *Blood 22*: 477–484, 1963.

63. ———, Leader, R.W., Gorham, J.R., and O'Mary, C.C.: The Familial occurrence of the Chediak–Higashi syndrome in mink and cattle, *Genetics 49*: 505–512, 1964.

64. Padgett, G.A.: Personal communication, 1966.

65. Tietz, W.: A syndrome of deaf-mu-

tism associated with albinism, showing dominant autosomal inheritance, *Amer. J. Hum. Genet. 15*: 259–264, 1963.

66. Keeler, C.D.: Albinism, xeroderma pigmentosum, and skin cancer, *Nat Cancer Inst.* (Monograph 10): International Conference of the Biology of Cutaneous Cancer, U.S. Department of Health, Education, and Welfare, Public Health Service, 1963; pp. 349–259.

67. Bloom, G.E., Warner, S., Gerald, P.S., and Diamond, L.K.: Chromosome abnormalities in constitutional aplastic anemia, *New Eng. J. Med. 274*: 8–14, 1966.

68. Todaro, G.J., Green, H., and Swift, M.R.: Susceptibility of human diploid fibroblast strains to transformation by SV40 virus, *Science 153*: 1252–1254, 1966.

69. Hitch, J.M.: Dyskeratosis congenita, *Cutis 4*: 1229–1232, 1968.

70. Cole, H.N., Rauschkolb, J.E., and Toomey, J.: Dyskeratosis congenita with pigmentation, dystrophia unguis and leukokeratosis oris, *Arch. Derm. Syph. 21*: 71–95, 1930.

71. Bryan, H.G., and Nixon, R.K.: Dyskeratosis congenita and familial pancytopenia, *JAMA 192*: 203–208, 1965.

72. Swift, M.M., and Hirschhorn, K.: Fanconi's anemia: susceptibility to chromosome breakage in various tissues, *Ann. Intern. Med. 65*: 496–503, 1966.

73. ten Bensel, R.W., Stadlan, E.M., and Krivit, W.: The development of malignancy in the course of the Aldrich syndrome, *J. Pediat. 68*: 761–767, 1966.

74. Pearson, H.A., Shulman, N.R., Oski, F.A., and Eitzman, D.V.: Platelet survival in Wiskott–Aldrich syndrome, *J. Pediat. 68*: 754–760, 1966.

75. Peterson, R.D., Cooper, M.D., and Good, R.A.: The pathogeneses of immunologic deficiency diseases, *Amer. J.*

Med. 38: 579–604, 1965.

76. Page, A.R., Hansen, A.E., and Good, R.A.: Occurrence of leukemia and lymphoma in patients with agammaglobulinemia, *Blood 21*: 197–206, 1963.

77. Resiman, L.E., Mitani, M., and Zuelzer, W.W.: Chromosome studies in leukemia: I. Evidence for the origin of leukemic stem lines from aneuploid mutants, *New Eng. J. Med. 270*: 591–597, 1964.

78. Dungal, N.: The Special Problems of Stomach Cancer in Iceland, *JAMA 178*: 789–798, (Nov.), 1961.

79. Videbaek, A., and Mosbech, J.: The Aetiology of Gastric Carcinoma Elucidated by a Study of 302 Pedigrees, *Acta. Med. Scand. 149*: 137–159, 1954.

80. Woolf, C.M.: Further Study on the Familial Aspects of Carcinoma of the Stomach, *Amer. J. Hum. Genet. 8*: 102–109, (June), 1956.

81. Gorer, P.A.: Genetic Interpretation of Studies on Cancer in Twins, *Ann. Eugen. 8*: 219–232, (May) 1938.

82. Buckwalter, J.A., Wohlwend, C.B., Colter, D.C., Tidrick, R.T., and Kowler, L.A.: The Association of the ABO Blood Groups to Gastric Carcinoma, *Surg. Gynec. Obstet. 104*: 176–179, 1957.

83. Mosbech, J.: ABO Blood Groups in Stomach Cancer, *Acta Genet.* (Basel), 8: 219–227, 1958.

84. Mosbech, J.: *Heredity in Pernicious Anemia: A Proband Study of the Heredity and the Relationship to Cancer of the Stomach*, Copenhagen: E. Munksgaard, 1953.

85. Wright, P.D., Venables, C.W., and Dawber, R.P.R.: Vitiligo and Gastric Carcinoma, *Brit. Med. J. 3*: 148, (July) 1970.

86. Allison, J.R. and Curtis, A.C.: Vitiligo and Pernicious Anemia *A.M.A. Arch. Derm. 72*: 407–408, (Nov.) 1955.

87. Howel–Evans, W., McConnell, R.B., Clarke, C.A., and Sheppard, P.M.: Carcinoma of the Esophagus with Keratosis Palmaris et Plantaris (Tylosis): A Study of Two Families, *Quart. J. Med. 22*: 413–429, 1958.

88. Harper, P.S., Harper, R.M.J., and Howel–Evans, A.W.: Carcinoma of the Oesophagus with Tylosis, *Quart. J. Med. 39*: 317–333, 1970.

89. Shinc, I., and Allision, P.R.: Carcinoma of the Oesophagus with Tylosis (Keratosis Palmaris et Plantaris), *Lancet 1*: 951–953, 1966.

90. Mosbech, J., and Videbaek, A.: On the Etiology of Esophageal Carcinoma, *J. Nat. Cancer Inst. 15*: 1665–1673, 1955.

91. Huriez, C., Deminatti, M., Agache, P., and et al: Une Génodysplasie non Encore Individualisée: La Génodermatose Scléro–atrophiante et Kératodermigue des Extrémités Freuqemment Dégénérative, *Sem. Hop. Paris 44*: 481–488, (Feb.) 1968.

92. Dobson, R.L. Young, M.R., and Pinto, J.S.: Palmar Keratoses and Cancer *Arch. Derm.* (Chicago), 92: 553–556, (Nov.) 1965.

93. Bean, S.F., Foxley, E.G., and Fusaro, R.M.: Palmar Keratoses and Internal Malignancy: A Negative Study, *Arch. Derm.* (Chicago), 97: 528–532, 1968.

94. Rhodes, E.L.: Palmar and Plantar Seed Keratoses and Internal Malignancy, *Brit. J. Derm. 82*: 361–363, (April) 1970.

95. Butterworth, T. and Strean, L.P.: Clinical Genodermatology, Baltimore, The Williams and Wilkins Company, 1962, p. 22.

96. Eraux, L.P. and Schopflocher, P.: Familial Primary Self–healing Squamous Epithelioma of Skin, *Arch. Derm. 91*: 589–594, 1965.

97. Beare, J.M.: Molluscum Sebaceum, *Brit. J. Surg. 41*: 167–172, 1953.

98. Muller, S.A., et al: Adenoid Squamous Cell Carcinoma (Adenoacanthoma of Lever): Report of Seven Cases and Review, *Arch. Derm. 89*: 589–597, 1964.

99. Anderson, N.P.: Abstract of Discussion, *Arch. Derm. 75*: 219–223, 1957.

100. Hadida, E., and Sayag, J.: Keratoacanthome et epithelioma baso–cellulaire, *Bull. Soc. Franc. Derm. Syph. 71*: 404–405, 1964.

101. Einaugler, R.B., et al: Keratoacanthoma With Basal Cell Carcinoma, *Amer. J. Ophthal 65*: 922–925, 1968.

102. Burge, K.M. and Winklemann, R.K.: Keratoacanthoma: Association With Basal and Squamous Cell Carcinoma, *Arch. Derm. 100*: 306–311, 1969.

103. Epstein, N.N., Biskind, G.R., and Pollack, R.S.: Multiple Primary Self–healing Squamous–cell "Epitheliomas" of the Skin: Generalized Keratoacanthoma, *Arch. Derm. 75*: 210–223, 1957.

104. Sommerville, J. and Milne, J.A.: Familial Primary Self–healing Squamous Epithelioma of the Skin, *Brit. J. Derm. 62*: 485–490, 1950.

105. Davision, B.C.C.: Epidermolysis Bullosa, *J. Med. Genet. 2*: 223–242, 1965.

106. Allen, A.C.: The Skin: A Clinicopathological Treatise, 2nd ed., New York, Grune and Stratton, 1967, p. 303.

107. Andrews, G.C. and Domonkos, A.N.: Diseases of the Skin, 5th ed., Philadelphia, W.B. Saunders Company, 1963, p.

108. Wechsler, H.L., et al: Polydysplastic Epidermolysis Bullosa and Development of Epidermal Neoplasms, *Arch. Derm. 102*: 374–380, 1970.

109. O'Brien, P.H. and Brasfield, R.D.: Kaposi's Sarcoma, *Cancer 19*: 1497–1502, 1966.

110. Ackerman, L.V.: Symposium on Kaposi's Sarcoma, *Univ. Internat. Contra. Cancrum 18*: 320–511, 1962.

111. Packs, G.T. and Davis, J.: Concomitant Occurrence of Kaposi's Sarcoma and Lymphoblastoma, *Arch. Derm. Syph. 69*: 604–611, 1954.

112. Oettlé, A.G.: Geographical and Radical Differences in the Frequency of Kaposi's Sarcoma as Evidence of Environmental or Genetic Causes, *Acta Un. Int. Cancr. 18*: 330–363, 1962.

113. Miller, R.W.: Down's Syndrome (Mongolism), Other Congenital Malformations and Cancers Among the Sibs of Leukemic Children, *New Eng. J. Med. 268*: 393–401, 1963.

114. Rosner, F.: Dermatoglyphics of Leukaemic Children, *Lancet 2*: 272–273, 1969.

115. Wertelecki, W., Plato, C.C., and Fraumeni, J.F., Jr.: Dermatoglyphics in Leukemia, *Lancet 2*: 806–807, 1969.

116. Verbov, J.L.: Dermatoglyphics in Leukemia, *J. Med. Genet. 7*: 125–130, 1970.

117. Heath, C.W., Jr. and Maloney, W.C.: Familial Leukemia; Five Cases of Acute Leukemia in Three Generations, *New Eng. J. Med. 272*: 882–887, 1965.

118. Steinberg, A.G.: The Genetics of Acute Leukemia in Children, *Cancer 13*: 985–999, 1960.

119. Fraumeni, J.F., Jr., Vogel, C.L., and DeVita, V.T.: Familial Chronic Lymphocytic Leukemia, *Ann. Intern. Med. 71*: 279–284, 1969.

120. Freeman, R.G.: Carcinogenic Effects of Solar Radiation and Prevention Measures, Cancer 21: 1114–1120, 1968.

121. Blum, H.F.: Carcinogenesis by Ultraviolet Light, Princeton: University Press, Princeton, N.J., 1959.

122. Silverstone, H.: sited as a personal communication by Urbach, F. et al: Ultraviolet Radiation and Skin Cancer in Man, Ch. 12, pp. 195–214, in Montagna, W. and Dobson, R.L. (ed): *Advances in Biology of Skin. Carcinogenesis,* Pargamon Press, Oxford, 1965, Vol. 7.

123. Silverstone, H. and Searle, J.H.A.: The Epidemiology of Skin Cancer in Queensland: The Influence of Phenotype and Environment, *Brit. J. Cancer 24*: 235–252, 1970.

Chapter 15

GENETIC COUNSELING

by Henry T. Lynch, M.D.

INTRODUCTION AND PHILOSOPHY

In the ideal clinical setting, genetic counseling should be viewed and practiced in context with usual medical practice which includes diagnosis and therapy, as well as discussion of the natural history and prognosis of the particular disease.[1] However, traditionally, genetic counselors who have not received medical training have ignored the multifaceted medical and emotional components of genetic diseases and have been concerned primarily with a stereotyped dissemination of mathematically factual information about inheritance. These genetic counselors have been comprised primarily of members of zoology and genetic departments at colleges and universities. Of course, they have necessarily emphasized areas in which they were proficient, namely, the specific mode of inheritance for a particular disorder when this information was known and when it wasn't available, they provided the patient with empiric risk figures for the possibility of a repeat occurrence of a particular disease or trait in the family. When cytogenetic factors were important they could explain these particular mechanisms. Unfortunately, however, this type of genetic counseling, if indeed it could be termed counseling, does not sufficiently meet the basic needs of the patient, namely his underlying anxieties about the disease and his quest for a better understanding of the natural history of the particular disease in his family.

Part of the reason for the persistence of this situation, noteworthy for a lack of medical involvement, has been because medical genetics is a relatively new discipline, having only recently appeared in some medical school curricula; thus many physicians have not been knowledgeable about medical genetics in general and genetic counseling in particular.

McKusick[2] has taken strong issue with a non–medical approach to the problem. Specifically, he believes that genetic counseling should be performed by the physicians who are closest to the patient's problem. A summation of his views is crystalized in the following statement: "Too long genetic counseling has, by default, fallen to the province of the college professor of genetics, who is informed that the diagnosis is Humpty Dumpty's disease, who looks up the usual mode of inheritance of H–D disease in a book and on the basis of this and the specific pedigree, gives advice. Genetic counseling, like other medical diagnoses, should be integral in the practice of clinical medicine. The physician is in the best position to meet (the needs of genetic counseling)...(and) with improved education in medical genetics, sound genetic counseling should become the rule in medical practice."

If genetic counseling were a simple endeavor it might be possible to resolve the patient's problems concerning the specific "family disease" through the mere provision of salient genetic facts about his condition. Unfortunately, however, it is quite evident that such an approach will only be successful when the genetic problem is devoid of any significant feeling content, that is when it involves a problem that is of only casual concern to the patient, such as the genetics of eye color, hair color, or blood type, or of a mere passing intellectual concern such as *another* person's genetic problem.

However, when the family problem is relatively serious, either concerning the potential risk for a significant disease, or the possibility of its occurrence in children, siblings, or other members of the family, it takes on a magnitude and character which goes well beyond the realm of a superficial fact–oriented stereotyped approach. As a matter of fact, the latter approach may only aggravate the situation when the patient realizes that his anxiety is not relieved but possibly intensified because of his dissatisfaction which often results from an incomplete discussion of his deeper worries and concerns. Indeed, in our own experience, we have found that when the genetic problem is serious, the patient rarely worries *only* about genetic risk information. Obviously, then, a mere recitation of statistics regarding risk factors is just *one* part of the counseling problem; and we feel that it is of less importance than an exposition of the natural history of the disorder in context

with his present comprehension of the problem; to achieve this end we must permit the patient to relate his *own* fears and anxieties regarding these serious diagnoses. In short, letting the patient talk and providing him with an empathetic "listening ear" and in turn interpreting and reflecting these fears and anxieties are the essence of genetic counseling.[1]

Our philosophy of genetic counseling is person–centered and psychodynamically oriented. In context with this philosophy the manifold *psychologic* (feelings, emotions, and attitudes) and *medical* problems (natural history of the disease, diagnosis, prognosis, and treatment) are brought to the forefront.[3, 4] Thus, our objectives are broad in scope embracing the total needs of the patient, obviously a challenging task! We believe that this can be expediently and realistically managed by the family physician, who is closest to his patient's problem; he will usually be more acutely aware of the available resources for the patient and it is he who in the end analysis must assume responsibility for managing the patient's hereditary disease, and assist the patient in coping with it.

Physical Examination

It is essential when performing a physical examination that the physician be aware of the wide–range of expressivity of clinical findings in many genetic diseases. A typical example is the finding of only *café au lait* spots or axillary freckling in patients with von Recklinghausen's neurofibromatosis. Though a patient may manifest only this single physical sign, if neurofibromatosis is known to be present among his relatives then he must be considered to harbor the gene for this dominantly inherited disease. The potential for this patient to develop more serious sequelae of this disease, namely, sarcoma, meningiomas, pheochromocytomas, and other lesions must also be considered.[5] Thus, any physical examination of patients suspected of having a hereditary disease should include a careful search for *minimal* stigma which may be consistent with reduced penetrance or variable expressivity of the gene. At the conclusion of the physical examination, the physician will often have gained new insight into the manifestations of the hereditary disease in the family, especially when he queries his patient about the presence or absence of physical signs of the disease in his relatives. Of course, he should also constantly appraise attitudes and feelings towards the "family disease."

One of the most gratifying experiences for a physician is to exclude the existence of a hereditary disease in his patient! Thus, the doctor may be dealing with a situation in which his patient had assumed for many years that he was affected, but a careful medical examination, might, with augmentation by specialized diagnostic studies, reveal that the patient is *unaffected*! Indeed, this may be the patient's first realization that he is not at genetic risk for the family disease and that he cannot transmit the gene and hence the disease or trait to any of his children.

Psychologic Approach: Family Oriented

In genetic counseling we believe that a sensible approach to the patient's genetic disease should include an integrative psychologic appraisal. This implies total medical and psychosocial evaluation of the patient and his family. This is obviously in contradistinction to a piece-meal approach to the problem such as compartmentalizing the physical sequelae, the anxiety about being at genetic risk, depression from observing serious disease in relatives, impotency, frigidity, and pregnophobia because of fear of transmitting the disease to progeny. In the integrative psychologic approach, we assume that *all* of these factors may be present to some degree, depending upon the particular circumstances, the patient's emotional and social background, and the seriousness of the disease. This approach is essential in genetic counseling because of the often complex and multifaceted aspects of genetic problems which are interrelated with the total psychosocial and physical problems caused by the "family disease."[3, 4] Thus in genetic counseling, we must continually observe the patient in the context of his family. Moreover, we must appraise fully the attitudes and feelings and amount of acceptance of the particular trait or disease in members of the family who may be at risk for the disease since these factors may interact significantly with psychotherapeutic efforts of genetic counseling with the particular patient. Actually, emphasis upon the family as a unit in general medicine and psychiatry is by no means a new concept since it has been fostered for at least the past two decades.[6] Certainly, in dealing with a hereditary disease wherein a varying quantity of genes is shared in common with blood relatives, determined by their degree of relationship to the proband, it is only logical and practical that the family be viewed as a functioning and therapeutically concerned unit. Thus, in the family oriented approach to genetic counseling the focus is shifted to the patient's interpersonal relationships within the family unit rather than viewing him as an independent and discrete psychological and disease entity. Therefore, the genetic counselor will be concerned with resolving psychological conflicts which might have been generated by the presence of the disease in the family as well as developing a program of preventive medical care whenever this might be indicated.[3, 4] Indeed, progress in genetic counseling may be totally defeated if the family milieu is not evaluated in context with the patient receiving genetic counseling.

It is important that we differentiate family oriented genetic counseling from so–called group therapy. In the former, we are dealing with the family as a natural group of people who have shared a relatively common history and who also share a variable percentage of genes in common. On the other hand, group therapy differs in that the group is comprised of individuals who are not necessarily selected for any similarity in their heritage and certainly, do not in the usual case share any genes in common.

With respect to responses to the genetic counseling process, it is obvious that the family per se will become an acutely critical issue wherein decisions are made between husband and wife relevant to whether they will take the "chance" on another pregnancy, should significant genetic disease already have occurred to one or more of their children. It would obviously be ludicrous for the physician counselor to focus his entire attention upon just one of the marital partners without bringing the other spouse into the issue with full recognition of his or her role, feelings, attitudes, identifications and responsibility for future progeny. Thus, if homeostasis within the family unit is to be obtained, the physician must look beyond his patient and

be willing to involve other significant members constituting the family milieu. In general the more significant the particular genetic trait is from the standpoint of such factors as cosmetically disfiguring diseases, psychiatric, chronic, and progressively debilitating diseases, the more disturbed the family unit may become.[3, 4, 6] And in turn, there may be greater difficulty in achieving homeostasis within the family.[6] However, by the same token, there is an increasingly greater need for the physician to involve the family in genetic counseling as the medical significance of the particular disease increases.[4]

It is in just such cases as these that the family physician may be best equipped to engage in a psychodynamically oriented approach to the family unit with the goal of achieving maximum therapeutic gain for the patient and his relatives.

Methods of applying family oriented genetic counseling may vary depending upon the particular disease being considered and the character of the family from the standpoint of acceptance of the disorder, presence of hostility and consternation pertaining to the genetic fault, as well as upon physical factors pertinent to the availability of the immediate relatives of the affected patient. Thus, in certain situations the physician may find it more desirable to see relatives individually, but at the same time, evaluate their behavior as they describe it in context with their family milieu. In other situations, the physician may find it more desirable to see several of the relatives together in a conjoint family therapy session wherein patterns of interaction may be managed with respect to the hereditary disease. Patterns of adaptation to the family disease as well as interaction of family members may not become recognized until a conjoint family session is held. After one or more of these sessions, the physician may choose to see selected relatives individually or even continue with a variety of group sessions since relatives may not be aware of their various interactions until they have had an opportunity to express their attitudes and feelings in such a group setting.

A family–oriented approach, as proposed here, could promote preventive measures with control for an increasingly large number of genetic disorders, the reason being primarily the advantage of tailoring a diagnostic follow–up of close relatives at genetic risk for the particular hereditary disease.[7] Examples of this will be given shortly for xeroderma pigmentosum and familial malignant melanoma.

In our experience in counseling over 1,000 families with genetic diseases, we have been impressed with the success of a non–directive psychotherapeutic approach permitting the patient to discuss at length important issues as he sees them.[1] The role of the physician is primarily that of a good listener with the ability to interpret pertinent medical and socio–psychological material to the patient in a comprehensible manner which the patient can accept. We believe that this approach, while admittedly time–consuming in certain cases, may actually be time–saving in the long run. Anxieties and fears surrounding the possibility of transmitting a deleterious gene may be incredibly intense and may require considerable time for discussion. This requires a full measure of empathy and acceptance by the physician.

In short, it should become obvious that genetic counseling must embody all of the trust and confidence which is inherent in a physician–patient relationship. The following summarizes what we consider ro be of particular importance to genetic counseling:

1. It implies that we are dealing with an ego–involved patient.
2. It is medically oriented in that the counselor has a deep interest in and obligation to explore the disease status of his patients. Therefore it follows that the counselor will use all available diagnostic, preventive medicine, and therapeutic regimens available in his medical armamentarium. Thus, for example, a patient at risk for multiple polyposis coli, a serious aspect of Gardner's syndrome, should have benefit of proctosigmoidoscopy; if found to be affected, he should be advised, and in fact urged to undergo colectomy as a preventive measure if the diagnosis is made early enough.
3. It implies case finding in the family for the presence of hereditary diseases in other family members when this is indicated; again polyposis coli in Gardner's syndrome is a classical example of such a necessity.
4. It is psychodynamically and family oriented; this implies that the counselor is sufficiently versed in psychology and psychiatry to recognize and deal effectively with emotional content which may be prevalent in the family in general and in the patient in particular. In short, the counselor must appraise fully the emotional factors and he must be sympathetic to them, providing "an empathetic listening ear."

5. The counselor must provide accurate genetic information to the patient only at a time when the patient is emotionally capable of grasping its importance and significance.[1-5, 7]

Clinical Examples

Case 1, Xeroderma Pigmentosum

In order to illustrate our approach to genetic counseling in context with the subject of this book, we shall present appropriate cases involving genetics, skin lesions, and cancer. We have personally counseled and followed each of the two families we will be discussing, for a relatively long period of time.

The first example is that of a family showing xeroderma pigmentosum. (This is the same patient and family presented in chapter 5). In summary, the proband was first seen by us at age 17. He was referred for evaluation of malignant melanoma and was known to have had a previous diagnosis of xeroderma pigmentosum (xdp) established at age 13. Two sisters and two brothers were similarily affected. (See pedigree in Chapter 5).

Psychosocial Interviews

The parents' first knowledge of the disorder in the family occurred in 1956, when their second–born child, a daughter, then aged 13, was treated for what appeared to them to be a "cold sore" on her lip following exposure to the sun while swimming. This lesion did not heal normally. She was referred to a plastic surgeon, who recommended insertion of radon which, though painful, would not be disfiguring. This procedure was accepted and the result was excellent. This physician, aware of the genetic aspects of this disorder, immediately made the diagnosis in the other siblings and has since assumed total medical management of the family. He informed the family of the carcinogenic role of sunlight exposure in this disease and advised total restriction of exposure to sunlight for the three affected children. (Twin sons born later, in 1959, are also affected.)

This advice led to a complete transformation of activities for the three children to an environment sheltering the children from sunlight. They had a library and many kinds of creative art materials in the home. The children who had been avid swimmers were encouraged to swim in the evenings or to use indoor pools. Other athletic activities (tennis, baseball, etc.) were performed in the evening under artificial lights. Riding in automobiles necessitated sitting away from the windows. Clothing requirements included wide–brimmed hats and long sleeves and high–necked blouses or shirts at all times. Special creams were used on exposed skin areas. Continual vigilance was obviously necessary on the part of the mother since the children would "forget" about the restrictions in pursuing the normal activities of childhood. Since they felt well physically, it only added to their dilemma. A strong motivational force was their physician, whom the children respected and revered.

The father apparently found the total situation extremely difficult to accept and for several years was so emotionally disturbed that he developed numerous psychosomatic complaints and became depressed. He was hospitalized and after electric shock treatments and many psychotherapy sessions was able to gain some degree of insight into his problem.

The parents assumed the responsibility for worry and watchful waiting to enable the children to lead as normal lives as possible within the limitations imposed on them. An overprotective atmosphere was inevitable; however, the parents have accepted the need for transferring responsibilities for their own physical protection to the children.

Both parents expressed concern about the oldest affected daughters, ages 22 and 23. Although both daughters are attractive, popular and intelligent, neither had accepted offers of marriage, fearing that they may pass the disorder on to their children. Both have seemingly sublimated by concentrating on academic training. One was teaching art and the other was studying for a Ph.D. In one of the genetic counseling sessions, (see subsequent discussion) the unlikelihood of an affected member having an affected child was pointed out. One daughter has since married.

Initially, neither parent accepted the fact that the twin sons, born two years after the condition had become known to the family, also had the disorder; however, they used the same precautions against sunlight with these boys "because they have freckles, dry skin, and might possibly develop the condition." (However, following genetic counseling they have now fully accepted the fact that these children are affected.)

Feelings of guilt were apparent in both parents. Both have asked after learning that each was a heterozygous carrier of the recessive gene, "How did we happen to come together when there were so many other persons we *might* have married?" However, each parent has spoken of the close family relationships and of the "outside" help each has received from his religious faith and from the empathetic physician who has help-

ed them during the past 10 years.

Genetic Counseling

After detailed background material was obtained, physical examination and laboratory studies completed, and the social worker had completed a series of interviews with the family, genetic counseling was begun. Two one–hour counseling sessions were held with the parents on successive days.

The initial concern of the parents related to the history of malignant melanoma in their son (proband). This concern was tempered by the fact that their family physician gave them a frank appraisal of the possibility of metastatic malignant melanoma. It was obvious that they were cognizant of and accepted all eventualities. Since all laboratory studies and physical examinations of their child (other than the skin changes) were within normal limits, the parents were advised that there was no evidence of malignant melanoma at present; however, they were told that this was no assurance against the subclinical presence of malignant melanoma, the seriousness of which was reemphasized. Hope, albeit restrained, was fostered. They accepted this sword of Damocles and both avowed to their strong religious faith.

Both parents expressed intense interest in the inheritance of xdp in the family. They stated that in spite of numerous inquiries to their physicians, they had never received a full and satisfying explanation of the heritable factors in this disease. They and their children had harbored major misconceptions, namely that this disorder would most likely be passed on by their affected children should they marry and that it could also occur in the progeny of their unaffected children. They repeated in detail the grave concern and fears of their adult daughters who until that time had rejected the thought of marriage and children because of their concern about "passing the disease on."

The first phase of genetic counseling of the parents was to appraise critically their attitudes, feelings, and knowledge about their "family disease". We then began to acquaint them in lay terminology with the basic fundamentals of genetics with particular emphasis upon probability figures for "passing on genes." Further emphasis was placed upon the rarity of the XDP gene and the unlikli-hood of two *unrelated* carriers of this gene meeting and marrying. The parents were told that in their case, each being a carrier, the statistical probability of having affected children was 25% even though five of their seven children were affected. They were shown how this was still in the realm of statistical probability.

A pedigree of the family was constructed only after it was believed that the parents understood the above-mentioned rudimentary material. They were relieved, almost ecstatic, to realize the small likelihood of their affected children transmitting the disease and the impossibility of the unaffected children transmitting it. This information rested of course upon the statistical rarity of the gene and the unlikelihood of an affected child marrying an individual heterozygous for this condition; however, they were also told that transmission would indeed be possible and with increased odds if one were to marry a cousin.

Case 2, Malignant Melanoma

The second case involves a family with malignant melanoma. This family is also discussed along with the pedigree in Chapter 6. In summary, the proband was a 51-year-old white woman with a diagnosis of malignant melanoma, whose sister and son also had this disease.

The proband's son was unusually interested in discussing various aspects of this disease including his family's attitudes toward medical problems in general. He stated that he had always been objective about his problem of recurrent melanoma. The medical facts had been clearly presented to him several years previously by the then attending surgeon. He had accepted this risk and was determined to do everything possible to detect lesions in their earliest stages. He also stated that he was sympathetic to his relatives' feelings concerning medical care, but wished they could be more objective. After the family history was explored with this patient, his pedigree was constructed and the inheritance was explained in detail.

This patient understood and fully appreciated and accepted the possible risk to his future offspring. He was concerned about the risk to his siblings (Chapter 6, Fig. I, III-3, 4, 5) who had multiple nevi; in particular, he discussed his sister's (Chapter 6, Fig. I, III-3) complete disregard for this disease. While on vacation and visiting this sister, aged twenty-four, he observed a lesion which appeared to be similar to one which was recently excised from him, diagnosed as CM. He urged her to see her physician immediately. However, because of her deep fear of physicians she adamantly refused to follow his advice. After considerable persuasion during a period of several months, she finally consented to see a surgeon, who excised a skin lesion from her left anterior chest wall. Histological diagnosis was benign compound pigmented nevi with active junctional activity. He wrote, "We will continue to observe this patient, though it is really a problem to determine which lesions to remove."

From the standpoint of genetic counseling, important aspects in this family are the unusual objectivity, acceptance, and understanding in one member of the family, and the repression and suppression of its significance, i.e., so-called ostrich-with-head-in-the-sand phenomenon in another.

Undoubtedly much of the positive attitude seen in the patient treated at the Anderson Hospital was abetted by some of the key physicians who saw him initially and made him aware of the danger signals of malignant melanoma without causing excessive fear.

In genetic counseling of families with malignant melanoma, one is afforded an unusual opportunity for early cancer detection since more favorable prognosis can be offered a patient with this disease when the lesion is discovered and treated before it enlarges significantly and metastasis occurs. With metastases the outlook becomes exceedingly dismal. In our experience, malignant melanoma is one of the most dreaded cancers by *both* patient and physician. Unfortunately, physicians appear to be more pessimistic about this disease than is warranted if one considers its natural history and, particularly its prognosis when detected early and adequate therapy undertaken.[8]

When counseling with the hereditary form of this disease we advise relatives at risk of the possibility that the disease may be transmitted as an autosomal dominant; we show them how the penetrance of the gene may be reduced so that gen-

erations may appear to be "skipped." We take special care to make certain that they understand the danger signals which appear in nevi, by a sudden increase in rate of growth, darkening of pigmentation, and bleeding. In the case of intraocular melanoma, we alert patients to be aware of any visual impairment or symptoms suggestive of glaucoma, and to report these immediately to their ophthalmologist.

In the light of present evidence it appears, for the most part, that the inheritance of these lesions will be on a site-specific basis in families, i.e. cutaneous or intraocular malignant melanoma, but not both. However, we have observed families with melanoma who also showed an increased occurrence of cancer of other histologic varieties.[9] Further genetic studies will, hopefully, clarify this problem.

GENETIC COUNSELING INTERNATIONALLY

It has been estimated that approximately one-third of *all* diseases have a genetic etiology to some degree. This obviously has important implications for genetic counseling. Therefore, it is not surprising that the Expert Committee on Human Genetics of the World Health Organization has stressed not only the importance of genetic counseling but also the need for a compilation of an international directory of genetic counseling services.[10]

An *International Directory of Genetic Services* was first published by us in 1968, with a second edition published the following year.[11] Recently, using the above directory as a reference source, a questionnaire survey was made of all genetics units identified as offering genetic counseling services.

Of the 404 genetics units which offer counseling services throughout the world, 324 (80%) responded to the questionnaire. These responses included 140 of 179 sent to directors of units in the United States (83%) and 175 of 225 units in foreign countries (78%).

Results of this study showed the following: 1) Full responsibility for genetic counseling is assumed by the genetics units in a majority of instances (92% in the United States, and 91% in foreign units).

2) In spite of the number of genetic units engaged in genetic counseling, about one-half of all of the genetic units (76 in the United States and 89 in foreign countries) provide genetic counseling services only to one to nine patients per month, and only approximately 18 per cent of the genetics units in the United States and 16 per cent of the foreign units see more than twenty patients per month. Finally, only 3 units in the United States and 2 in foreign countries see more than 1,000 patients per year.

3) Physicians assumed responsibility for practically all of the genetic counseling. A significant number of pediatricians assume this responsibility both in the United States (75 per cent) and in foreign countries (56 per cent) and more than one specialist may be involved with genetic counseling in any single unit.

4) A recently inaugurated diagnostic procedure in units throughout the world is amniocentesis. It is therefore noteworthy that 77 units in the United States and 51 in foreign countries offer this service.

5) Financial support for genetic counseling is provided by both private and public means in the United States and in foreign countries. However, a significantly greater number of genetic units receive public support in foreign countries (62 per cent as opposed to 31 per cent in the United States).

6) A large number of public and private health and welfare organizations were listed by the various genetic units as agencies with which cooperation was sought. By far the largest number of referrals were made to public health organizations such as city, county, state, provincial, and national or governmental health services (152 in the United States and 101 in foreign countries). A large number of private health organizations were listed with small number of referrals to each.

From the above information it is obvious that with the relatively small number of worldwide genetics units which offer genetic counseling, and with the relatively small number of patients seen annually by these units, the large number of patients requiring this service cannot possibly be met. Therefore, the only logical way to meet this responsibility for genetic counseling would be for the family physician to accept this challenge. After all, it is he who knows the family best and is responsible for its medical care. Undoubtedly, as medical genetics courses become a part of the curricula of medical schools and postgraduate education, family physicians will be better prepared to offer this essential service to their patients.

Specialized training in genetics for paramedical personnel would allow the physician more time for genetic counseling of individuals and families. For example, in our own department, a medical social worker has assumed responsibility for practically all medical and genealogical data collection as well as pedigree construction and literature review, all integral, but nevertheless time-consuming aspects of genetic counseling. She also ascertains the family's emotional reactions to and understanding of the hereditary disorder present among its members. She may then assist the family with their planning for the services of community health and welfare agencies for amelioration of problems surrounding the presence of the disease, and with physical and vocational rehabilitation plan for affected members. If family members have misconceptions or misunderstandings about the genetic disorder they are directed to the medical geneticist, or family physician for further discussion and clarification.

Finally, genetic registries, with appropriate data available to practicing as well as to clinical investigators could aid in identification of high genetic risk families and earlier diagnosis.[12]

REFERENCES

1. Lynch, H.T.: *Dynamic Genetic Counseling For Clinicians,* Springfield, Illinois, Charles C. Thomas, 1969. pp. 354.

2. McKusick, V.A.: Genetics in Medicine and Medicine in Genetics, *Amer. J. Med. 4*: 594–599, 1963.

3. Lynch, H.T., Krush, T.P., Krush, A.J.

and Tips, R.L.: Psychodynamics of Early Hereditary Deaths, *Amer. J. Dis. Child. 108*: 605–610, 1964.

4. Tips, R.L., and Lynch, H.T.: The Impact of Genetic Counseling Upon the Family Milieu, *JAMA 184*: 183–186, 1953.

5. Lynch, H.T.: Hereditary Factors in Carcinoma, In *Recent Results in Cancer Research,* New York, Springer–Verlag, 1967, Vol. 12.

6. Sholevar, G.: Family Therapy, *J. Albert Einstein Med. Ctr. 13*: 61–66, 1970.

7. McKusick, V.A.: Family–Oriented Follow–up, *J. Chron. Dis. 22*: 1–7, 1969.

8. Hendrix, R.C.: Unusual Survival Patterns of Patients with Metastatic Melanoma, *Cancer 24*: 574–, 1969.

9. Lynch, H.T., and Krush, A.J.: Heredity and Malignant Melanoma: Implications for Early Cancer Detection, *Canad. Med. Ass. J. 99*: 17–21, 1968.

10. World Health Organization Technical Report Series, 1969, Number 411.

11. Lynch, H.T. (ed.): *International Directory of Genetic Services,* (2nd ed.), New York, The National Foundation, 1969.

12. Emery, A.E.H. and Smith, C.: Ascertainment and Prevention of Genetic Disease, *Brit. Med. J.* 2: 636–637, (Sept.) 1970.

Epilogue

by Henry T. Lynch, M.D.

An attempt has been made throughout this book to focus attention upon dermatologic signs, which when coupled with genetic information, can provide clues to the existence of cancer in a variety of genetically determined conditions. A major objective of this pursuit is, of course, improved cancer control.

The reader may well ask, "Why spend so much time delving into the family history, when many of the conditions discussed, such as xeroderma pigmentosum, multiple nevoid basal cell carcinoma syndrome, keratosis palmaris et plantaris (tylosis) with esophageal cancer, are so exceedingly rare that the doctor may never encounter a case in his entire lifetime?" The answer to such a question is not easy because if we were concerned only with rarely occurring diseases such as those mentioned, it would probably not be profitable to discuss these diseases as we have. However, certain facts reveal that the aggregate of these so-called "rare" diseases constitutes a considerable proportion of cancers in man. Recall the listings in Tables 1 to 4 and one will appreciate the extent of this involvement. However, another factor which has received little attention is the role of heterozygous carriers in some of the rare recessive diseases and the question as to whether these individuals may have an increased susceptibility for the development of cancer. As a matter of fact, certain data indicate that heterozygous carriers of the gene for Fanconi's aplastic anemia and ataxia telangiectasia are more susceptible to the development of cancer than those individuals without this gene. It is quite apparent that it is of great importance to learn more about heterozygotes in the other recessively inherited cancer-predisposing diseases. Finally, rare as a disease may be, if a physician has in his practice a family with one of these conditions, the disease may turn out to be relatively "common" so far as his own experience is concerned. Recall the family presented in Chapter 5 with xeroderma pigmentosum wherein five individuals were affected in a sibship of nine. In this case, knowledge of the family history led to prompt diagnosis in all of the affected individuals and cancer control was prompted through the strict avoidance of exposure to solar radiation. This, in turn, has led to an unusually mild clinical course with only occasional occurrences of skin cancer.

In these days of advanced technology in medicine, increased use of automated laboratory studies, improved radiological surveys, use of a variety of radioactive materials and other diagnostic advances. our chances for earlier cancer diagnosis should be improved. However, relatively few patients utilize these specialized diagnostic facilities since for the most part they are found only at major medical centers. In turn, these highly specialized diagnostic studies may be expensive, time consuming, and in some cases not without hazard. However, available within every physician's grasp is a truly simple approach and guide to the diagnosis of hereditary cancer, namely that of the family history! Indeed the family history may lead immediately to the recognition of specific disease entities which are associated with cancer in a manner which few available diagnostic studies could duplicate. In spite of this potential, it is surprising that accurate family histories are infrequently obtained and utilized for individuals at genetic risk for specific traits and diseases. In addition, it is a known fact that the busy physician often neglects to observe the patient's integument critically. The pressure of a busy practice often results in a rather restricted physical examination which is directed toward the patient's specific complaint, i.e. an "earache," "sore throat," a "boil on the neck," or a "cut finger." However, while attention is being focused upon such discrete areas of the body, a mere glance at a patient's skin in a well–lighted area could provide clues to the possibility of an underlying cancer, which in fact, may literally be staring the physician in the face. It has therefore been the goal of this book to call attention to these relatively simple and straight–forward measures in the hope that their more frequent use will result in improved cancer control.

Dr. Arnold Kaplan has provided a chapter on the basic fundamentals of genetics which is designed to assist the clinician in a fuller comprehension of genetic principles. This short discourse presents a stream of thought which will have implications for many of the unresolved genetic problems, particularly those concerned with the possibility of genetic interrelatedness or distinctiveness as in the neurocutaneous syndromes and other diseases discussed in this book; thus we might better appreciate the problems involved in a single gene hypothesis versus differing genes at distinct chromosomal loci. In addition, Dr. Kaplan has provided succinct discussion with excellent reference sources for perusal in depth of these basic genetic issues.

The chapter by Drs. Ricardi and Cleaver pertaining to DNA repair synthesis in tissue culture studies of patients with xeroderma pigmentosum (xdp) presents a completely unique experimental model in the search for an explanation of the basic defect in this disease. Thus, we are provided with insight into pathogenetic mechanisms occurring at the molecular level in this hereditary disease. While the significance of this work is of crucial importance for xeroderma pigmentosum, it may be of importance in the future understanding of other hereditary diseases associated with cancer. Indeed, further work on the model could provide methods for overcoming the enzyme deficiency (endonuclease) in xeroderma pigmentosum. When present, endonuclease cleaves a damaged, but unbroken DNA chain which is integral to the initiation of the process of excision of the damaged regions. Thus, when cleavage does not occur the subsequent steps involved in the incision–repair process cannot be carried out. In accordance with the defective excision repair process in xeroderma pigmentosum, UV irradiation is found to be associated with a decrease in cell proliferation (in–vitro), or the development of new growth patterns, i.e. dysplasia and neoplasia (in–vitro).

The chapter by Lynch on the clinical aspects of xeroderma pigmentosum is a logical sequel to the work on basic mechanisms concerning the defect in this disease. A family with xdp is described wherein squamous and basal cell carcinomas of the skin as well as malignant melanoma (in two siblings) were found. Of chief interest in this family, however is the fact that relatively few skin cancers have occurred in affected siblings, which appears to be a result of stringent prevention of exposure to sunlight.

The next chapter treats the subject of malignant melanoma and includes several families which have been under investigation by Lynch and his associates. Although hereditary factors occur in only approximately 3 percent of patients with malignant melanoma, it is important for the physician to understand that the familial form of melanoma appears to behave as an autosomal dominant. In addition, cancer of other histologic sites also appears to occur in excess in such melanoma families though data on this aspect of the problem at the present time is rather limited because of incomplete reporting in most family studies. A review of the literature also has shown that malignant melanoma may be associated with xeroderma pigmentosum and with von Recklinghausen's neurofibromatosis.

The chapter on ataxia telangiectasia by Dr. John Jackson reviews the myriad disorders associated with this rarely occurring autosomal recessively inherited disease. Thus, we find cerebellar ataxia, ocular cutaneous telangiectasia, telangiectasias of the ears and butterfly area of the face and bridge of the nose and periorbital region, and an absence or deficiency of IgA which is undoubtedly associated with the manifestations of recurrent and occasionally severe sinopulmonary infections in this disease. Increased occurrences of malignant neoplasms are found in this condition particularly of lymphoid tissue and the central nervous system; others include multiple basal cell carcinomas of the skin, reticulum cell sarcoma, Hodgkin's disease, cerebellar medulloblastoma, frontal lobe glioma, and bilateral ovarian dysgerminomas.

The chapter by Drs. Haruo Okazaki and William Harlan on the neurocutaneous syndromes focuses attention upon the complex interrelationships between such phakomatoses as tuberous sclerosis (Bourneville's disease), Sturge–Weber Dimitri disease, von Recklinghausen's neurofibromatosis, ataxia telangiectasia, melanosis cerebri, and the multiple nevoid basal cell carcinoma syndrome. A commonly occurring clinical finding in all of these conditions is *café au lait* spots. Skeletal anomalies and mental subnormality are also frequently present. Cancer occurs in all of these conditions, and thus, we have substantive support for the possible existence of a unifying carcinogenic factor. Intracranial neoplasms are known to occur in excess in each of these disorders. The interrelatedness of clinical findings is impressive in these authors' support for a unifying concept for these diseases; however, it is nevertheless readily apparent that these data are insufficient at this time to confirm the presence of a single gene showing variable expressivity or for alternative hypotheses, i.e. that modifying genes and/or environmental interactions account for variations in clinical expressions in kindreds. Indeed we see that in at least one of these, namely ataxia telangiectasia, an entirely distinct mode of inheritance, namely autosomal recessive, can account for the overwhelming majority of occurrences of this disease while on the other hand, autosomal dominant inheritance patterns prevail in the remaining conditions.

Dr. R. Neil Schimke's paper on "The Mucosal Neuroma Syndrome" presents a recently described syndrome in which the mucocutaneous hallmarks include mucosal neuromas in association with peripheral neurofibromas. In addition, an interesting cancer association occurs in the increased occurrence of medullary thyroid carcinoma with bilateral pheochromocytomas. Dr. Schimke describes in detail some of the features of this disorder which appear to be similar to those found in von Recklinghausen's neurofibromatosis. However, Schimke classifies this syndrome as distinct from neurofibromatosis and indeed he has also distinguished the syndrome from other endocrine neoplasia syndromes. Thus, in the chapter on neurocutaneous diseases by Okazaki and Harlan, we find a good case for the "lumpers" while in Schimke's chapter, we find an equally convincing case for "splitters." Perhaps, in due time, as we learn more about the biochemistry, pathology, and genetics of these fascinating diseases, we might arrive at a greater degree of orderliness and clarity with respect to their final classification.

An extensive historical and clinical review of the multiple nevoid basal cell carcinoma syndrome is presented by Dr. Gorlin. This syndrome bears his name in some of the medical literature, since he was one of the first individuals to clearly describe it and correlate it with hereditary mechanisms. The reader is provided with a clear differential diagnosis of this autosomal dominantly inherited disorder.

Gardner's syndrome is brought up to date by Dr. Alvin Watne. This condition is now known to be associated with an increasingly large spectrum of malignant neoplasms in addition to the commonly occuring adenocarcinoma of the colon as part of the polyposis coli complex in this disease. Specifically, other neoplasms have included fibrosarcomas, lipomyosarcomas, desmoid tumors, and thyroid carcinomas.

Dr. Woodbury presents a survey of diseases and tumors involving the gastrointestinal system, relevant to the theme of this book, skin, genetics, and cancer. A variety of entities are described which have a clear delineation of gastrointestinal manifestations.

The chapter by Drs. Villacorte and Townley deals with the general problem of immunology with specific reference to skin, genetics, and cancer. In light of the intensive investigations in the area of cancer immunology which are being carried out in many laboratories throughout the world at this time, we thought it would be timely to present a survey of those conditions with cutaneous manifestations and underlying cancer wherein immunological mechanisms are involved. Implications for susceptibility to cancer on an immuno–genetic basis, when relevant, are discussed in this chapter.

The chapter by Dr. Lynch on disorders with a known or presumed genetic basis, wherein skin and cancer occur, is in the strict sense "miscellaneous." Specifically, a number of conditions, any one of which could have merited a separate chapter, are presented collectively in this chapter for the purpose of completeness. It is not implied that those conditions which were treated as separate entities elsewhere in the book were necessarily the most "important" subjects so far as cancer control or for their relevance to a better understanding of genetics and carcinogenesis. Although many of the subjects in this chapter have been given special attention by individual authors in separate texts and journals our plan nevertheless was to bring together under one cover the general theme of skin, malignant neoplasms, and genetics.

Finally, the chapter on genetic counseling is designed primarily to assist the clinician to apply genetic information to families in his clinical practice. Practical information is provided concerning each of the clinical examples such as xeroderma pigmentosum and malignant melanoma in the chapters devoted to

these entities. These particular clinical problems were chosen not only because they represent our own personal experience, but also because they present challenging problems in cancer control. As a sequel to this chapter we have provided a listing of genetic units throughout the United States and other countries of the world wherein genetic counseling is offered; a separate listing is given of units which conduct cancer genetic research. However, inclusion of this material does not in any way detract from our general theme that ideally the physician who is caring for the particular family is the most capable person to perform genetic counseling. We believe that the availability of information contained in this registry of genetic units could help the physician should he wish additional assistance with genetic problems in his practice.

Appendix

GENETIC COUNSELING AND CANCER GENETIC UNITS IN THE UNITED STATES AND OTHER COUNTRIES OF THE WORLD

GENETIC COUNSELING AND/OR CANCER GENETICS IN THE UNITED STATES
A "G" following the name of the unit denotes Genetic Counseling
A "C" denotes Cancer Genetics

ALABAMA

Paul C. Bailey — C
Department of Biology
Birmingham Southern College
Birmingham, Alabama 35201

Wayne H. Finley — CG
Laboratory of Medical Genetics
University of Alabama Med. Center
Birmingham, Alabama 35233

ALASKA

Edward M. Scott — G
Public Health Service
Arctic Health Research Center
College, Alaska 99701

ARIZONA

Charles M. Woolf — G
Department of Zoology
Arizona State University
Tempe, Arizona 85281

ARKANSAS

Robert E. Merrill — G
Birth Defects Center
Univ. of Arkansas
4301 Markham
Little Rock, Arkansas 72201

CALIFORNIA

Donna Daentl — G
Kern County Health Dept.
Bakersfield, California 93305

Curt Stern — G
Dept. of Zoology
University of California
Berkeley, California 94720

David E. Comings — CG
Department of Medical Genetics
City of Hope Medical Center
Duarte, California 91010

Patricia H. Henderson — G
Fresno County Health Dept.
515 So. Cedar Avenue
Fresno, California 93702

E. David Weinstein — G
Kaiser–Permanente Medical Center
Department of Pediatrics
1050 W. Pacific Coast Hwy.
Harbor City, California 90710

Kenneth W. Dumars — CG
Department of Pediatrics
University of Calif. at Irvine
Irvine, California 92650

Oliver W. Jones — CG
Medical Genetics Unit
Univ. of California School of Med.
La Jolla, California 92037

William L. Nyhan — G
Biochemical Genetics Lab.
Univ. of Calif. School of Med.
La Jolla, California 92037

Lawrence J. Schneiderman — G
Dept. of Community Medicine
School of Medicine
Univ. of Calif., San Diego
La Jolla, California 92037

Willard R. Centerwall — G
Genetics, Birth Defects &
  Chromosome Services
Loma Linda University Med. Center
Loma Linda, California 92354

George N. Donnell — G
Dept. of Ped. and Biochem.
Children's Hospital
Los Angeles, California 90054

Allan J. Ebbin — G
L.A. County–USC Med. Center
Genetics Birth Defects Center
1200 N. State Street
Los Angeles, California 90033

Robert S. Sparkes — CG
Dept. of Med. & Ped.
UCLA School of Medicine
760 Westwood Place
Los Angeles, California 90024

Miriam G. Wilson — G
Dept. of Pediatrics
Univ. of So. Cal. Med. School
1200 No. State Street
Los Angeles, California 90033

S.W. Wright — G
Depts. of Ped and Med.
University of California
Center for Health Sciences
Los Angeles, California 90024

Ronald Bachman   G
Dept. of Ped. & Gen.
Kaiser Foundation Hospital
280 West MacArthur Blvd.
Oakland, California 94611

Arnold Nurock   G
Dept. of Birth Defects
Children's Hos. Med. Center
Oakland, California 94609

Harold N. Bass   G
Kaiser–Permanente Medical Center
Department of Pediatrics
13652 Cantara Street
Panorama City, California 91402

Charles J. Epstein   G
Ross General Hospital
1150 Sir Francis Drake Blvd.
Ross, California 94957

Robert S. Stempfel, Jr.   G
Birth Defects Center
Sacramento Medical Center
2315 Stockton Blvd.
Sacramento, California 95817

Irving E. Allen   G
Dept. of Pediatrics
St. Bernardine's Hospital
San Bernardino, California 92404

Dominic A. De Santo   G
Mercy Hospital and Medical
  Center Clinic
4077 Fifth Avenue
San Diego, California 92103

Frederick A. Frye   G
Birth Defects Center
Children's Health Center
San Diego, California 92123

Louis Gluck   G
University Hospital
San Diego County
P.O. Box 3548
San Diego, California 92103

Charles J. Epstein   G
Dept. of Pediatrics
University of California
  Medical Center
San Francisco, California 94122

Melvin M. Grumbach   G
Dept. of Pediatrics
Univ. of California
San Francisco Medical Center
San Francisco, California 94122

Charles Epstein   G
Santa Barbara Co. Health Dept.
4440 Calle Real
Santa Barbara, California 93105

John Mann   G
Kaiser Hosp. Ped. Clinic
900 Kiely Boulevard
Santa Clara, California 95051

Leslie M. Holve
St. John's Hospital
1328 22nd Street
Santa Monica, California 90404

Howard M. Cann
Dept. of Pediatrics
Stanford Univ. School of Medicine
Stanford, California 94605

Luigi Luzzatti
Dept. of Pediatrics
Stanford Univ. Med. Center
Birth Defects Clinic
Stanford, California 94305

David L. Rimoin
Div. of Med. Genetics
Harbor Gen. Hospital
1000 W. Carson Street
Torrance, California 90509

Felice Weber
Ventura Cty. Health Dept.
Ventura, California 93001

COLORADO
Donough O'Brien
Dept. of Pediatrics
Univ. of Colorado
4200 East 9th Avenue
Denver, Colorado 80220

C.W. Reiquam
Presbyterian Med. Center
Dept. of Pathology
Denver, Colorado 80218

Arthur Robinson
Depts. of Ped. and Biophy.
Univ. of Col. Med. Center
4200 East 9th Avenue
Denver, Colorado 80220

George J. Siemens
Dept. of Human Genetics
Univ. of Colorado
1100 Fourteenth Street
Denver, Colorado 80202

CONNECTICUT
Robert M. Greenstein
University of Connecticut
  Medical School
Dept. of Pediatrics
2 Holcomb Street
Hartford, Connecticut 06112

Merton S. Honeyman
Dept. of Health
Connecticut Twin Registry
79 Elm Street
Hartford, Connecticut 06115

Leon Rosenberg
Dept. of Ped. & Med.
Yale Medical School
New Haven, Connecticut 06520

George Mickey   G
Dept. of Cytogenetics
P.O. Box 308
New England Inst. for Med. Res.
Ridgefield, Connecticut 06877

DISTRICT OF COLUMBIA

Luis F. Arias–Bernal   CG
Dept. of Ob. & Gynecology
Columbia Hospital for Women
2324 L Street, N.W.
Washington, D.C. 20037

Mihaly Bartalos   G
Medical Genetics Unit
Howard University
College of Medicine
Washington, D.C. 20001

Robert J. Clayton   G
Depts. of Ped. and Obstet.
Georgetown Univ. Hospital
3800 Reservoir Rd., N.W.
Washington, D.C. 20007

Cecil B. Jacobson   CG
Reproductive Gen. Unit
The Geo. Washington Univ. Clinic
2150 Penn Ave., N.W.
Washington, D.C. 20037

Marvin C. Mengel, Capt.   G
Malcolm Grow USAF Med. Center
Human Genetics Service
Washington, D.C. 20231

Robert F. Murray, Jr.   G
Dept. of Pediatrics
Howard Univ. Col. of Med.
Washington, D.C. 20001

N. C. Myrianthopoulos   G
Gen. Counseling & Res. Center
George Washington Univ. Hosp.
Washington, D.C. 20037

Beale H. Ong   G
Dept. of Neurology
Children's Hosp.
2125 13th Street, N.W.
Washington, D.C. 20009

FLORIDA

Mark V. Barrow   G
Dept. of Medicine
University of Florida
Gainesville, Florida 32601

Arlan L. Rosenbloom   G
Birth Defects Center
J. Hillis Miller Health Center
Gainesville, Florida 32601

Richard J. Warren   G
University of Miami
Mailman Center for Child Dev.
P.O. Box 6, Biscayne Annex
Miami, Florida 33152

GEORGIA

Arthur Falek   G
Dept. of Psychiatry
Emory Univ.
Georgia Mental Health Inst.
Atlanta, Georgia 30306

Malcolm Freeman   G
Div. of Perinatal Pathology
Emory Univ. School of Med.
80 Butler Street, S.E.
Atlanta, Georgia 30303

John T. Godwin   G
St. Joseph's Hospital
Dept. of Pathology
265 Ivy Street, N.E.
Atlanta, Georgia 30303

J. Rogers Byrd   G
Dept. of Endocrinology
Med. College of Georgia
Augusta, Georgia 30902

Clyde Keeler   G
Central State Hospital
Milledgeville, Georgia 31062

HAWAII

Sharon Bintliff   G
Dept. of Birth Defects
Kauikeolani Children's Hosp.
Honolulu, Hawaii 96817

Newton E. Morton   G
Population Genetics Lab.
University of Hawaii
2411 Dole Street
Honolulu, Hawaii 96822

IDAHO

J. R. Marks   G
Idaho M.R. Program
Boise, Idaho 83701

R. S. McKean   G
Mental Retard Program
Idaho State School & Hosp.
Box 47
Nampa, Idaho 83651

ILLINOIS

William Alpern   G
Amniocentesis Service
Michael Reese Hosp. & Med. Center
530 E. 31st Street
Chicago, Illinois 60616

Anthony P. Amarose   CG
Univ. of Chicago
Dept. of Obst. & Gynec.
5841 S. Maryland Avenue
Chicago, Illinois 60637

Paul E. Carson   G
Dept. of Medicine
University of Chicago
Chicago, Illinois 60601

Carl Cohen   G
Center for Genetics
University of Illinois
Medical Center, Chicago
1853 W. Polk Street
Chicago, Illinois 60612

Albert Dorfman   G
Dept. of Pediatrics
Univ. of Chicago
950 East 59th Street
Chicago, Illinois 60637

David C. Garron   G
Presbyterian–St. Luke's Hosp.
1753 W. Congress Parkway
Chicago, Illinois 60091

Eva Krompotic   CG
Dept. of Exptl. Pathology
Mt. Sinai Hosp. Med. Center
Chicago, Illinois 60608

H. L. Nadler   G
Dept. of Genetics
Children's Memorial Hosp.
Chicago, Illinois 60614

Samuel Pruzansky, D.D.S.   G
Center for Craniofacial Anomalies
University of Illinois
Medical Center, Chicago
1853 W. Polk Street
Chicago, Illinois 60612

Ira M. Rosenthal   G
Dept. of Pediatrics
Cook County Hospital
700 S. Wood Street
Chicago, Illinois 60612

Jeanette Schulz   G
Illinois State Ped. Inst.
1640 West Roosevelt Road
Chicago, Illinois 60608

Donald C. Burns   G
Dept. of Res.
Evanston Hospital
2650 Ridge Avenue
Evanston, Illinois 60201

David Yi-Yung Hsia   G
Dept. of Pediatrics
Loyola Medical Center
Hines, Illinois 60141

INDIANA

A. Donald Merritt   CG
Dept. of Med. Genetics
Indiana Univ. Med. Sch.
Indianapolis, Indiana 46207

IOWA

Hans Zellweger   G
Dept. of Pediatrics
University Hospital
Iowa City, Iowa 52240

KANSAS

R. N. Schimke   CG
Dept. of Medicine
Kansas Univ. Med. Center
Kansas City, Kansas 66103

Leo P. Cawley   CG
Dept. of Clinical Pathology
Wesley Med. Res. Foundation
Wichita, Kansas 67214

KENTUCKY

C. C. Mabry   G
Dept. of Pediatrics
Univ. of Kentucky Med. Center
Lexington, Kentucky 40506

Bernard Weisskopf   G
Child Evaluation Center
Univ. of Louisville Med. Sch
540 South Preston Street
Louisville, Kentucky 40202

LOUISIANA

H.W. Kloepfer   CG
Dept. of Anatomy
Tulane University
New Orleans, Louisiana 70112

Richard C. Juberg   G
Birth Defects Center
Dept. of Pediatrics
L.S.U. Sch. of Med. in Shreveport
Shreveport, Louisiana 71101

MAINE

John C. Van Pelt   G
Genetic Counseling Center
50 Union Street
Ellsworth, Maine 04605

MARYLAND

Richard Heller   G
Dept. of Pediatrics
Sinai Hospital
Baltimore, Maryland 21215

R. Rodney Howell   G
The Johns Hopkins Univ.
School of Medicine
601 North Broadway
Baltimore, Maryland 21205

Victor A. McKusick   G
The Moore Clinic
The Johns Hopkins Hospital
Baltimore, Maryland 21205

George H. Thomas   G
Human Genetics Lab.
John F. Kennedy Inst.
707 No. Broadway
Baltimore, Maryland 21205

MASSACHUSETTS

Howard P. Baden   G
Massachusetts General Hosp.
Dermatology Genetics Clinic
Boston, Massachusetts 02114

Murray Feingold   G
Birth Defects Center
20 Ash Street
Boston, Massachusetts 02115

P. S. Gerald   G
Clinical Gen. Div.
Children's Hosp. Med. Center
Boston, Massachusetts 02115

John W. Littlefield   G
Dept. of Pediatrics
Massachusetts Gen. Hosp.
Boston, Massachusetts 02114

Peter V. Tishler   G
Channing Laboratory &
  Thorndike Memorial Lab.
Harvard Medical Unit
Boston City Hospital
Boston, Massachusetts 02118

MICHIGAN

James Neel   G
Dept. of Human Genetics
Univ. of Michigan
Ann Arbor, Michigan

Roy Schmichel   G
Dept. of Pediatrics
Univ. of Michigan Med. Center
Ann Arbor, Michigan 48104

Paulinus F. Forsthoefel   G
Dept. of Biology
University of Detroit
Detroit, Michigan 48221

Lester Weiss   G
Dept. of Pediatrics
Henry Ford Hospital
2799 W. Grand Blvd.
Detroit, Michigan 48202

Fred A. Baughman, Jr.   CG
Blodgett Mem. Hosp.
Ped. Neuro–Muscular Dis. Clinic
1810 Wealthy S.E.
Grand Rapids, Michigan 49506

James V. Higgins   G
Dept. of Zoology
Michigan State Univ.
Lansing, Michigan 48901

Isak O. Berker   G
Lapeer State Home & Train. Sch.
Medical Dept.
Lapeer, Michigan 48466

Homer Weir   G
Dept. of Mental Health
Plymouth St. Home & Train. Sch.
Northville, Michigan 48167

MINNESOTA

Robert J. Gorlin   G
Human Genetics Clinic
University of Minnesota Hospital
Minneapolis, Minnesota 55455

F. Patrick Maloney   G
Kenny Rehabilitation Assoc.
1800 Chicago Avenue
Minneapolis, Minnesota 55404

Sheldon C. Reed   G
Dight Inst. for Human Gen.
Univ. of Minnesota
Minncapolis, Minnesota 55455

Lee F. Schacht   G
Human Genetics Unit
Minnesota Dept. of Health
Minneapolis, Minnesota 55440

Carl Witkop   G
School of Dentistry
Univ. of Minn. Dent. Sch.
Minneapolis, Minnesota 55415

Jorge J. Yunis   G
Medical Genetics Div.
Dept. of Lab. Med.
Univ. of Minnesota Hosp.
Minneapolis, Minnesota 55415

Hymie Gordon   CG
Genetics Consulting Service
Mayo Clinic
Rochester, Minnesota 55901

MISSISSIPPI

John F. Jackson   CG
Dept. of Preventive Med.
Univ. of Mississippi Med. Cen.
Jackson, Mississippi 39216

MISSOURI

Clement E. Brooke   G
Dept. of Pediatrics
Univ. of Missouri Med. Center
Columbia, Missouri 65201

C. B. Francisco   G
Neurology Dept.
Children's Mercy Hospital
Kansas City, Missouri 64108

Patricia L. Monteleone   G
Cardinal Glennon Hosp.
1465 S. Grand Boulevard
St. Louis, Missouri 63104

William S. Sly   G
Div. of Med. Gen.
Dept. of Ped. & Med.
Washington Univ. Med. Sch.
St. Louis, Missouri 63110

NEBRASKA

R. Stephen Amato   G
Molecular Gen. Lab.
Dept. of Pediatrics
Univ. of Nebraska Med. Center
Omaha, Nebraska 68105

James D. Eisen   G
Univ. of Nebraska Med. Center
42nd & Dewey Avenue
Omaha, Nebraska 68105

H. T. Lynch   CG
Dept. of Preventive Med.
Creighton Univ. Sch. of Med.
Omaha, Nebraska 68131

T. R. Pfundt   G
Birth Defects Clinic
Children's Memorial Hosp.
Omaha, Nebraska 68105

NEW HAMPSHIRE

D. Hoefnagel   G
Dept. of Path. & Med.
Dartmouth Medical School
Hanover, New Hampshire 03755

NEW JERSEY

Phoebe Hudson   CG
Hackensack Hosp. Assn.
Child Evaluation Center
243 Atlantic Street
Hackensack, New Jersey 07602

Theodore Kushnick   G
Dept. of Ped., Col. of Med.
   of New Jersey at Newark
100 Bergen Street
Newark, New Jersey 07103

NEW MEXICO

Thomas McConnell   G
Dept. of Pathology
Univ. of New Mexico Med. Sch.
Albuquerque, New Mexico 87106

NEW YORK

Ian H. Porter   G
N.Y. State Dept. of Health
Birth Def. Inst.
Albany Med. Col.
Dept. of Ped. Room K116
Albany, New York 12208

Autub H. Aqzi   G
Downstate Med. Center
Dept. of Pediatrics
450 Clarkson Avenue
Brooklyn, New York 11203

Harvey Dosik   C
Div. of Hematology
Jewish Hosp. of Brooklyn
555 Prospect Place
Brooklyn, N.Y. 11238

Felix Feldman   G
Pediatric Service
Coney Island Hosp.
Ocean Parkway and Ave. Z
Brooklyn, New York 11235

Irving B. Wexler   G
Dept. of Pediatrics
Jewish Hosp. and Med. Center
   of Brooklyn
Brooklyn, New York 11238

Alexander S. Wiener   C
64 Rutland Road
Brooklyn, New York 11225

R. M. Bannerman   C
Dept. of Med.
Buffalo General Hosp.
100 High Street
Buffalo, New York 14203

Jean A. Cortner   C
Dept. of Pediatrics
State Univ. of New York
Children's Hospital
Buffalo, New York 14222

Ronald G. Davidson   •
Dept. of Pediatrics
State Univ. of New York
   at Buffalo
Children's Hospital
Buffalo, New York 14222

Jack Sherman
Gen. Unit Ped. Clinic
Meadowbrook Hospital
P.O. Box 175
East Meadow, New York 11554

John R. Whittier
Med. Services Div.
Creedmoor Inst., Sta. 60
Jamaica, New York 11427

Arthur E. Mirkinson
Genetics Lab.
North Shore Hosp.
Manhasset, L.I., New York 11030

Alexander G. Bearn
Human Gen. (Med.)
New York–Cornell Med. Center
525 East 68th Street
New York, New York 10021

Louis Z. Cooper
Dept. of Pediatrics
Rubella Birth Def. Eval. Proj.
New York Univ. Med. Sch.
New York, New York 10006

Edward Gendel
Dept. of Pathology
New York Med. Col–Metro. Hosp.
97 St. and First Avenue
New York, New York 10029

J. German   G
The New York Blood Center
310 East 67th Street
New York, New York 10021

Kurt Hirschhorn   CG
Dept. of Pediatrics
Mt. Sinai Sch. of Med.
New York, New York 10029

H. P. Klinger   G
Dept. of Gen.
Albert Einstein Col. of Med.
1300 Morris Park Avenue
New York, New York 10461

Ernest Lieber   G
Medical Genetics
Beth Israel Med. Center
10 Nathan D. Perlman Place
New York, New York 10003

O. J. Miller   CG
Columbia University
New York, New York 10032

Harold M. Nitowsky   G
Gen. Counseling Program
Albert Einstein Col. of Med.
Bronx Municipal Hosp. Center
New York, New York 10461

Kiyoshi Oikawa   G
Dept. of Ped. and Gen.
Hosp. for Joint Diseases
1919 Madison Avenue
New York, New York 10035

John D. Rainer   G
Dept. of Med. Gen.
N.Y. State Psychiatric Inst.
New York, New York 10032

Richard Boies Stark   G
Cleft Palate Clinic
St. Luke's Hosp. Center
New York, New York 10025

Salome Gluecksohn Waelsch   G
Albert Einstein Col. of Med.
Eastchester Road & Morris Park Ave.
New York, New York 10461

Dorothy Warburton   G
Presbyterian Hospital
New York, New York 10032

Sandra R. Wolman   CG
Dept. of Pathology
N.Y. Univ. Med. Center
550 First Avenue
New York, New York 10016

Philip L. Townes   G
Div. of Genetics
Rochester Univ. Med. Sch.
Rochester, New York 14620

David Tiersten   CG
Rt. 25A
St. John's Episcopal Hospital
Smithtown, New York 11787

George A. Jervis   G
New York State Inst. for
    Research in Mental Retardation
1050 Forest Hill Road
Staten Island, New York

L. I. Gardner   G
Dept. of Ped.
Upstate Medical Center
Syracuse, New York 13210

Lawrence R. Shapiro   G
Director of Cytogenetics
Letchworth Village
Thiells, New York 10984

NORTH CAROLINA

Dept. of Pediatrics   G
Birth Defects Clinic
Chapel Hill, N. Carolina 27515

A. C. Christakos   G
Dept. of Obstet & Gynec.
Duke Med. Center
Box 3274
Durham, N. Carolina 27706

William W. McLendon   CG
Moses H. Cone Memorial Hosp.
1200 North Elm Street
P.O. Box 13227
Greensboro, N. Carolina 27405

James J. Thomas   G
Birth Defects Eval. Clinic
Western Carolina Center
Morganton, N. Carolina 28655

C. N. Herndon   G
Bowman Gray Sch. of Med.
Genetics Sec.
Dept. of Ped.
Wake Forest Univ.
Winston–Salem, N. Carolina 27103

NORTH DAKOTA
W. A. Wasdahl   C
Dept. of Pathology
Univ. of North Dakota
Grand Forks, N.D. 58202

OHIO
Josef Warkany   G
Dept. of Ped.
Children's Hosp. Res. Found.
Cincinnati, Ohio 45229

Arnold R. Kaplan   G
Dept. of Med. Gen.
Cleveland Psychiatric Inst.
1708 Aiken Avenue
Cleveland, Ohio 44109

Irwin A. Schafer   G
Dept. of Ped.
Case Western Reserve Univ.
Cleveland Metrop. Gen. Hosp.
Cleveland, Ohio 44109

A. G. Steinberg   G
Dept. of Biology
Case Western Reserve Univ.
Cleveland, Ohio 44106

Richard M. Goodman   G
Dept. of Med.
University Hospital
Ohio State University
410 W. 10th Avenue
Columbus, Ohio 43210

Stella B. Kontras   G
Dept. of Ped.
Children's Hospital
Columbus, Ohio 43205

Audrey Pfefferle   C
Dept. of Gen. Serv.
Metagen Lab., Inc.
4035 Roberts Road
Columbus, Ohio 43228

Meinhard Robinow   G
Birth Defects Eval. Center
1735 Chapel Street
Barney Children Med. Center
Dayton, Ohio 45404

OKLAHOMA
J. R. Seely   G
Dept. of Ped.
Univ. of Oklahoma
Children's Hospital
Oklahoma City, Oklahoma 73104

OREGON
Gerald H. Prescott   CG
Dept. of Pediatrics
Sacred Heart Hospital
Eugene, Oregon 97401

Ronald R. Stuart   CG
Crippled Child Div.
  Gen. Clinic
Rogue Valley Mem. Hosp.
2825 Barnett Road
Medford, Oregon 97501

Frederick Hecht   CG
Gen. Clinic
Crippled Child Div.
Univ. of Oregon Med. Sch.
Portland, Oregon 97201

PENNSYLVANIA
John A. Malcolm   G
Dept. of Path.
Geisinger Med. Center
Danville, Pennsylvania 17815

K. R. Dronamraju   G
Lancaster Cleft Palate Clin.
24 North Lime Street
Lancaster, Pennsylvania 17604

Angelo M. Digeorge   G
St. Christopher Hosp.
  for Children
2600 N. Lawrence Street
Dept. of Ped.
Philadelphia, Pennsylvania 19133

Laird G. Jackson   CG
Div. of Gen.
Jefferson Med. College
1025 Walnut Street
Philadelphia, Pennsylvania 19107

B. N. Kaufmann   G
Dept. of Anatomy
Section of Genetics
Hahnemann Medical College
Philadelphia, Pennsylvania 19102

William J. Mellman   G
Dept. of Ped.
Children's Hospital
Philadelphia, Pennsylvania 19146

Mark W. Steele   G
Children's Hospital
Pittsburgh, Pennsylvania 15213

J. Howard Turner   G
Dept. of Obstet. & Gyn.
Magee–Women's Hospital
Pittsburgh, Pennsylvania 15213

RHODE ISLAND
Paul H. Lamarche   CG
Dept. of Pediatrics
Rhode Island Hospital
Providence, Rhode Island 02902

SOUTH CAROLINA
Vladimir Wertelecki   CG
Medical Univ. of S.C.
80 Barre Street
Charleston, South Carolina 29401

TENNESSEE
Carmen B. Lozzio   G
Birth Defects Eval. Center
University of Tennessee
Knoxville, Tennessee 37916

Robert L. Summitt   G
Dept. of Pediatrics
Univ. of Tennessee
860 Madison Avenue
Memphis, Tennessee 38103

E. Perry Crump   CG
Hubbard Hospital
Dept. of Pediatrics
1005 18th Ave. No.
Nashville, Tennessee 37208

Eric Engel   G
Dept. of Medicine
Vanderbilt Hospital
Nashville, Tennessee 37203

Saburo Hara
Dept. of Pediatrics
Meharry Med. College
Nashville, Tennessee 37208

TEXAS

E. J. Arganaras   C
Chief of Laboratory
Vet. Admin. Hosp.
Big Spring, Texas 79720

Norman G. P. Helgeson   G
Dir. of Clin. Path.
Baylor Univ. Med. Center
3500 Gaston Avenue
Dallas, Texas 75246

Lillian Lockhart   G
Dept. of Ped. & Human Gen.
Univ. of Texas Med. Branch
Galveston, Texas 77550

Felix L. Haas   CG
Dept. of Biology
M.D. Anderson Hospital
Houston, Texas 77025

Dan G. McNamara   G
Dept. of Pediatrics
Baylor Univ. Col. of Med.
Houston, Texas 77025

Rebecca P. Schwanecke   G
Birth Defects Center
Texas Children's Hospital
6621 Fannin Street
Houston, Texas 77025

Anil K. Sinha   G
Birth Defects Center
Texas Children's Hospital
6621 Fannin Street
Houston, Texas 77025

Robert Tips   G
Dept. of Med. Gen.
Pasadena Gen. Hosp.
Pasadena, Texas 77501

Jose M. Louro   G
Section of Gen. & Cytogenet.
Dept. of Ped.
Univ. of Texas Med. Sch. at San Antonio
7703 Floyd Curl Drive
San Antonio, Texas 78229

Wallace McNutt   G
Dept. of Anatomy
Univ. of Texas Med. Sch.
7703 Floyd Curl Drive
San Antonio, Texas 78229

UTAH

Eldon J. Gardner   CG
Dept. of Zoology
Utah State University
Logan, Utah 84321

Garth G. Myers   G
Birth Defects Clinic
320-12th Avenue
Primary Children's Hosp.
Salt Lake City, Utah 84103

Charles D. Scott   G
Department of Internal Medicine
College of Medicine
University of Utah
Salt Lake City, Utah 84112

VERMONT

William E. Hodgkin   G
Dept. of Pediatrics
Mary Fletcher Hospital
Burlington, Vermont 05401

David S. Newcombe   G
Dept. of Med. & Anatomy
Univ. of Vermont Col. of Med.
Burlington, Vermont 05401

VIRGINIA

Johnson T. Carpenter   G
Dept. of Internal Med.
Univ. of Virginia Hosp.
Charlottesville, Va. 22901

James Q. Miller   G
Chromosome Res. Lab.
Univ. of Virginia Med. Sch.
Charlottesville, Virginia 22901

A. Ray Goodwin   CG
Dept. of Pathology
DePaul Hospital
Norfolk, Virginia 23505

Roscoe D. Hughes   G
Dept. of Bio. & Gen.
Med. Col. of Virginia
Richmond, Virginia 23219

Reuben B. Young   G
Dept. of Pediatrics
Med. Col. of Virginia
Richmond, Virginia 23219

WASHINGTON

Arno G. Motulsky   CG
Dept. of Medicine
University of Washington
Seattle, Washington 98105

David W. Smith   G
Dept. of Pediatrics
Sysmorphology Unit
Univ. of Washington, Med. Sch.
Seattle, Washington 98105

Robert G. Scherz   G
Dept. of Pediatrics
Madigan General Hospital
Tacoma, Washington 98431

WISCONSIN

Wm. J. Dewey   G
Dept. of Medical Genetics
University of Wisconsin
Madison, Wisconsin 53706

Elisabeth Kaveggia   G
Central Wisconsin Colony
  and Training School
317 Knutson Drive
Madison, Wisconsin 53704

John Opitz   G
Dept. of Med. Gen.
Univ. of Wisconsin Med. Sch.
Madison, Wisconsin 53706

Frank A. Walker   G
Cytog. Lab. and Gen. Clinic
The Milwaukee Children's Hosp.
1700 W. Wisconsin Avenue
Milwaukee, Wisconsin 53233

PUERTO RICO

A. A. Cintron–Rivera   G
Dept. of Clin. Res.
Univ. of Puerto Rico
San Juan, Puerto Rico

GENETIC COUNSELING AND/OR CANCER GENETICS IN OTHER COUNTRIES
A "G" following the name of the unit denotes Genetic Counseling
A "C" denotes Cancer Genetics

ARGENTINA

Herman Bleiweiss   G
Genetica Medica
Sarmiento 2569, 2DO. P. DP. 4
Buenos Aires, Argentina

Diego Brage   C
Neurology Clinic
Carlos Pellegrini 1336
Univ. of Buenos Aires
Buenos Aires, Argentina

Julio C. Ortiz de Zarate   G
Div. of Neurology
Fac. de Medicina del Salvador
Balcace 900 San Martin
Buenos Aires, Argentina

Nestor O. Bianchi   G
Dept. of Cytogenetics
Comision de Investigacion de la
  Provincia de Buenos Aires
La Plata, Argentina

AUSTRALIA

J. H. Bennett   G
Dept. of Genetics
University of Adelaide
Adelaide 50001, Australia

Neville Davis   C
Queensland Melanoma Project
Princess Alexandra Hosp.
Ipswich Rd. Woolloongabba, S.2
Brisbane, Queensland, Australia

D. C. Wallace   CG
Human Gen. Unit
Queensland Inst. for Med. Res.
Brisbane, Australia

C. B. Kerr   CC
Dept. of Prev. Social Med.
Univ. of Sydney
Royal Alexandra Hosp. for Child.
Camperdown 2006, Australia

R. L. Kirk   G
Dept. of Genetics
John Curtin Sch. of Med. Res.
Box 334, GPO
Canberra, Australia

R. J. Walsh   G
Sch. of Human Gen.
Univ. of New South Wales
P.O. Box 1, Kensington
N.S.W., 2033, Australia

David M. Danks   G
Univ. of Melbourne & Royal
  Children's Hosp. Res. Found.
Melbourne, Australia

Denys W. Fortune   G
Dept. of Pathology
Royal Women's Hospital
Melbourne, Australia

Brian Turner   G
Oliver Latham Lab.
Psychiatric Center
North Ryde, 2113
N.S.W., Australia

A. G. Baikie   C
Dept. of Medicine
Univ. of Tasmania
Royal Hobart Hospital
Tasmania, Australia

G. J. L. Hamilton   G
Dept. Men. Health Ser. of W.A.
Irrabeena Diagnostic Center
84 Thomas Street
West Perth 6050, Australia

J. A. Kirkland   C
Dept. of Obstet. & Gynec.
Queen Elizabeth Hosp.
Woodville, 5011, Australia

BELGIUM

Ludo Van Bogaert   G
Dept. of Neurogenetics
Foundation Born-Bunge
Antwerp, Belgium

   G

J.G. Leroy
Dept. of Genetics
Medical Genetic Unit
Antwerp State Univ.
Antwerp, Belgium

Marie L. Destine   G
Rue Antoine Gautier, 65
1040 Brussels, Belgium

A. Govaerts   G
Dept. of Immunology
Hosp. St. Pierre
322 Rue Haute
1000 Bruxelles, Belgium

J. Francois   G
Dept. of Ophthalmology
135, De Pintelaan
9000 Gent, Belgium

Herman Van Den Berghe   G
Dept. of Human Gen.
University of Leuven
Minderbroederstraat
Leuven, Belgium

Jacques Frederic   G
Lab. of Cytogenetics
University of Liege
Liege, Beligum

P. Dodinval   G
Dept. of Human Gen.
University of Liege
Liege, Belgium

BRAZIL

M. Ayres   G
Laboratorio de Genetica
Generalissimo Deodoro 413
Ciencias e Letros
Belem, Para, Brazil

Ademar Freire-Maia   G
Departamento de Genetica
Facul. Cienc. Medicas e Biol.
Botucatu, Sao Paulo, Brazil

Bernardo Biguelman   G
Dept. of Med. Gen.
University of Campinas
Campinas, Sao Paulo, Brazil

Newton Freire-Maia   G
Dept. of Gen.
Federal Univ. of Parana
Curitiba, Parana, Brazil

Judith Viegas Centeno   G
Lab. de Genetica Humana
Fac. de Medicina de Pelotas
Ipesse C.P. No. 464
Pelotas, RS, Brazil

Francisco M. Salzano   G
Universidade Federal
   do Rio Grande do Sul
Dept. of Gen.
Caixa Postal 1953
Porto Alegre, RS, Brazil

Jose Carneiro Leao   G
Inst. de Medicina Infantil
   de Pernambuco Coelhos
Recife, Brazil

Cassio Bottura   CG
Dept. of Hema. and Cytology
Med. Sch. of Ribeirao Preto
Ribeirao Preto, Sp., Brazil

Iris Ferrari   G
Medical Genetics II
Fac. Medicina-Ribeirao Preto
Cx301 Ribeirao Preto (SP)
Brazil

H. Krieger   G
Dept. of Genetics
University of Sao Paulo
Ribeirao Preto, SP, Brazil

J. C. Cabral de Almeida   G
Lab. Radiobiologia Celular
Instituto Biofisica
Av. Pasteur 458
Rio de Janeiro, GB, Brazil

Eliane S. Azevedo   G
Dept. of Preventive Med.
Hosp. Prof. Edgard Santos
Salvador, Bahia, Brazil

Jorge Paulete   CG
Fac. Regional de Medicina
Caixa Postal, 659
Sao Jose do Rie Preto, Sp, Brazil

Cora de Moura Pedreira   G
Lab. de Gen. Humana
Hospital Prof. Edgard Santos
60 Andar
Salvador, Bahia, Brazil

Willy Becak   G
Dept. of Genetics
Instituto Butantan
Sao Paulo, Brazil

O. Frota–Pessoa   G
Lab. de Genetica Humana
Dept. Biologia, Univ. Sao Paulo
C.P. 8105
Sao Paulo, Brazil

P. H. Saldanha   G
Faculty of Medicine
Lab. of Med. Genetics
P.O. Box 2921
Sao Paulo, Brazil

BULGARIA

Jordan Stoytchkov   C
Inst. of Haematology
  and Blood Transfusion
Sofia 56, Bulgaria

CANADA

Peter Bowen   G
Dept. of Pediatrics
4–120 Clinical Sciences Bldg.
Edmonton 7, Alberta, Canada

J. Philip Welch   G
Dept. of Pediatrics
Dalhousie Univ.
Halifax, Nova Scotia, Canada

Nancy E. Simpson   G
Dept. of Pediatrics
Queen's University
Kingston, Ontario, Canada

F. R. Sergovich   CG
Dept. of Cytogenetics
Children's Psych. Res. Inst.
London, Ont. Canada

Andre Barbeau   G
Dept. of Neuro–Biology
Clin. Res. Inst. of Montreal
110 W. Pine Ave.
Montreal, Canada

Louis Dallaire   G
Medical Gen. Section
Sainte Justine Hospital
3175 Chemin Ste-Catherine
Montreal, 250, P.Q., Canada

F. Clarke Fraser   G
Dept. of Med. Gen.
Montreal Children's Hospital
Postal Zone 108
Montreal, Quebec, Canada

Leonard Pinsky   G
Div. of Medical Gen.
Jewish General Hospital
Montreal, Canada

C. R. Scriver   G
Dept. of Biochem. Gen.
The Montreal Children's Hosp.
Postal Zone 108
Montreal, Canada

Maureen H. Roberts   G
Dept. of Paediatrics
University of Ottawa
Ottawa, Ont., Canada

Elizabeth J. Ives   C
Dept. of Pediatrics
University Hospital
Saskatoon, Sask, Canada

A. Axelrad   C
Div. of Histology
Dept. of Anatomy
University of Toronto
Toronto, Ont., Canada

A. G. Bell   C
Dept. of Zoology
Univ. of Toronto
Toronto, Ont., Canada

J. M. Berg   C
Research Department
Mental Retardation Center
Toronto, Ont., Canada

L. Siminovitch   C
Dept. of Genetics
Hospital for Sick Children
Toronto, Ont., Canada

James R. Miller   C
Div. of Medical Gen.
Dept of Pediatrics
Univ. of British Columbia
Vancouver, Br. Col., Canada

John Hamerton
Dept. of Med. Gen.
Children's Hosp. of Winnipeg
Winnipeg, Manitoba, Canada

S. B. Hrushovetz
Western Cytogenetic Lab.
P.O. Box 3687
Winnipeg 4, Manitoba, Canada

CHILE

Manuel J. Aspillaga
Dept. of Pediatrics
Hospital Luis Calvo Mackenna
Santiago, Chile

Edmundo Covarrubias
Dept. of Human Genetics
University of Chile
Santiago, Chile

R. Cruz–Coke
Dept. of Med. Gen.
Hospital J.J. Aguirre
Santiago, Chile

COLOMBIA

Efraim Otero–Ruiz
Inst. Nacional de Cancerologia
Dept. of Research
Bogota, Colombia

B. Rafael Elejalde   CG
Dept. of Pathology
Universidad de Antioquia
Apartado Aereo 1226
Medellin, Colombia

ECHOSLOVAKIA
Andrej Getlik   G
Pediatric Clinic
Postgraduate Medical Inst.
Kramare
Bratislava, Czechoslovakia

Zdenek Brunecky   G
Institute of Ped. Res.
Cernopolni 9
Brno, Czechoslovakia

Karel Krajca   G
Dept. of Neurology
Dubnica Nad Vahom
Czechoslovakia

NMARK
A. J. Therkelsen   G
Inst. of Human Gen.
Inst. of Medical Microbiology
University of Aarhus
8000 Aarhus C, Denmark

Petrea Jacobsen   G
Inst. for Mental Defec.
  for South East Jutland
Brejning, Denmark

Jan F. Mohr   G
Tagensvej 14
2200 Copenhagen, N., Denmark

John Philip   G
Lab. of Cytogenetics
Rigs Hospitalet
Univ. of Copenhagen
Copenhagen, Denmark

Erik Wamberg   G
John F. Kennedy Inst.
Gl. Landevej 7–5
Glostrup, Denmark

Anders Froland   G
County Hosp. of Copenhagen
Hellerup, Denmark

Johannes Nielsen   G
The Cytogenetic Lab.
Arhus State Hospital
DK–8240 Risskov, Denmark

'PT
Fouad M. Badr   G
National Res. Center
Human Genetics Unit
N. R. C. Cairo, Egypt

Nemat Hashem   CG
Dept. of Pediatrics
Medical Genetics Unit
Ain–Shams Medical Col.
Cairo, Egypt

ENGLAND
D. G. Harnden   C
Dept. of Cancer Studies
Univ. of Birmingham
Birmingham 15, England

J. Insley   G
Children's Hospital
Birmingham B16 8ET, England

Herman Lehmann   G
Med. Res. Council
40 Univ. Dept. of Biochem.
Cambridge Cambs, England

L.S. Penrose   G
Kennedy–Galton Center
Harperbury Hospital
Hertfordshire, England

M. D'A. Crawford   CG
Dept. of Genetics
Stead House
The University of Leeds
Leeds 2, England

C. A. Clarke   CG
Dept. of Medicine
Univ. of Liverpool
Liverpool, England

C. O. Carter   G
Clin. Gen. Res. Unit
Inst. of Child Health
London, England

Wm. M. Davidson   G
Dept. of Haematology
King's Col. Hosp. Med. Sch.
London W.E.5, England

Harry Harris   G
The Galton Lab.
Univ. College London
Wolfson Hse., 4 Stephenson Way
London, N.W.1, England

Barrie Jay   G
Genetic Clinic
Moorfields Eye Hospital
City Road
London E.C.1, England

P. C. Koller   C
Chester Beatty Res. Inst.
Inst. of Cancer Res.
Royal Cancer Hospital
London, S.W.3, England

P. E. Polani   G
Paediatric Res. Unit
Guy's Hosp. Medical Sch.
London S.E.1, England

G. Pontecorvo   C
Imperial Cancer Res. Fund
Lincoln's Inn Fields
London W.C.2, England

James H. Renwick   CG
London Sch. of Hyg. & Trop. Med.
Keppel Street
London W.C.1, E. 7HT, England

R. S. Wells   G
Dept. of Genetics
St. John's Hospital
Lisle St., Leicester Sq.
London W.C.2, England

Rodney Harris   CG
Dept. Medical Genetics
Royal Infirmary
Manchester, England

N. B. Atkin   C
Dept. of Cancer Research
Mt. Vernon Hosp., Northwood
Middlesex, England

D. F. Roberts   G
Lab. of Human Gen.
Univ. of Newcastle–Upon–Tyne
19 Claremont Place
Newcastle–Upon–Tyne, England

A. C. Stevenson   G
Population Gen. Res. Unit
Medical Research Council
Oxford, England

C. E. Blank   G
Centre for Human Gen.
117 Manchester Road
Sheffield S. 10 5DN, England

V. Dubowitz   G
Dept. of Child Health
Univ. of Sheffield
Sheffield, England

FINLAND
Albert de la Chapelle   G
Folkhalsan Inst. of Gen.
Apollogatan 1, Helsinki 10,
Finland

Pertti Aula   G
Chromosome Lab.
Children's Hospital
Univ. of Helsinki
Helsinki, Finland

Ulla Gripenberg   G
Dept. of Genetics
Univ. of Helsinki
Pohj. Rautatiekatu 13
Helsinki 10, Finland

FRANCE
C. Ropartz   G
Center Dept. of Transfus. Sang.
609 Chemin de la Creteque
76 Bois–Guillaume, France

C. Mouriquand   C
Univ. of Grenoble
Faculte de Medicine
38 La Trouche, France

Collete Laurent   G
Institute Pasteur
Section of Cytogenetics
69 Lyon, France

Andre Stahl   C
Dept. D'Embryologie et
   Cytogenetique, Fac. de Medecine
27 Boulevard Jean–Moulin
13 Marseille, France

George Barski   C
Tissue Culture & Virus Lab.
Inst. Gustave–Roussy
Paris 94–Villejuif, France

Jean De Grouchy   C
Clinique de Genetique Medicale
Hosp des Enfants Malades
Paris XV, France

Ingrid Emerit   C
Lab. de Cytogenetique
Clinique de Cardiologie
Hopital Broussais
Paris, France

Jerome LeJeune   C
Lab. de Cytogenetique
Hopital des Enfants–Malades
149 Rue de Severes
Paris XV, France

Pierre Royer
Medical Genetics
Hospital Enfants–Malades
149 Rue de Sevres
Paris, France

Senecal
Serire Pediatrie B
Centre Hospitelier Univ.
Rennes, France

GERMANY
Herbert Luers
Institut fur Genetik
Freie Universitat
Berlin, Germany

R. Widmaier
Inst. of Cancer Research
German Acad. of Sci. of Berlin
1115 Berlin–Buch, G.D.R., Germany

A. Gropp   C
Professor of Pathology
Pathologisches Inst.
Univ. of Bonn
Bonn, Germany

Gerhard Koch   G
Inst. fur Humangenetik and Anthr.
Der Univ. Erlangen–Nurnberg
852 Erlangen Bismarckstrasse 10
Erlangen, Germany

K. H. Degenhardt   G
Inst. fur Humangenetik und
   Vergleichende Erbpatologie
Paul-Ehrlichstr. 41–43
Frankfurt, Germany

Ulrich Wolf   G
Inst. of Human Genetics
   of the University
78 Freiburg 1, Br., Germany

Walter Fuhrmann   G
Ins. fur Humangenetik
Universitat Giessen
D63 Giessen, Germany

Peter E. Becker   G
Inst. fur Humangenetik der
   Universitat
Nikolausberger Weg 23
Gottingen, Germany

H. Werner Goedde   G
Inst. fur Humangenetik
Univ. Hamburg, Martinistra. 52
Hamburg, Germany

Lothar Loeffler   G
Obsterstrasse 57
Hannover, Germany

F. Vogel   G
Inst. fur Anthropologie U.
Humangenetik D. Univ.
Heidelberg, Germany

W. Lehmann   G
Inst. fur Humangenetik
   der Univ. Kiel
Hospitalstr. 42
23 Kiel, Germany

Herman Adolf Hienz   C
Path Inst. Stadt Krankenanstalten
Luther-Platz 40
415 Krefeld, Germany

B. Wittwer   G
Human and Med. Gen. Unit
Medizinische Akademie
301 Magdeburg, Germany

G. G. Wendt   G
Dept. of Human Genetics
Univ. of Marburg
Marburg, Germany

Fritz H. Lampert   C
Dept. of Pediatrics
Universitats-Kinderklinik
Munich, Germany

Jan Murken   G
Dept. of Pediatrics
Kinderpoliklinik der Univ.
Pettenkoferstrasse 8A
Munich, Germany

Klaus D. Zang   CG
Dept. of Neuropathology
Max-Planck-Inst. of Psychiatry
Munich, Germany

Edith Zerbin-Rudin   G
Dept. of Genealogy & Demography
Max-Planck-Inst. of Psychiatry
Munich, Germany

W. Lenz   G
Dept. of Human Genetics
Inst. of Human Genetics
Munster, Germany

L. Pelz   G
Dept. of Cytogenetics
Pediatric Hospital (Univ.)
Rostock, GDR, Germany

H. Kirchmair   G
Pediatric Hospital (Univ.)
Rostock, GDR, Germany

W. Bethmann   C
Klinik F. Gesichtschirurgie
7251 Thallwitz, GDR, Germany

GHANA

Felix I. D. Konotey-Ahulu   G
Dept. of Med.
Ghana Med. Sch.
P.O. Box 4236
Accra, Ghana

GREECE

Spyros A. Doxiadis   G
Inst. of Child Health
Aghia Sophia Children's Hosp.
Athens 608, Greece

N. Matsaniotis   G
St. Sophi's Children's Hosp.
Athens 608, Greece

HUNGARY

S. F. Eckhardt   C
Dept. of Chemotherapy
National Cancer Institute
Budapest, XII, Rath Gy. U7, Hungary

George Lenart   G
Janos Korhaz Clinic
Budapest XII, Diosarok-U.1
Hungary

D. Schuler — CG
Med. Sch. of Budapest
Second Dept. of Ped.
Budapest IX Tuzolto–U.7
Hungary

G. Szabo — G
Biological Institute
Medical Univ.
Debrecen 12, Hungary

F. Varga — G
Dept. of Pediatrics
Univ. Medical School
Pecs. Jozsef All, Hungary

Gyorgy Kiszely — G
Biologiai Intezet
Szote
Szeged, Hungary

INDIA

G. Sadasivan — G
Dept. Anatomy
College, Hyderab
1–A.P., India

L. D. Sanghvi — C
Epidemiology Div.
Cancer Res. Inst.
Tata Memorial Center
Bombay 12, India

J. V. Undevia — CG
Epidemiology Division
Cancer Research Inst.
Tata Memorial Centre
Parel, Bombay 12, India

Amala Chaudhuri — G
Hon. Director
The Chaudhuri Cen. for Med. Gen.
Calcutta 14, India

Chamara R. Puttana — G
Inst. of Cell Biology
No. 2 Yadavgiri 1 Main Road
Vanivilaspuram, Mysore 2, India

R. K. Gulati — C
Dept. of Anthropology
Deccan College
Poona, India

IRELAND

Norman C. Nevin — G
Human Gen. Unit
Dept. of Med. Statistics
Queen's Univ. and Royal Hosp.
Belfast, North Ireland

ISRAEL

T. Cohen — G
Dept. of Human Gen.
Hadassah University Hosp.
P.O. Box 499
Jerusalem, Israel

Kalman Fried — G
Dept. of Human Gen.
31 Habanai, Beth–Hakerem
Jerusalem, Israel

Isaac G. Halbrecht — G
Fetal Devel. & Gen. Unit
Hasharon Hospital
Petah Tiqua, Israel

Juan Chemke — G
Dept. of Pediatrics
Birth Defects Centre
Kaplan Hospital
Rehovot, Israel

Ramot Bracha — C
Chief, Dept. of Haematology
Tel–Hashomer Government Hosp.
Tel–Hashomer, Israel

Cyril P. Legum — G
Child Devel. Assess. Centre
14 Balfour Street
Tel–Aviv–Yaffo, Israel

Arieh Szeinberg — G
Dept. of Chemical Path.
Tel Hashomer Hospital
Tel Aviv Univ. Med. Sch.
Tel Hashomer, Israel

ITALY

Umberto Bigozzi — G
Centro Genetica Medica
c/o Clinica Medica–Viale Morgagni
50139 Firenze, Italy

Marco Fraccaro — CG
Euratom Unit for Human Rad.
  and Cytogenetics
Via Forlanini, 14
27100 Pavia, Italy

Luigo Gedda — G
1st. di Genetica Medica e
  Gemellologia G. Mendel
Piazza Galeno 5
00161 Rome, Italy

Angelo Serra — G
Univ. Cattolica del Sacro Cuore
1st. di Genetica Umana
Via Della Pineta Sachetti, 644
Rome, Italy

Ezio Silvestroni — G
Centro di Studi D. Microcitemia
Citta Universitaria
Rome, Italy

Ruggero Ceppellini — G
Dept. of Med. Gen.
University of Turin
Torino, Italy

B. Chiarelli — G
Dept. of Anthropology
Via Accademia Albertina 17
10123 Torino, Italy

JAPAN

Hiroshi Fujino   G
Dept. of Oral Surgery
Kyushu University
Fukuoka, Japan

Yoshigoro Kuroiwa   G
Dept. of Neurology
Kyushu University
Fukuoka, Japan

Isamu Awano   C
Dept. of Internal Med.
Fukushima Medical College
4-45 Sugitsuma-Cho
Fukushima-Shi, Japan

Yoshito Tsuji   CG
Dept. of Public Health
Fukushima Medical College
Fukushima, Japan

Atsushi Fujiwara   CG
Dept. of Obstet. & Gynec.
Hiroshima University
Hiroshima, Japan

Norio Fujiki   G
Dept. of Genetics
Res. Inst. & Central Hosp.
Aichi Col. for Men. & Phys.
Kasugai City, Aichi Pref., Japan

Sadanabu Miyao   C
Dept. of Geriatrics
Inst. of Constitutional Med.
Kumamoto University
Kumamoto City, Japan

Masasuke Masuda   G
Div. of Hemat. & Gen.
Dept. of Internal Med.
Kyoto Pref. Univ. of Medicine
Kyoto, Japan

Ei Matsunaga   G
Dept. of Human Gen.
Nat. Inst. of Genetics
Mishima, Japan

Ujihro Murakami   G
Res. Inst. of Environmental Med.
Nagoya University
Furo-Cho, Chikusa-Ku
Nagoya, Japan

Kinzaburo Watanabe   G
Dept. of Obstet. & Gynec.
Kawasumi-Cho Mizuho-Ku
Nagoya, Japan

Iwao Luchi   C
Dept. of Clin. Path.
Kawasaki Hosp. & Tumor Inst.
Okayama City, Japan

Hisatoshi Mitsuda   G
Dept. of Neuropsychiatry
Osaka Medical College
Takatsuki, Osaka, Japan

Motomichi Sasaki   CG
Chromosome Research Unit
Faculty of Science
Hokkaido University
Sapporo, 060, Japan

Michihiro C. Yoshida   C
Chromosome Research Unit
Faculty of Science
Hokkaido University
Sapporo, Japan

Kazuo Miyoshi   G
Dept. of Medicine
Tokushima University
Tokushima, Japan

Tanemoto Furuhata   C
Nat. Res. Inst. of Police Sci.
6 Sanban-Cho, Chiyoda-Ku
Tokyo, Japan

Akira Hidano   G
Genetic Coun. Section
Tokyo Metro. Police Hosp.
Fujimi, Chiyodaku
Tokyo 102, Japan

Eiji Inouye   G
Dept. of Human Gen. & Criminology
Inst. of Brain Research
Univ. of Tokyo Fac. of Med.
Tokyo, Japan

Akira Nakajuma   G
Dept. of Ophthalmology
Juntendo University
Tokyo, Japan

N. Shinozaki   G
Dept. of Population Quality
Inst. of Population Problems
Tokyo, Japan

Katumi Tanaka   CG
Dept. of Human Genetics
Tokyo Med. & Dental Univ.
Tokyo, 113, Japan

Akira Tonomura   G
Dept. of Human Cytogenetics
Tokyo Med. and Dental Univ.
Tokyo, Japan

Shunzo Konishi   G
Dept. of Pediatrics
Yamaguchi University
School of Medicine
Ube, Japan

Yoshitoshi Handa   G
Dept. of Anatomy
Wakayama Medical College
Wakayma-Shi, Japan

Ichiro Matsui G
Dept. of Ped. & Cytogen. Lab.
Kanagawa Children's Med. Centre
Mutsukawa 2-138-4, Minamiku
Yokohama, Japan

MEXICO
Salvador S. Armendares G
Dept. of Med. Gen.
Hospital de Pediatria
Mexico City, Mexico

A. L. De Garay G
Dept. of Gen. Programs
Com. Nacional de Energia Nuclear
Apdo. Postal No. 27-190
Mexico 18, D.F., Mexico

Ruben Lisker G
Dept. of Genetics
Instituto Nacional de la Nutricion
Mexico 22, D.F., Mexico

Mario Gonzalez Ramos G
Unidad de Genetica
Hospital Infantil de Mexico
Dr. Marquez No. 162
Mexico 7, D.F., Mexico

Raul Garza Chapa G
Dept. of Genetics
Univ. Autonoma de Nuevo Leon
Apartado Postal 1563
Monterrey, N.L., Mexico

NETHERLANDS
A. De Froe G
Dept. of Human Bio. and Gen.
Anthropobiological Lab.
Mauritskade 61
Amsterdam, The Netherlands

B. J. M. Aulbers G
Dept. of Gen. Counseling
Hof. Van Delftlaan 126
Delft, The Netherlands

G. J. P. A. Anders G
Dept. of Human Genetics
Anthropogenetic Institute
Groningen, The Netherlands

Hemophilia Clinic G
Flevolaan 71, Huizen (H.H.)
The Netherlands

G. A. Fraser G
Dept. of Human Genetics
University of Leiden
Leiden, The Netherlands

S. J. Geerts G
Dept. of Human Gen.
Fac. Med.
University of Nymegen
Nymegen, The Netherlands

P. H. Jongbloet G
Inst. for Mental Retardates
Ottersum, The Netherlands

H. K. A. Visser G
Dept. of Ped., Med. Sch.
Sophia Children's Hosp.
Neonatal Unit
Rotterdam, The Netherlands

John Huizinga G
Dept. of Human Biology
State Univ. of Utrecht
Utrecht, The Netherlands

NEW ZEALAND
Robin W. Carrell G
Biochemistry Unit
Christchurch Hospital
Christchurch, New Zealand

Peter H. Fitzgerald CC
Dept. of Cytogenetics
Christchurch Hospital
Christchurch, New Zealand

A. M. O. Veale CC
Human Gen. Res. Unit
Univ. of Otago Med. Sch.
Dunedin, New Zealand

NORWAY
Kare Berg C
Inst. of Med. Gen.
University of Oslo
Oslo, Norway

O. H. Iversen C
Dept. of Pathology
Rikshospitalet
Oslo, Norway

PERU
Teresa Perez Nunez G
Dept. of Path.
Univ. Peruana Cayetano Heredia
Box 6195, Lima, Peru

PHILIPPINES
Pelagia S. Bayani-Sioson C
Basic Sciences & Res. Sec.
College of Dentistry
Univ. of Philippines, Padre Faura
Manila, D-406, Philippines

POLAND
K. Boczkowski C
Dept. of Endocrinology
Medical Academy
Warsaw, Poland

Ignacy Wald C
Dept. of Genetics
Psychoneurological Inst.
Warsaw, Pruszkow, Poland

RUMANIA

St. M. Milcu G
Dept. of Endocrinology
Institute de Endocrinology
Bucarest, Rumania

G. Scripcaru G
Dept. of Forensic Med.
Institute of Medicine
Iassy, Rumania

SCOTLAND

A. W. Johnston G
Aberdeen Royal Infirmary
Aberdeen, AB9 2ZB Scotland

Alan Emery G
Univ. Dept. Human Gen.
Edinburgh, Scotland

Malcolm A. Ferguson-Smith CG
Medical Genetics Unit
Queen Mother's Hospital
Glasgow, C.3, Scotland

SOUTH AFRICA

Ralph E. Bernstein CG
Metabolic Res. and
   Human Biochem. Gen. Unit
S. African Inst. for Med. Res.
Johannesburg, South Africa

Eugene Wilton G
Cytogenetic Unit
So. African Inst. for Med. Res.
P.O. Box 1038, Hosp. St.
Johannesburg, South Africa

Ingram F. Anderson G
Dept. of Medicine
Pretoria General Hospital
Pretoria, South Africa

J. D. J. Hofmeyr G
Dept. of Genetics
University of Pretoria
Pretoria, South Africa

SPAIN

Jaime Antich G
Dept. of Human Genetics
Inst. Provincial de Bioquimica
Barcelona C-Roberto Bassas 1
Barcelona 14, Spain

Jorge Prats Vinas CG
Hosp. Infantil, Seguridad
Barcelona, Spain

Andres Sanchez Cascos G
Dept. of Human Gen.
Fundacion Jimenez Diaz
Madrid, Spain

Luis Izquierdo Gongora G
Dept. de Genetica
Hospital Clinico
Madrid, Spain

Emilia Barreiros Miranda G
Dept. de Genetica Humana
Clinica Infantil
La Paz
Madrid, Spain

Geronimo Forteza Bover G
Dept. de Invest. Citologicas
De La Caja de Ahorros
Jorge Juan, 15
Valencia 4, Spain

Rafael Baguena Candela G
Dept. of Med. Gen.
Faculty of Medicine
Paseo Valencia Al Mar 17
Valencia 5, Spain

SWEDEN

Hans Olof Akesson G
Dir. of Med. Gen. Div.
Psychiatric Research Center
St. Jorgens Hospital
Lillhagen, Sweden

Carl A. Larson G
Dept. of Med. Gen.
Institute of Genetics
Lund, Sweden

J. Lindsten G
Dept. of Clin. Gen.
Karolinska Hospital
10401, Stockholm 60, Sweden

Jan A. Book G
Uppsala U., Inst. for Med. Gen.
24 V. Agatan
TS-75220 Uppsala, Sweden

K. H. Gustavson G
Dept. of Pediatrics
Akademiska Sjukhuset
750 14 Uppsala 14, Sweden

SWITZERLAND

G. R. Stalder G
Univ. Children's Hospital
Romergasse 8
Basel, Switzerland

Tadashi Kajii G
Lab. of Embryology &
   Cytogenetics, Univ. Clinic
   of Gynec. & Obstet. 1211
Geneva 4, Switzerland

David Klein CG
Dept. of Med. Gen.
University of Geneva
Chemin Thury 8
Geneva, Switzerland

Werner Schmid G
Dept. of Paediatrics
Univ. Children's Hosp.
Steinweisstr. 75
Zurich, Switzerland

THAILAND

    Supa Na–Nakorn   G
    Dept. of Hematology
    Siriraj Hospital
    Bangkok, Thailand

TURKEY

    Burhan Say   G
    Dept. of Pediatrics
    Hacettepe University
    Ankara, Turkey

    Bekir Sitki Sayli   G
    Univ. of Ankara
    Medical Faculty
    Cebeci–Ankara, Turkey

USSR

    N. P. Bochkov   G
    Inst. of Medical Gen.
    Acad. of Med. Sciences
      of the USSR
    Baltiyskaya U1., 8
    Moscow, A–315, USSR

    Jul I. Kerkis   CG
    Radiation Genetics Lab.
    Inst. of Cytology & Gen.
    Novosibirsk–90, USSR

    R. P. Martynova   C
    Lab. of Cancer Genetics
    Inst. of Cytology & Gen.
    Siberian Dept. USSR Acad Sci.
    Novosibirsk 630090, USSR

VENEZUELA

    Luis A. Muro   G
    Dept. de Medicina 3
    Lab. de Investigaciones
    Hospital Univ.
    Caracas, Venezuela

WALES

    K. M. Laurence   G
    Dept. of Child Health
    Llandough Hospital
    Penarth, Glamorgan, Wales

WEST INDIES

    Gerrit Bras   G
    Univ. of the West Indies
    Mona, Kingston 7
    Jamaica, West Indies

YUGOSLAVIA

    Marij Avcin   G
    Dept. of Pediatrics
    Univ. Children's Hospital
    Ljubljana, Yugoslavia

    Ljiljana Zergollern   G
    Dept. of Pediatrics
    Univ. of Zagreb–Rebro
    Zagreb, Yugoslavia

SUBJECT INDEX

AUTHOR INDEX

Abrahams, I., 154
Academy of Dermatology, the, 1964, 83
Ackerman, L. V., 234
Agatston, S. A., 223
Aisenberg, A. C., 199
Alexander, P., 196, 200
Allen, A. C., 233
Allison, A. C., 196, 197
Allison, J. R., 230
Almb, D., 199
Alpert, M. E., 195
Alvarez, E., 124
Anderson, D. E., 79, 87, 126, 131, 151, 153–156, 158
Anderson, N. P., 233
Andrews, G. C., 225, 228, 233
Andrews, J. C., 87
Arundell, F. D., 225
Ashbury, H. E., 153
Attie, J. L., 69
August, C. S., 194
Austad, W. I., 184
Bachus, H. L., 185
Balfour, D. C., 176
Ballard, H. S., 215
Bang, G., 151, 154, 156
Barnes, R. D., 224
Barr, M., 199
Bartholomew, L. G., 187
Basten, A., 226
Bataille, R., 153, 155
Batchelor, J. R., 196
Batschwarov, B., 157
Baughman, F. A., 176, 177
Bazex, A., 156
Beahrs, O. H., 157
Bean, S. F., 182, 232
Beare, J. M., 233
Becker, M. H., 153, 154, 156, 157
Beickert, A., 224
Benedict, P. H., 105
Benson, G. D., 184
Benziger, K., 79
Berenbaum, M. C., 197

Berlin, N. I., 59, 153, 156, 158
Bernier, J. J., 213, 214, 217
Bielschowsky, M., 121, 197
Binkley, G. W., 154–157
Black, P. H., 59
Blinstrub, R. S., 98
Block, J. B., 150, 154, 156, 158
Bloom, D., 98, 100, 227
Bloom, G. E., 59, 229
Bloom, R. A., 153
Blum, H. F., 236
Boatwright, H., 223
Boder, E., 94, 96, 198
Bopp, C. L., 157
Bourneville, D. M., 104
Bowen, S. F., 88
Boyd, M. W. J., 221, 223
Boyden, S., 193
Boyer, B. E., 149, 153, 154, 156
Bramley, P. A., 153, 154
Brinkley, G. W., 149
Broughton, R. B.K., 126
Brunjes, S., 224
Bruyn, 154
Bryan, H. G., 56, 59, 229
Buckton, K. E., 100
Buckwalter, J. A., 230
Bundey, S., 123, 131
Burdette, W. J., 25
Burge, K. M., 226, 233
Burk, P. G., 63
Burnet, F. M., 197
Butler, W. T., 194
Butterworth, T., 7, 69, 233
Cabot, R. C., 165, 167, 175, 176
Cacchione, A., 80
Cairns, R. J., 153, 154, 157
Calnan, C. D., 151
Camiel, M. R., 176
Cammarata, R. J., 197
Canada, W. J., 176, 185
Canale, D., 120
Capps, W. F., 175, 176
Carney, R. G., 151